D0990872

LIFE IN THE WOMB

LIFE IN THE WOMB:

The Origin of Health and Disease

Peter W. Nathanielsz

PROMETHEAN PRESS
ITHACA, NEW YORK
1999

ISBN 0-916859-56-8

PROMETHEAN PRESS
P.O. Box 6827
Ithaca, NY 14851
U. S. A.
www.lifeinthewomb.com

Prenatal care is a cooperation between you and your medical caregiver. The information given here is correct to the best of my knowledge, but the ultimate responsibility for you and your baby lies with yourself, your partner and your physician. Everyone is unique. —P. W. N.

LIBRARY OF CONGRESS
Library of Congress Catalog-in-Publication Data

PRINTED IN THE UNITED STATES OF AMERICA
01 00 99 5 4 3 2 1

For tomorrow's children.

Contents

List of Figures

Further Reading and Notes

PREFACE

Life in the Womb resumes the fascinating and awesome story of human development where my book *Life Before Birth* left off. Recent research provides compelling proof that the health we enjoy throughout our lives is determined to a large extent by the conditions in which we developed in the womb. How we are ushered into life is the major factor that determines how we leave it.

The quality of life in the womb, our temporary home before we were born, programs our susceptibility to coronary artery disease, stroke, diabetes, obesity and a multitude of other conditions in later life. *Programming* is the buzzword for the determination of health and disease by life in the womb. There is mounting evidence that programming of lifetime health by the conditions in the womb is equally, if not more important, than our genes in determining how we perform mentally and physically during life. *Gene myopia* is the term that best describes the current all-pervasive view that our health and destiny throughout life are controlled by our genes alone. I have tried to reverse this gene myopia by showing how the deck of cards we are dealt in our genes can be beneficially or adversely impacted by our home in the womb. We should be reassured by the remarkable findings discussed in this book since, while our genetic makeup is fixed at the time of the fusion of the sperm and egg that began our life in the womb, what happens thereafter as we develop can be improved and supported by providing the best possible home in the womb. In contrast to the relative fatalism of gene myopia, understanding the mechanisms that underlie programming by the quality of life in the womb, we can improve the start in life for our children and their children.

Understanding programming will also enable each of us to live in ways that will improve the rest of our lives. Although we cannot go back and undo our own past, each of us will be in a better position to lessen the potential adverse effects of our own life in the womb on our own future health during the remainder of our lives.

The evidence for programming is overwhelming. The story is compelling because it receives powerful support from three major sources: human epidemiology, clinical observations and from animal studies. These three approaches tell us, each in its own distinct and powerful way, how all the parts of our bodies work together under adverse as well as optimal conditions. Our bodies are more than the sum total of their parts.

Darwin led the way in showing us how we are related structurally and functionally to other life forms. Once our own species became aware of our close biological relationship to the other forms of life on planet earth—both plant and animal—human life changed dramatically and permanently. Many myths and philosophies required permanent alteration. It was not necessary to abandon the faiths of our past, but our beliefs and understanding of who we are needed to be reworked. In the same way, knowing how life in the womb can program how our liver, heart, kidneys and especially our brain function throughout our lives, will permanently alter our perception of how we function as individuals and as a society.

The word *programming* has a ring of finality, but there is no reason to be fatalistic. In the preface of *Life Before Birth*, I recounted the story of a high school student, a twelfth grader from Long Island, who asked me, "If the baby does not grow properly before birth, is it the mother's fault?" Each of us, not just pregnant women, has a responsibility to generations as yet unborn, whose names we do not know and whose faces we have not seen, to ensure that their lives are as healthy and fulfilled as possible. Only by knowing the way our bodies developed before birth and made their preparations for life after birth will we be able to optimally match the preparation we each made at this critical time of our lives in the womb with the world in which we now find ourselves living. We need to improve this match between past preparation and present function for our children by addressing the critical biological issues both during pregnancy and after it. Only by understanding the mechanisms that underlie programming of lifetime health and disease can we improve the health of tomorrow's children.

There are many revolutionary, iconoclastic ideas discussed in this book. The research that strongly supports them shows that we must reevaluate some basic concepts. For example, the transgenerational passage of characteristics by nongenetic means does occur. Lamarck was right, although transgenerational transmission of acquired characteristics occurs by mechanisms that were unknown in his day. Like many revolutionary thinkers, he was before his time. His failing was that, although he was right, he was unable to provide the firm, reproducible, scientific evidence that showed the existence of transgenerational passage of enjoyment of good health and susceptibility to illness. That evidence is here in this book.

Several friends and colleagues who I acknowledge later, read and constructively criticized early drafts of this book. They advised me on my errors of commission and omission. I have tried to follow their advice, but since no book can cover every area of this fascinating subject, I am solely responsible for the selection of evidence, examples and areas of interest. I have striven to convey the wonder and poetry of human development. Programming of lifetime health and disease by the conditions under which we developed in the womb is our own personal history.

Peter Nathanielsz
Ithaca, New York
November 1998

ACKNOWLEDGMENTS

This book relates the work of many outstanding researchers who have revealed the mysteries of life in the womb. I have been fortunate to know most of them personally. I am particularly indebted for the many hours of discussion I have had over the years with dedicated researchers all over the world who are trying to understand the underlying principles and mechanisms that make programming a feature of the biology of all mammalian species. Some of these are clinicians, and some are basic scientists: David Barker, Otto Blekker, John Challis, Gautam Chaudhuri, Jorge Figueroa, Peter Gluckman, Keith Godfrey, Robert Goldenberg, Dino Giussani, Nicholas Hales, Mark Hanson, Jane Harding, Michael Heymann, Barbera Honnebier, Thomas Kirschbaum, Janna Koppe, Mont Liggins, Charles Lockwood, Larry Longo, Stephen Lye, Thomas McDonald, Majid Mirmiran, Murray Mitchell, Leslie Myatt, William Oh, David Olson, Lucilla Poston, Jeffrey Robinson, Roberto Romero, Maria Seron-Ferre, "Buddy" Stark, Dick Swaab, Andre Van Assche, Charles Wood, Wen Wu and many, many others. All are dedicated to a better understanding of programming in order to provide a better life for future generations. I am grateful for their enthusiasm, learning and energy

Researchers in this field know that we could not study these important events without the tireless help of those who direct the various programs of the National Institutes of Health in the United States and equivalent bodies such as the Wellcome Trust in the United Kingdom. This work would not be possible without the financial and intellectual support that comes from society through these institutions. I would like to add my own very special thanks to those smaller charities and foundations who help young researchers to get started. We all owe a great debt to those who work in any capacity with the more specialized granting agencies such as Tommy's Campaign, The Lalor Foundation, WellBeing and many other such bodies.

Other friends who are not among the scientific community have encouraged me in this effort to put this story before the general reader. None more so than my dear friends Linda and Robert Lloyd, who encouraged me in my task in moments of uncertainty and when I had my doubts. To Linda in particular I owe many thanks for ideas that have made many concepts more accessible. Mark Nijland who helped set up information about this book on its web site. I would also like to thank Karen Moore, Susan Jenkins (who drew many of the figures) and Toni Coon for their invaluable help with many details of the text, figures and notes. Last, and most importantly, this book would not be possible without the help of Diana Nathanielsz in a thousand ways.

I would like to acknowledge the sources of some of the information presented here. The "Further Reading and Notes" section contains entries into the subject for the reader who wishes to go into more detail. However, there are many other sources that can be accessed through these publications as well as by other means. Many researchers have contributed to this field, and it is impossible to acknowledge everyone's contribution. Figure 1.1 was taken by Helmuth H. Prinz and kindly provided by Drs. Christa Einspieler and Heinz Prechtl. Figure 1.2 was kindly provided by Dr. Catherine Husa. I am also deeply indebted to Dr. Husa for help with the images on the cover. Figure 1.3 is modified from data presented in *Mothers, Babies and Health in Later Life* (D. J. P. Barker, Churchill Livingstone, 1998). Figure 1.4 is reproduced with permission from *Smith's Recognizable Patterns of Human Malformation* (fourth edition, Saunders, 1988). Figure 1.6 is adapted from Tanner, J. M., "Earlier maturation of man," *Scientific American*, 1968, Number 1, 21–27. Figures 2.2, 2.3, 2.4 and 2.8 are reproduced with permission of the Dutch War Museum. Figure 2.5 is drawn from data in Ravelli, G. P., et al., "Obesity in young men after famine exposure in utero and early infancy," *New Engl. J. Med.* 295 (1976): 349–353. Figure 2.7 was kindly provided by Dr. Janna Koppe. Figures 3.1, 10.2 and 10.3 were previously published in my book *Life Before Birth* (W. H. Freeman, 1996). Figure 3.2 is drawn using data from *Mothers, Babies and Health in Later Life* and G. Melvyn Howe in *Man, Environment and Disease in Britain* (Harper & Rowe, 1972). Figure 3.3 was kindly provided by Dr. Xiu Ying Ding. Figure 4.1 is reproduced with permission from the Arizona Historical Society. Figures 5.2 and 5.3 are reproduced with the kind permission of Dr. Steven Ford. Figure 5.4 is redrawn from data from Yellon, S. M. and Longo, L. D., "Effect of maternal pinealectomy and reverse photoperiod on the circadian melatonin rhythm in the sheep and fetus during the last trimester of pregnancy," *Biol. Reprod.* 39 (1988): 1093–1099. Figure 8.1 is redrawn from Bassett, J. M., et al., "Photoperiod: An important regulator of plasma prolactin concentration in fetal lambs during late gestation," *Q. J. Exp. Physiol.* 73 (1988): 241–244. Figures 9.1 and 10.1 were kindly provided by Dr. Thomas McDonald. Figure 9.3 is reproduced with permission from Stewart, R. J. C., et al., "Twelve generations of marginal protein deficiency," *British Journal of Nutrition* 33 (1975): 233–253. Figures 9.4 was kindly provided by Charles Mecenas. Figure 9.5 is modified from an original provided by Dr. Dick Swaab. Figure 10.4 was kindly provided by Brian Smistek. Figure 10.6 was kindly provided by Biex Inc., Dublin, CA. Figure 10.7 was kindly provided by Dr. James McGregor. Figure 11.1 is modified from *Bright Air, Brilliant Fire: On Mind and Matter*, by Gerald Edelman (Basic Books, 1992). Figure 1 in the "Notes" is redrawn from Prentice, A., et al., "Birth, life and death in rural Africa." *MRC News* 77 (1988): 12–16. Figure 2 in the "Notes" was kindly provided by Dr. Andrew Prentice. Finally, I am grateful to Susan Jenkins for drawing Figures 1.5, 2.1, 2.6, 4.1, 5.1, 5.5, 5.6, 6.1, 9.2 and 10.5.

ONE

THE ORIGIN OF HEALTH AND DISEASE

There are more things in heaven and
earth, Horatio,
Than are dreamt of in your philosophy.

William Shakespeare, *Hamlet, Prince of Denmark*

Recent research into the lifetime health records of babies born in the early part of this century show that the health we enjoy throughout life is markedly affected by the conditions we experience in the womb before we even enter this world. The consequences of an unfavorable environment in the womb may even be passed across many generations. This prenatal determination, or ***programming,*** *of the quality of our lives is a fascinating human story with vital consequences for each and every one of us. The concept of programming of lifelong health and disease by prenatal life has important health implications for future generations of our children and the society in which they will live.*

During development in the womb, there is a constant interplay between our genetic inheritance and the environment in which we develop. We are the products of both ***nature****—our genes—and*

***nurture**—the environment. When nurture is suboptimal, we pay a lifelong price. However carefully investigated, information from human health records can never yield the secrets of how unfavorable conditions before birth adversely affect us for the rest of our lives. These records cannot determine cause and effect, but they are firmly supported by clinical observations and experimental studies on fetal and newborn development in several different species of animals.*

*In my earlier book, **Life Before Birth: The Challenges of Fetal Development**, I told the fascinating story of how developing babies can respond to adverse conditions in the womb in order to protect their growing brain and heart. The methods babies use to do this are truly marvelous. However, there is a long-term price to pay if the baby has to take this protective action over an extended period of time during life before birth. Babies who have developed in unfavorable conditions before birth are more prone to heart disease, diabetes, obesity and altered stress responses during life after birth.*

This is not a how to book. Instead, I have provided the information on how and what researchers have learned about programming of health and disease. You, the reader, must assess the validity of the ideas and determine the consequences for yourself and your children. Then you must decide what you intend to do about it.

Biological Rules of Fetal Development

There is an old Bill Cosby act that takes a lighthearted approach to the baby's activities as she or he develops in the womb. Cosby sets up the routine by speaking as if the baby were living in a one room apartment. The baby bangs about, writing on the walls of the uterus, complaining of the awful conditions inside his temporary living quarters and generally raising a ruckus. Cosby suggests this is because the baby is confined, unhappy, recalcitrant, even mischievous. All this activity, he implies, indicates the baby's earnest wish to get out. I am afraid I must take issue with this media guru of family life. Although his description makes a good comedy act, the picture he paints of life before birth is downright wrong. When a pregnant woman is healthy, the womb is not an adverse environment, even though it is temporary housing. Normal pregnancy is a healthy biological situation, and the uterus of a healthy mother is simply the best place for the fetus to be in order to complete the critical preparations for life after birth. It is up to the parents, up to society—that's you and me—to ensure that the accommodations available for this critical period of life are of the very best quality.

The body of each newborn baby needs to be well-prepared and -constructed during all the stages of development in the womb. Preparation depends not only on the blueprint plans contained in our genes but also the materials from which our *body machine* is constructed and the conditions in which the production is carried out. Each human fetus should be given the proper environment her or his body needs to conduct extensive predelivery trials. It goes without saying that after birth, everything possible must be done to ensure adequate maintenance, but if predelivery construction was performed poorly, maintenance will naturally be more difficult. If there are problems with the temporary housing in the womb, the immediate and long-term consequences for the developing fetus can be substantial.

We ignore the biological rules by which we live at our peril. Every individual in every species faces similar challenges: obtaining enough food and oxygen, maintaining a normal body temperature, and excreting waste products that the body no longer needs. Essentially, our bodies are machines that function according to a precise set of biological rules, rules that are as fundamental as the physical laws of geology or astronomy.

How the heart functions is a good example of these fundamental biological rules in action. The heart is a pump that beats about once every second to circulate blood through our blood vessels to all the tissues in the body. When the blood vessels become constricted due to spasm of the muscle in their wall or clogged by plaques of cholesterol, the flow of blood around the body is impeded, and blood pressure is raised. When this happens, the heart has to work harder to pump the same amount of blood. If the heart is unable to increase the force with which it pumps, the flow of blood will decrease, just as an electrical current decreases if the electrical resistance in a circuit rises. The biological laws that govern the flow of blood through the body are as incontrovertible as the laws of conduction of electricity in the wires around your home.

The implication of these specific biological rules for the fetus developing in the womb are not minor. These biological rules control the development of the brain and our capacity to reason and hold down a good job when we grow up; they control the formation of the pancreas and our susceptibility to diabetes in later life; these rules control the development of the heart and cardiovascular system and the likelihood that we will die an early death due to heart disease; most importantly, we will see that these laws of fetal development affect our emotional life and how we relate to our friends and loved ones.

This lifetime alteration of biological function by the conditions that are present during development has been called *programming.* In order to appreciate how prenatal biological rules affect us, we must be aware of two concepts that are fundamental to the maturation of each and every human: the presence of critical periods of development at which programming takes place and the potentially permanent nature of programming. During fetal and newborn life, there are critical periods in the growth and development of each organ in our bodies. At these critical times, each individual organ is especially sensitive to challenges that have the potential to permanently alter the development of that organ and hence the whole body. Abnormal development at these critical periods may program the body for long-term adverse consequences to the overall health and function of the individual.

The first of these two features, the existence of critical periods of opportunity and vulnerability, will be of little surprise to anyone who has been involved in the growth and development of young children. During childhood, there are critical milestones when children are able to make the next step forward in their developmental profile. The critical period for each major developmental milestone cannot be significantly advanced in time by environmental or educational influences. Educationalists agree on the importance of identification of children who are at risk of falling behind in class before they begin to fail. It is equally important that we understand the progression of the normal milestones that occur before birth. Biologists have long known that each baby passes a greater number of important developmental milestones before birth than after birth. Yet we continue to ignore the importance of life before birth for good, long-term health of both body and mind.

The second characteristic of programming is that failure to complete or unsatisfactory completion of specific milestones may be permanent. In addition, when a critical phase in a child's development is missed or even significantly delayed for any reason, the next step may be impeded. In the development of language, a child cannot begin to formulate meaningful sentences until she has developed an adequate vocabulary of individual words. Normal development requires each critical milestone to be achieved in a specific order and with appropriate time delays between them. This is largely because each milestone interacts with the next one. Timing is everything.

Critical Periods of Development

During the development of the fetus, there are critical periods at which each specific process must occur if it is ever going to happen. Experiments conducted forty years ago in newborn female rats powerfully illustrate this point. The mature female rat will ovulate several eggs every four days. This short reproductive cycle corresponds to the longer, monthly menstrual cycle of women. However, if newborn female rats are injected with a single dose of male sex hormones on day five of their life, they will *never* ovulate. When they reach the age of puberty, their ovaries will still contain a normal complement of egg-containing follicles, some of which are completely mature and look as if they will release their egg any minute. But these ripe follicles are forever arrested at this point. In these rats, all the stages of development that prepare for the release of the eggs at the time of ovulation have been satisfactorily completed. However, because their brains were exposed to male sex hormones at a critical moment of development, their reproductive brain centers have been permanently altered and will never deliver the sharp periodic signals that occur every four days in the brain of a normal female rat to provoke ovulation. Instead of their normal cyclic function, the brains of these female rats have been programmed to function in the steady, continuous, noncycling male fashion. Female rats given the injection of male sex hormones on day twenty of newborn life are perfectly normal and completely fertile when they pass puberty. By twenty days of life, the critical window of susceptibility to programming by male hormones is past, and exposure to the male hormone has no long-term effects on the developing brain.

These classical studies show that there is a critical window during the first few days of newborn life in the female rat when the characteristic rhythmical nature of female reproduction is laid down in the brain. This effect of male hormones on the developing brain was one of the first examples of two general principles of developmental programming: the existence of a critical time frame during development in which programming occurs and the permanence of some, though not necessarily all, developmental programming. I can understand an initial reluctance to accept the concept of programming. So, as we look at evidence for more widespread and general effects of programming on lifelong health, I ask you constantly to bear in mind this key example of programming of the sexual rhythmicity of the female brain. This well-established example supports the theme to which we will repeatedly return: that normal development in the womb requires that the genetic program be played out under favorable environmental conditions. If unusual, excessive, or unwanted factors exist in the environment during prenatal life or if certain indispensable nutrients or conditions are absent, the program contained in our genes may not be able to unfold normally. When abnormal programming occurs, we may carry through life the consequences of any adverse conditions that existed in our prenatal life, our intrauterine history.

The Gene Is Not Necessarily Dominant

Our current understanding of how our bodies develop and function throughout life is firmly based on the view that the genetic blueprint we obtain from our parents determines our abilities, both mental and physical. The amazing discoveries of modern genetics and molecular biology are often taken to show that who we are is determined almost entirely by the specific genetic deck of cards that we have been dealt. Each cell in our bodies functions differently, according to which genes are switched on in that particular cell. The integration of the activity of all the genes in all the different cell types will regulate how we function as individuals. In this way, our genes do determine how we perform in the physically and mentally challenging world around us. However, genes are not the only determining factors. The environment in which we grow also influences our development and function. The level of nutrition available to all the cells of our bodies determines which specific genes are active at any particular time. For example, when our bodies are short of food, we activate the genes that control the mechanisms of conservation of food and energy. So to understand how our bodies work, we must ask how the mix of genes that are active at any moment is controlled. Are genes totally in control, or does the environment significantly influence which specific genes are switched on at any one time? Does the world around us during development in the womb affect the level of activity of critical genes? In relation to the origins of health and disease, the fundamental question we must ask is, "Can environmental influences permanently alter the way different cells in the body work?"

The nature-nurture controversy impacts our understanding of the origins of good health. It also addresses the course of diseases that afflict us and how malfunction impairs our lives. Some diseases are clearly inherited. We each have twenty-three pairs of chromosomes. Twenty-two pairs of the chromosomes are called autosomes and carry the genes for the vast majority of our characteristics: one gene from mother, one gene from father. The sex chromosomes are not paired. Thus, there are a few characteristics, those located on the sex chromosomes, for which we do not have two active genes.

Genes are unquestionably the fundamental units by which our bodies are constructed. They are the intricate, coded, transgenerational language that we pass on to our children. However, pure genetic determinism does not adequately explain the varied capabilities of our biology. Numerous human epidemiologic studies and a wide range of observations in a variety of animal species provides a broader view of the interplay of genes and the environment in determining our lifetime health and our susceptibility to disease. Recently available information clearly demonstrates that during development in the womb, genetically driven processes are modified by available maternal nutrition, alterations in blood supply to the uterus, changes in placental function and other environmental factors such as sensory stimulation to the fetus. The information in this book will show why it is no longer possible to consider fetal and newborn development as solely the result of the activities of the gene dominant.

A more accurate view of the role of the genome is to see the genes as providing the overall plan for the developmental pathways of the embryo and fetus. The actual pathway selected by any one fetus will be modified by the environment to which that individual fetus is exposed. Wide variation in prevailing environmental conditions has been present over the recent centuries of human history, changing climates, cycles of plentiful food alternating with famine and exposure to epidemics of infectious diseases. A generation takes, on average, about twenty years before a new set of humans is firmly established on the world stage. The mixing of genes in each generation can produce only small, incremental changes. For this reason, the collective gene pool of the human race can only change very gradually over many generations. The recent rise in the incidence of many human diseases such as diabetes has occurred far too fast for the fundamental basis of the increase to be solely genetic. We shall see that rapid changes in the environment, especially the diet we consume, have clearly played a key role.

Determinism, whether of the genes dominant or programming by the environment during development, strikes hard at our desire for free will. We humans find it hard to accept that we are just creatures of circumstances, unable to control our destinies. We find it much more appealing to our sense of personal worth and purpose to feel that we can influence the path of our lives even in a minor way. Surely, we believe the things we do during our lives also have a pervasive influence on who we are. Surely both our lives and how society works are impacted by the ability to educate our children, to pass on knowledge about how to control complex interactions with our environment such as building dams to provide water at times of shortage. In these and other ways, we feel we have the power to modify our development and improve our health and, as a result, the quality of our lives. We can each of us provide plentiful examples of how nurture of the individual plays a role and alters the way the genetic program is uniquely expressed in each human being. Clearly, genes are not the only factors responsible for the origins of lifetime health or disease. The story told in this book of how programming works can be seen as a story of optimism. If we understand programming better, we will be able to do more for tomorrow's children. In addition, we will learn some things that will be of use to us.

THE RELATIVE ROLE OF GENES IN THE CONSTRUCTION OF OUR BODIES

The currently conceived wisdom of biological science emphasizes the dominant position of our genetic inheritance in determining who we are, how we live our lives, the health we enjoy and the illnesses that afflict us. To question this dogma is to incur the wrath, the disdain and even the wan and patronizing smiles of some segments of the biomedical establishment. It is not my intention to question the fact that genes play a key role in determining the structure and function of all organisms including ourselves. I wish to redress the balance and focus attention on how the script written on the genes is altered by the prevailing dynamic positive and negative influences of the environment in the womb. By positive, I mean those conditions that set us up for a lifetime of good health; by negative, I refer to influences that predispose to disease and shorten lifespan. The complete story in the evolving drama that is your life or mine will depend on the whole production, set design, resources and other players, in addition to the genetic script. There is more to how the body develops and functions than the genes. A wide range of recent human and animal research studies presents an exciting new vista on the complexity of interaction of the genes and the environment in the control of development.

The 100,000 genes contained within the human chromosomes carry the architectural plans for the building that is our body. The final appearance of the building will depend on many factors other than the blueprints. Two builders given the same plans for a building but using different-quality materials and labor skills may well produce outwardly similar structures, but the durability of the buildings will likely differ greatly. The quality of the materials the builder chose to put into the structure will determine the health of the building and its resistance to such insults as rain and winds.

The prevailing weather at the time the building is erected will also be of considerable importance. We all know that paint that has not been left to dry properly before it is exposed to rain will peel earlier than paint that has been properly prepared. A correct period of time is required for the successful completion of each step, if all the various structural components are to function optimally. The old saying, "Timing is everything," reflects the critical importance of the sequence in which events occur. If these issues of how the blueprint is implemented are important for static objects such as a house, it is clear that they will be much more important in building structures with moving parts such as the human body. The safety of modern airplanes compared with older models is a tribute to how moving parts can be made to function better by using higher-quality materials such as carbon fibers and a better production line on which to assemble them. There is more to a safe Boeing 747 than the engineer's blueprint.

Why Care? Is Programming a Critical Health Issue?

Programming is the term used to describe the lifelong change in function that follows a particular event in the life of the individual. One of the earliest and most quoted examples of a lifelong change in function is the bonding of newborn birds to the first moving object they see. The behavioral scientist Konrad Lorenz first described this

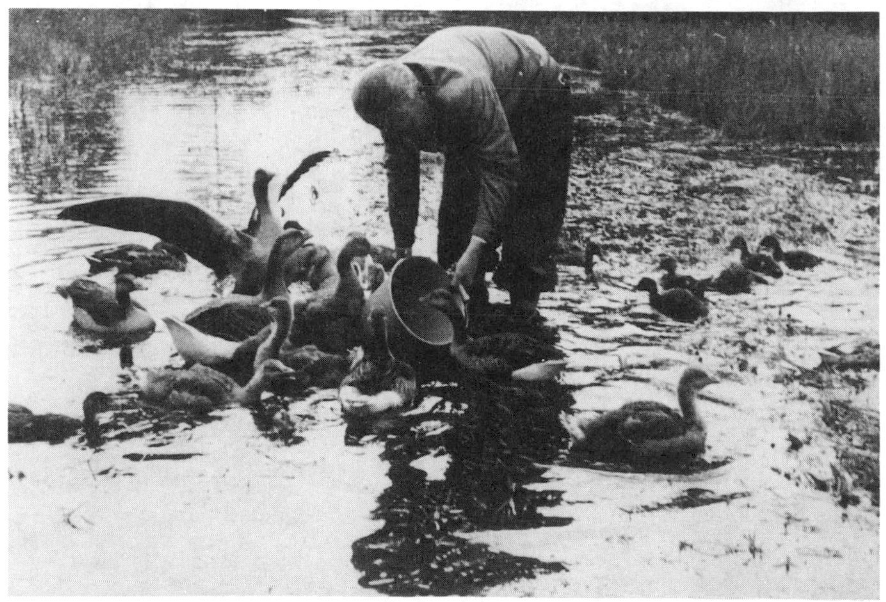

FIGURE 1.1

Konrad Lorenz feeding the geese that bonded with him because he was the first person they saw after they hatched.

process of bonding in geese. As soon as newborn geese emerge from their shell, they look for the first animal or bird moving in their immediate neighborhood. Fortunately, that individual is usually their mother. They fix on her and follow her continuously. Lorenz used the term *imprinting* for this lifelong fixation.

Babies who develop in a suboptimal environment in the uterus use very clever tricks to protect the development of their brain. If the placenta is not functioning properly or if the mother is poorly nourished, it is likely that the availability of oxygen and essential nutrients in the baby's blood will be less than optimal. In this event, the baby preferentially sends blood to the brain, cutting down the

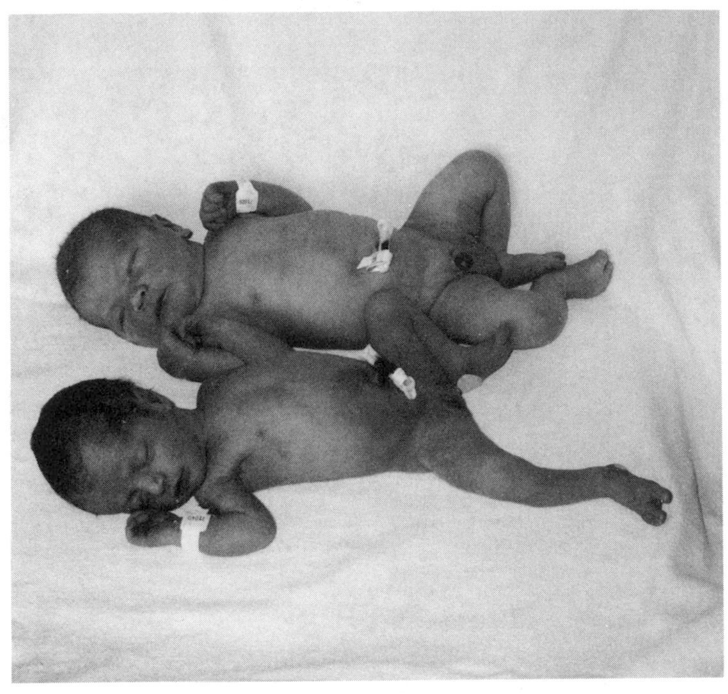

FIGURE 1.2

Two babies with very different body shapes at birth.

amount of blood going to other growing organs such as the gut and liver. As a result, a growth-retarded baby may have a relatively normal-sized head but has reduced abdominal girth. This reduction in girth can have far-reaching health implications throughout life. It is possible, for example, to relate the level of cholesterol in the blood of men at the age of fifty with the size of their abdomen at the time of their birth. The smaller a baby's abdominal girth at birth, the higher the cholesterol level in the blood in later life. I shall tell the full story of this intriguing discovery in chapter 3. For the moment, it is sufficient to note how men who were growth-retarded babies with small abdomens at birth are more likely to have high blood cholesterol later in life. Although this relationship may seem bizarre,

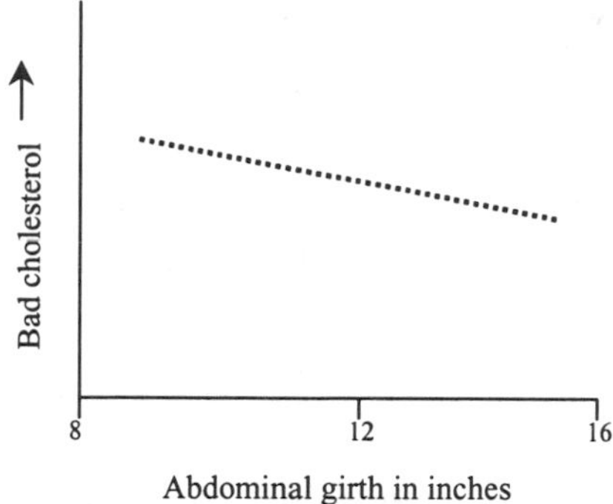

FIGURE 1.3

Level of the bad cholesterol at the age of fifty is higher in men and women who were growth retarded babies and had less girth around their abdomen at birth. Bad cholesterol is the LDL (low-density lipoprotein) cholesterol. Good cholesterol is the HDL (high-density lipoprotein) cholesterol. It is truly amazing that the conditions under which we developed in the womb can alter our blood cholesterol levels fifty years later.

it makes sense when we note that the liver is the largest organ in the abdomen. The abdomens of growth-retarded babies are small because their livers, as well as other abdominal organs, are small. Since the liver plays a central role in regulating cholesterol in the blood in later life, it is not too difficult to see how having grown a small liver before birth can result in high cholesterol levels in the blood in later life. Many growth-retarded babies have paid a price for protecting their brain against shortages of oxygen and nutrients. We don't get anything for free in this life, even before we reach the outside world. When I show these data to both scientists and to the general public, I try to remember to say that, in my view, this stunning piece of information should hang over the bathroom mirror of every politician. The numbers regarding abdominal size of babies are as important to the health of future generations as the Wall Street closing index. They are also equally important to our nation's economic future.

The redistribution of blood to the baby's head that occurs during times of nutrient or oxygen shortage in fetal life even alters the pattern of our fingerprints. The study of fingerprint patterns rejoices in the name *dermatoglyphics*. You, and law enforcement officers, would be forgiven for believing that the unique nature of your fingerprints is completely determined by your genes. However, that simple, gene-dominant view may not be true. Fingerprint ridges begin to form around the tenth week of fetal life. The actual pattern of these ridges is determined by the shape of the fingertip pad. If, at the critical period of development around the tenth week of life, the finger pad swells for any reason, the ridges are drawn out into a circular design (whorls), and when the tip is slim and flat, the ridges are more like arches. One recent study of babies eight weeks after birth reported an association between signs of impaired growth in the womb and the shape of their fingerprint ridges.

Under unfavorable conditions during fetal development, more blood is pumped into the arteries supplying the head. This increased blood supply may lead to swelling of the very deprived tissues to which the blood system is trying to provide extra nourishment. Swelling of the developing fingertips at the critical time the ridges are forming leads to an increase in the number of whorl patterns. There are more whorls on the fingertips of babies who show signs of growth retardation before birth. This explanation is supported by a very interesting difference in the fingerprint structures on the right and left hands in some individuals. In early fetal life, the blood in the artery feeding the developing right arm carries the same blood that supplies the head, while the artery supplying the developing left arm carries the same blood that feeds the legs. It is of considerable interest that studies of large groups of people show that the number of fingerprint whorls is greater on the right hand than those on the left. It is also of interest that the number of whorls on the babies' fingers can be related to the number of whorls in their mothers' fingerprints. The initial reaction to this observation of a similarity between mother and child is to consider the similarity to be genetically driven. However, as we shall see, the conditions a mother experienced when she herself

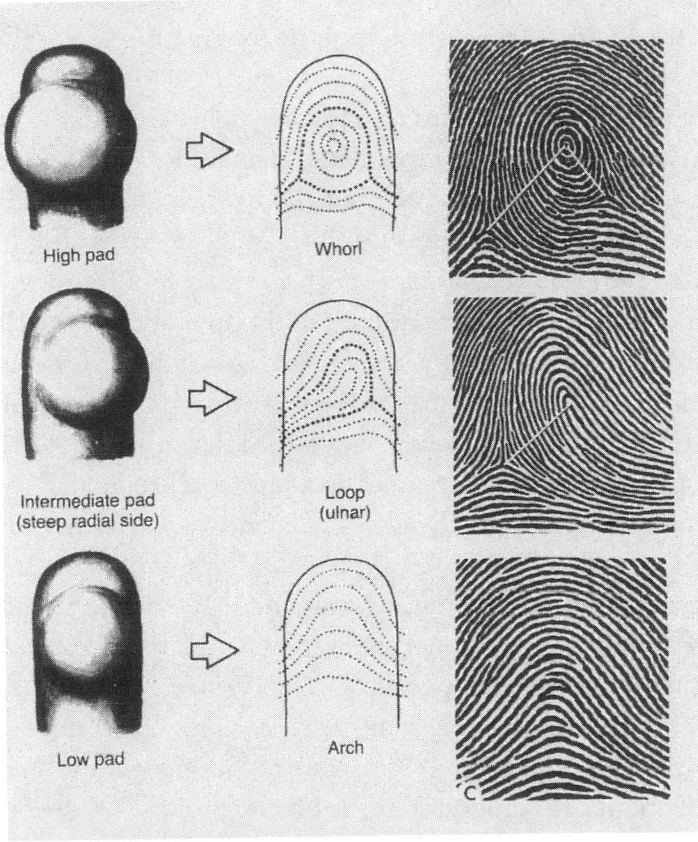

FIGURE 1.4

The formation of fetal fingertip ridges at sixteen to nineteen weeks of fetal life. Whorls and ridges form according to the degree of curvature and swelling of the fingertip as it develops.

Was developing as a fetus may help determine the environment in her own womb when she becomes pregnant.

Fingerprint patterns are dependent on a mix of genetic and prenatal environmental factors. The association of increased numbers of whorls, with characteristics such as a high ratio of head- to-abdominal circumference connects the fingerprint pattern to clear markers of increased susceptibility to heart disease in later life. Perhaps palmists are right, though why do they look only at the ridges on the palms and not at those on the fingertips? I also wonder whether we couldn't learn something by looking more closely at our toes.

There are two independent reasons why it is necessary to evaluate the evidence for programming. One reason is more directed at research investigators. The other speaks to society at large. For the biologist, understanding the mechanisms of programming can illuminate the role of factors that govern fetal and neonatal development and subsequent adult health. In addition, the effects of the environment on the way genes function may provide a better explanation of many features of evolution than a simple view governed by the straitjacket of genetic determinism. Putting the concept of programming in its appropriate place allows a better relation of how nature (the genotype) and nurture (the environment) combine to produce the very special phenotype that is each human being. The importance of programming must be factored in if we are to obtain the full biological picture of the life history of the individual and evolution of different species.

There is a more urgent human reason that urges us to understand programming. It is essential to incorporate the causes and consequences of programming into our thinking on the origins of health and disease. The spectacular technological advance of modern medicine has been based on an ever more detailed understanding of the physiology (normal function) of the body and the reasons it may go wrong. Within the last hundred years, modern medicine has largely put aside routine bleeding with leeches and anecdotal justification of therapies for which no scientific basis has been shown. These idiosyncratic and anecdotal remedies have been replaced by rational treatments based on a diagnosis that is supported by precise laboratory tests that give a better, though as yet often incomplete, understanding of disease processes.

There are two forms of diabetes. In one, the patient is not producing any insulin. In the other, the patient produces insulin, but the body is resistant to insulin's actions. Insulin treatment is essential for the first type of diabetes, but diet can often control the second form. The progress that has been made in prevention, diagnosis and treatment of diseases such as diabetes is truly remarkable. Similarly, understanding the mechanisms that result in programming and their consequences will lead to further improvement in diagnosis and treatment of many disease conditions. Information on how developmental events play out and impact the function of our bodies will help cope with problems that result from events long ago when we ourselves were in our own home in the womb. A better understanding of the nature of normal development of the fetus in the womb and the consequences of a suboptimal prenatal environment is the very frontier of knowledge of the origins of health and disease.

The biology of our bodies might well be called *cellular sociology.* Each organ in our bodies is made up of many different cell types that must live side by side as good neighbors, just as individual people in any human society must tolerate each other and work together if that society is to be harmonious. The different types of cells perform specialized functions. Some cells in the liver store glucose in times of plenty after a meal, while other close neighbors have the opposite job to do, releasing glucose into the blood when food is not available. Cells also talk to other cells nearby, suggesting to their neighbors that they increase or decrease their activities for the common good. At the end of this chapter I provide a list of ten principles of programming. The fourth of my list identifies the importance of developing the correct balance of cells during fetal life in all the organs that make up our bodies. Major problems can arise when the balance of key body functions is altered during suboptimal development. As in human society, the body works best when the correct balance is achieved between different activities, in this case the varying functions of different cells. Understanding how these complex interactions occur is as fascinating as the investigation of the features that govern human societies. The beauty of biology is as fascinating and awe inspiring as the beauty of the cosmos.

If we accept the concept of programming as true, we must pay attention to the health of our children, particularly our daughters, even before they reach childbearing years, since all the evidence from animal studies shows that the preconceptual health of the mother is critical to a normal pregnancy. In human society, action is often easier when the economic and commercial payoff comes rapidly. Farmers and horse breeders have long understood the consequences of programming in the womb. Animal scientists have incorporated these fundamental biological ideas into their commercial breeding practice for years. They know that the level of a mother's nutrition both before and after conception is critical to the health of a lamb or calf. This countryman's wisdom is strongly supported by recent human epidemiological studies that clearly demonstrate that women who are not well nourished *before* they become pregnant have smaller, less healthy babies. What is now known about the influence of programming on lifelong health shows that these smaller babies will enjoy less healthy lives and will be a greater economic and social cost to themselves, to their families and to society.

I fear that the initial response to my reference to application of animal breeding practices to humans is to presume that I am advocating genetic selection in humans. Not so. Quite the opposite. It is not deterministic genetic selection to which I refer but the need to pay attention to the quality of life before birth. It is unfortunate but true that we humans often pay more attention to the quality of the prenatal environment and nutrition provided for our broodmares and pedigreed dogs than in human pregnancy.

We must not penalize the unborn because the environment into which they are thrust before and immediately after birth is suboptimal. This view may seem very altruistic, but there are many completely selfish reasons why we should care about the consequences of programming and attempt to understand it better. Our society spends billions of dollars coring out coronary arteries and transplanting hearts, picking up the pieces produced by poor preventive medicine. Similarly, when it comes to the consequences of a suboptimal home in the womb, very little preventive medicine is carried out at the present time. The vast expenditures on critical medical care in later life are largely the result of a lack of understanding about how our bodies work under good conditions and how they may be abnormally programmed to work inefficiently by a particular prenatal environment. Many of the features of our modern

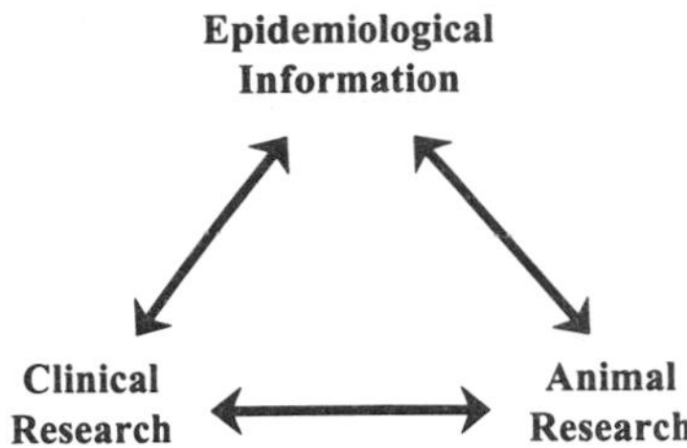

FIGURE 1.5

The interaction of different sources of information on programming during life in the womb.

lifestyles are very different from the biological society for which our bodies were prepared over the millennia of evolution. As a consequence, the health of both mother and fetus may suffer. When the fetus suffers, the consequences can be lifelong and very harmful to health in adult life.

The Triangle of Epidemiology: Clinical, Medical, and Animal Research

For some people, the view that the quality of life before birth is important to our health is self-evident. It is a well-known fact. However, even if you are already disposed to accept the view that programming occurs during development, it is necessary to evaluate the evidence in favor of this important biological principle. It is important to know which systems in the body, brain, heart and liver are affected, and to what extent, under different conditions. I hope this book will leave you with a better understanding of the magnitude and extent of the impact of unfavorable prenatal development on the health of the individual and the health of society.

The underpinning of these ideas comes from three main sources: epidemiological studies, clinical practice and observations in animals. Over the past thirty years, a mounting and overwhelming body of epidemiologic evidence has accumulated from many countries throughout the world. The evidence came to light slowly through the '60s, '70s and '80s. Much of the credit for bringing these issues to the forefront of scientific and medical thinking must go to Dr. David Barker and his Medical Research Council (MRC) Epidemiology Unit at Southampton University in England. As a result of his pioneering efforts, many researchers in this field call the concept of prenatal programming the Barker hypothesis. In chapter 3, we will see how Barker and his colleagues have studied birth records from babies born in the United Kingdom between 1910 and 1930 and related their weight at birth and other physical characteristics to the health these individuals enjoyed and the illnesses they endured during their lives. Many of the subjects of these studies have now died and it is possible to relate the cause of their death to their weight and body form when they were born.

David Barker has shown, for example, that the likelihood an individual will die as a result of heart disease is increased by over 50 percent in men whose birthweight was less than 5.5 pounds, compared with men with a birthweight of 9.5 pounds. The relationship of this increased risk of an early death from heart disease to poor early growth is further demonstrated by the fact that boys who weigh less than 18 pounds at one year of age have two and a half times the risk of dying of heart disease in adulthood when compared with boys who weigh more than 26 pounds at one year of age. The fact that boys show these correlations but girls do not is of considerable interest and reflects the tenth principle of programming listed at the end of the chapter. At all stages of development, male fetuses and infants grow faster than girls. We will see in chapter 5 that quickly growing cells are generally more vulnerable to the effects of inadequate supply of nutrition than slowly growing cells—part of our first principle of programming. When cells are growing faster, they need more resources. So, if the resources are cut off, cells that are growing rapidly are less able to survive the cutbacks. It is likely that this increased rate of growth is responsible for the greater vulnerability of boys than girls at all stages in life. So much for the weaker sex. "But," you may say, "these are only correlations, and any epidemiologist knows that it is very difficult to tell why things happen just from correlation alone." As Stephen Jay Gould warns us in his book *Full House,* we must not "conflate correlation with causation." True. A single instance of epidemiologic correlation between two events cannot define the mechanism that causes one or both of the events to occur. In some instances, when changes take place in the environment, looking at correlations before and after the change can help to discover the cause. To see how this type of study can provide useful information, it will pay us to look at the epidemiological evidence that links smoking to lung cancer.

The first epidemiologic correlation on the effect of smoking on lung cancer was reported in the 1940s. The report firmly indicated that smoking cigarettes greatly increased the likelihood that an individual would develop lung cancer. However, the tobacco industry was quick to use the limitations of epidemiologic research to exonerate cigarettes. Those with an interest in defending the smoking habit aggressively pointed out that there was a host of other factors in society in addition to smoking that correlated very well with the increased incidence of lung cancer in smokers. They acknowledged that the incidence of lung cancer had risen over the years in step with the increase in the number of cigarettes smoked but pointed out that the increase in lung cancer could also be correlated with other recent changes in society: the number of bananas eaten, for example, as the Western nations became more affluent. By pure correlation alone, it could be argued that the cause of the increase in lung cancer was not smoking cigarettes but the consumption of bananas.

However, a human experiment of sorts did take place. Not surprisingly, doctors are among the first to see the ravages caused by new forms of disease. At very close quarters, these doctors had seen large numbers of their patients who were smokers suffer the often agonizing deaths associated with lung cancer and other lung disease. The painful experience of seeing their patients die was enough for many physicians. They gave up smoking. Since not all physicians stopped smoking, those who stopped can be considered an experimental population while those who continued were the control population, thereby making it possible to compare the incidence of deaths from lung cancer in the two groups. The result was dramatic.

The death rate among those physicians who quit smoking dropped rapidly when compared with their colleagues who did not stop smoking.

You would think this comparison was powerful evidence for a causal relationship between smoking and lung cancer. However, the tobacco industry was still able to put up a plausible explanation to counter this second striking epidemiologic connection. The supporters of the tobacco industry argued that there was something different about the doctors who were able to give up smoking compared with those who were unable to stop smoking. They put forward the explanation that doctors who were able to give up smoking were individuals who, because they were different from those who could not give up smoking, were also less likely to get lung cancer. I suppose, according to this view, the same doctors who were able to quit might be less likely to get cancer from bananas or perhaps they just didn't eat bananas.

The ability of the tobacco industry to mount such a defense shows how difficult it is to come to firm conclusions about causation from epidemiologic studies. Epidemiologic studies using data often collected many years after the event can never give the certainty that is provided by carefully controlled, prospectively designed interventions. To counter this argument that the two groups of doctors differed, it would have been necessary to set up a carefully controlled, highly regulated experiment. The first step would be to get together a large group of cigarette smoking doctors (or other group of people who share a similar age, profession, sex and social class) who have not yet decided to stop smoking and then divide the group up randomly into two subgroups. One subgroup would then not be allowed to smoke and the other would be made to continue. Ideally, the subjects of the study should not be allowed to choose the group they wished to join. We can see that such a randomly assigned human trial would be very difficult, if not impossible, to set up.

In good experimental studies, it is necessary to rule out all possible factors that may affect the outcome under investigation other than the one factor under study. Epidemiologic studies generally attempt to rule out other potentially confounding or additive factors by having such large groups that these other factors such as diet, marital and economic status will be the same in both groups purely as a result of the large numbers. The other approach is to decide on other potentially confounding factors before the epidemiologic study is started and to include or exclude certain categories of subjects before the study starts. However, if for example, the study were confined to women between thirty and fifty, the conclusions reached by the study could only apply to women in that age range. While this is important information, the results would tell us nothing about the mechanisms by which smoking causes cancer.

Because of these difficulties and other requirements, it is impossible to learn everything we need to know about the cause of a clinical condition from human epidemiologic studies. So the second line of approach in understanding the causes of a disease is to look at how patients respond clinically to various forms of treatment. Collecting paticnts who do not have any other confounding factors in their medical history is very difficult. One of the major confounding factors is the change that occurs in society over the time that is necessary to collect together enough patients to make the results statistically sound. In addition, it is also impossible to evaluate the precise effects of the condition under study on particular body organs, such as lungs, liver, heart or kidneys. To do this, we would need samples of blood and specimens from the various tissues in two groups of individuals: a group that is suffering from the disease under study (the experimental group) and a second group who does not have the disease (the control group). Often, it is also necessary to have samples from individuals in both groups before, during and after exposure. In addition, as mentioned above, a good study ensures that all other factors and disease conditions than the one under study are the same in both groups. It is difficult to almost impossible to rigorously control for all these factors in human epidemiologic and clinical studies. It is particularly difficult to design epidemiological and clinical studies that control all the factors in a mother's environment both before and during pregnancy. The presence of the fetus complicates analysis of what is happening to the mother. We cannot do anything to control genetic differences among the fetuses in different human pregnancies. Such control would be necessary if epidemiologic and clinical studies are to provide a full mechanistic understanding of the effects of different prenatal conditions on long-term health. These shortcomings of epidemiologic studies in no way decrease their importance in identifying the cause of disease or the requirements for health.

At some stage, in every aspect of medical research, animal investigations are indispensable to understand health and disease at the organ and cell level. Study of critical biological processes in animals is particularly necessary when we try to understand what is happening in pregnancy. Pregnancy is a complex interaction between two independent organisms locked in the closest of biological embraces. The presence of a shared organ, the placenta, with unique capabilities to act as a lung, transporting oxygen, a gut transporting food, and a kidney, removing the body's waste products, further complicates the study of this fascinating and critically important period of life. The fifth of our principles of programming is the importance of the function of the placenta. We are extremely ignorant of the function of this most important structure. We need to know much more about how the placenta forms and functions. The placenta acts as a conduit between mother and fetus, protecting the baby from some harmful compounds but allowing others to pass freely. The placenta also has its own nutritional needs, which may at times conflict with those of the fetus.

In order to determine the extent to which prenatal programming lies at the heart of many diseases, it is necessary to study developing animals who have been exposed to different degrees and types of nutritional and other challenges during fetal development. Since part of the pathological mechanism may be due to interactive changes in the mother, placenta and fetus, it is impossible to study all the components of this system in a test tube. It is necessary to understand how placenta, brain, liver, pancreas and developing heart interact. Although study of cultures of these tissues does yield useful information, the only situation that allows study of the integrated interactions between the external world, mother, placenta and fetus is the intact pregnancy itself. If we are ever to understand how the placenta affects our lifetime health, there is ultimately no substitute for observing the whole complex situation.

It is often said that the computer can simulate these complex interactions. Again, just as there is need for information from studies on single cells, computer simulation can often provide useful information. However, the computer can only simulate situations that are based on data that have been entered into the computer. The value of any computer simulation will depend on the quality of the biological information that is provided. The data entered into the computer have to be obtained from real-life situations. There is an old and much-favored saying of computer specialists: "Garbage in, garbage out."

As I have already mentioned, Dr. David Barker has been the pioneer in calling attention to the overwhelming epidemiologic data that show the importance of prenatal events to lifetime health. He has expanded the human database on the connection of life in the womb to lifetime health to include populations throughout Europe, India and China. David Barker has produced a very sound basis for the overall thesis that our health and our susceptibility to disease in later life is in large measure programmed before birth. Yet, in spite of the power of his analyses, he has repeatedly called for experimental animal studies to elucidate the mechanisms by which these prenatal influences produce their effects. It is only by understanding the mechanisms at the cellular, organ and whole- animal level that it will be possible to both prevent the adverse outcomes in generations to come and to lessen the consequences for those of us who may have been exposed to suboptimal conditions prenatally but cannot turn back the clock and return to our home in the womb.

As we shall see, there is a clear correlation between the incidence of death from coronary heart disease and the conditions experienced in the womb before birth. At a recent meeting in New York, David Barker stated clearly that, in his view, an understanding of the cause of coronary heart disease will not come from cardiologists but from those who are researching the factors that regulate fetal development using animal models.

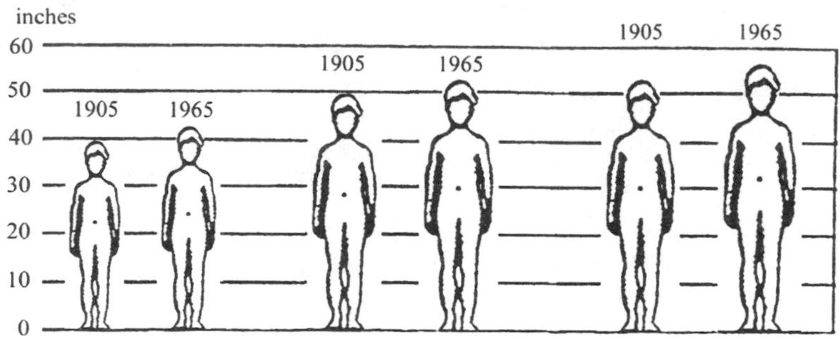

FIGURE 1.6

Increase of average height of European children between 1905 and 1965.

What Is Usual? What is Normal?

Nothing is more certain to raise the temperature of discussion than an attempt to introduce the concept of normality. For most people, the difference between normal and abnormal is a very subjective distinction. Normality is what is acceptable to us and abnormality is what is unacceptable. This approach provides a very easy personal solution to a very difficult question. The scientist solves the problem just as easily but in another way: by looking at the whole population, finding a marker for the characteristic under study and then looking at its statistical distribution. With most human characteristics, people range across the well-known bell curve. If we compare the distribution of the weight of pregnant women in the United States and India, they will be very different. The most common weight is at the center of the curve. However, it is clear that there is a very great difference in the most usual weight in these countries. Since people living in the subcontinent of India are smaller than in the Western world, the weight at the middle of the Indian bell curve will be lower than in the United States. But the question still remains, even within one group, "If we want to define *usual,* how far out from the center of the bell curve should we go? What proportion of the two tails of the curve should be acceptable as the norm, and who are the real outliers?"

Although the issue of prenatal programming involves considerations of normality, programming first and foremost is about how development is permanently modified by the environment to which an individual is exposed during life before birth. It is better to think in terms of optimal and suboptimal environments in which a particular individual may develop rather than normal or abnormal. An optimal environment in the womb is one in which babies develop to their full biological potential, both mental and physical. A good example of the effect of early development is the increase in height and weight in Japanese society as nutrition has improved over the last few decades. The average height of Japanese men has increased dramatically over the last two or three generations. What then is the *normal* height for the Japanese male? Whether the full biological potential of a particular individual is normal or abnormal will depend on the social and physical climate in which that particular individual will need to function.

The nature of the environment in which an individual has to function is of course critical to the success that individual will have in surviving and enjoying life. In the Darwinian sense, if individuals are not adequately prepared by their own development, both before and after birth, for survival in their species habitat, not only will they not survive, but their genes will not be passed on. In the extreme case, if the species cannot provide enough individuals to survive in an environment, particularly a changing environment, the whole species will fail in that environment.

So normality is really a question of interaction of the individual and the environment. Being born bigger may not always be better. When food is short, poor maternal nutrition leads to the delivery of smaller babies. It is of value to the species that smaller babies are born during a time of food shortage. These smaller babies will have smaller appetites, and decreased appetites will be easier to feed if food is in short supply. There is evidence that babies deprived of nutrition in the womb develop a thrifty dietary lifestyle and are more able to withstand situations of prolonged food shortage throughout their lives. It is difficult to determine the birthweight that constitutes normality in a situation of food scarcity. Are moderately growth-retarded babies normal in this situation? Certainly, small people are likely to have a greater chance of survival in a situation where food resources are limited. We need to fuse Darwinian concepts, genetic knowledge and an appreciation of environmental challenges (and their consequences) to understand the full implications of an individual's specific biology rather than define normality.

What Is Good Health?

When asked to define poetry, one famous critic is supposed to have replied, "It would be easier to define what isn't poetry." This is a clever way out but doesn't improve our understanding. Similarly, when asked to define health, it is tempting to say that we can identify disease more easily than health. In one respect, good health allows us to function at the level that fits reasonably within the normal distribution for our species. Therefore, health can be defined against the background of what each member of the species should be able to do to survive and perform the activities that allow the species to continue in its ecological niche and produce offspring that are also able to take advantage of their special survival skills. Thus, what constitutes good health is somewhat different for animals in the wild and the animals that have been bred for special functions. A cow that is not providing enough milk for her calf is unlikely to be healthy. She is certainly not producing enough for commercial purposes. For the cow, the commercial expectation of normality is set by the dairy farmer. A cow that produces little milk is not normal both according to commercial as well as evolutionary needs and expectations.

Normality of every single one of our bodily functions is not necessary for good health. Individuals with conditions such as spina bifida or those born without a limb can enjoy very good health. Expectations constitute a major feature of good health. You can be very healthy but not be able to compete on the tennis or basketball court. Indeed, to compete really well at basketball, you had better have the abnormal (or unusual) physical attributes necessary. You must be tall—very tall. Athletic physical fitness is certainly one aspect of good health, but it is not the same thing.

Holistic approaches to health have become very popular in recent years. There are many very good reasons for this development. Good health implies that all our various systems are functioning appropriately: muscles, gut, heart and, of course, the brain. What about the preparation of these structures during development? If we as individuals failed to prepare, we must be prepared to fail. If our immune system did not go through the correct preparatory stages during development, it is likely that we will not throw off infections as well and as quickly as we otherwise might. I shall describe studies in adult rats that clearly show that responses to stress differ according to the level of stress to which their mothers were exposed during pregnancy. Certainly, the way we handle stress is a major determinant of our overall health. For some people, stress just tones them up; for others, stress constitutes an intolerable burden.

Proper preparation for an event requires a clear and correct assessment of the needs of the event. For all animals, the event for which they are preparing in the womb is their life in the physical and social environment inhabited by their species. A major problem for the human race is that our social and physical environment is changing at a bewildering pace. The rate of change accelerates every year as society grows more complex. Our genetic complement just cannot change that fast. Rapid changes may render inadequate certain aspects of preparation based on previous evolutionary needs. Worse still, some preparations may even be inappropriate to the conditions the individual eventually encounters. As mentioned above, if a pregnant woman is short of nutrients, her baby in the womb can develop what is called a thrifty approach to food availability, thereby preparing for an outside world in which food may be scarce for prolonged periods of time. If, however, after the baby is born, food is not scarce and the individual has a plentiful supply throughout life, then the preparation the baby made before birth was unnecessary. Worse still, when food is available in excess, this incorrect preparation during life before birth may even be harmful. This is our seventh principle of programming.

Congenital Is Not The Same as Genetic

Almost every day, I pick up a newspaper or even a scientific report that assumes a condition that is present at birth is therefore automatically genetically determined. Perhaps the most glaring

Ten Principles of Programming

1. During development, there are **critical periods of vulnerability** to suboptimal conditions. Vulnerable periods occur at different times for different tissues. Cells dividing rapidly are at greatest risk. Factors that increase risk include:
   - Too much of a normal chemical such as a hormone, critical nutrient or vitamin
   - Deficiency of a normal chemical such as a hormone, critical nutrient or vitamin
   - Abnormal chemicals such as alcohol or nicotine
   - Abnormal physical forces, such as high blood pressure

2. Programming has **permanent effects** that alter responses in later life and can modify susceptibility to disease.

3. Fetal development is **activity dependent.** Normal development is dependent on continuing normal activity. Each phase of development provides the required conditions for subsequent development.

4. Programming involves several different **structural changes in important organs.**
   - The absolute numbers of cells in the organ may increase or decrease.
   - The relative proportions and distribution of different types of cell within the organ may be unbalanced.
   - The normal blood supply to the organ may not form.
   - Too many or too few hormone receptors may form with a resultant resetting of feedback and other control mechanisms.

TEN PRINICIPLES OF PROGRAMMING (CON'T)

5. The **placenta** plays a key role in programming.

6. **Compensation carries a price.** In an unfavorable environment, the developing baby makes attempts to compensate for deficiencies. Following compensation, birthweight may be normal or only slightly decreased. However, the compensatory effort carries a price.

7. **Attempts made after birth to reverse the consequences of programming may have their own unwanted consequences.** When postnatal conditions prove to be other than those for which the fetus prepared, problems may arise.

8. **Fetal cellular mechanisms often differ from adult processes.** Fetuses react differently to suboptimal conditions than do newborn babies or adults.

9. The **effects of programming may pass across generations** by mechanisms that do not involve changes in the genes.

10. Programming often has **different effects in males and females.**

example is the rush to conclude that because something is more common in identical twins than in single babies, then the cause *must* be genetic. It should never be forgotten that twins share the same world in the womb for nine months before birth. Since identical twins have exactly the same genetic composition, characteristics that occur in identical twins are often considered to be excellent indicators of genetically determined conditions. However, there are different types of identical twins. If the single egg that gives rise to identical twins splits within the first two days after fertilization each twin will have a separate placenta. This situation occurs in 20 to 30 percent of identical twins. In all the other sets, the identical twin fetuses share the same placenta. However, the situation is not as simple as it may seem. When twins share the placenta, each twin has a different portion, and the sharing may be unequal. When the placenta is shared, there are many factors that determine the amount of maternal blood that may pass to the areas accessed by the blood in the umbilical cord of each fetus. How much of the space in the womb and the exact location will also differ. It is very difficult to unravel the factors that are different from those that are similar in the environment shared by identical twins in the womb. Identical twins obviously have the same mother, but the proportion of the resources available in the womb that each baby receives will differ, as will the exact space they inhabit. To be correct, a condition that exists at birth must first be considered congenital, and not all congenital conditions are genetic. Some are due solely to the impact of the environmental conditions the baby has experienced during development.

It is vital to remember that the preparation in the womb is influenced by factors other than genes. During the nine months of life before birth, the developing baby is exposed to the conditions imposed upon her or him by the mother. The baby develops according to the constraints of both the genetic blueprint and the availability of food and a variety of other stimuli to which she or he has been exposed. The conditions that exist in the womb impact each of us at a critical period of our lives. The prenatal origin of health and disease is one of the most important issues that affects us and our children.

Two

The Dutch Hunger Winter
September 1944-May 1945

I keep six honest serving-men
(They taught me all I knew);
Their names are What and Why and When And How
and Where and Who.
I send them over land and sea,
I send them east and west;
But after they have worked for me,
I give them all a rest.

Rudyard Kipling, *The Elephant's Child*

Our bodies need good nutrition throughout life. This requirement is particularly important during the first nine months of our lives as we grow in the womb. It is a shameful fact that we know more about the requirements for good nutrition before and during pregnancy in animals than in pregnant women. However, there are some unfortunate historical periods of poor human nutrition from which we can learn. One such episode is the Dutch Hunger Winter. Between September 1944 and May 1945, the occupying German forces virtually starved the population of western Holland. The starvation was a reprisal for an ambitious air drop of paratroopers at Arnhem in Holland that the wartime Allies fighting Germany had hoped would end the war quickly.

The Hunger Winter had a lifelong effect on the health of children born to women who were pregnant during this period. The specific effects of the Hunger Winter on lifetime health depend on the stage of pregnancy at which the pregnant mother was deprived of adequate nutrition. Male children born during the Dutch Hunger Winter had a greater tendency to obesity if their mothers were only exposed to starvation in the first third of pregnancy. If their mothers were starved in the last third of pregnancy, male children had a decreased likelihood of becoming obese in later life. There is also a higher incidence of diabetes and schizophrenia among the children of the Dutch Hunger Winter.

Women who were themselves daughters of the Hunger Winter were more likely to have a growth-retarded baby when they became pregnant. Thus the effects of poor conditions during pregnancy can be transmitted across generations.

During the 872-day siege of Leningrad, there was a similar extreme shortage of food. Over two million people died. Babies born after the siege have a higher susceptibility to heart disease. These long-term effects on lifetime health caused by adverse circumstances during fetal life highlight the importance of the conditions in our earliest home in the womb.

Starvation Affects Those as Yet Unborn

Recent famines in Somalia and other parts of Africa, as well as harvest failures in some major crop-producing areas, show how vulnerable we inhabitants of this small globe are to shortages of food. Newspaper pictures and news footage of starving children and adults have become commonplace, and the feeding of whole populations has become a regular task for world aid organizations and charity groups. The problems posed by starvation are seen as immediate and pressing. And so they are for the victims. However, one recent starvation story has demonstrated that the consequences of poor nutrition are not confined to the need for survival for those exposed to the famine. Undernutrition has long-term implications across generations for children as yet unborn.

A Bridge Too Far: Punitive Starvation

The airdrop of British paratroopers at Arnhem in Holland in the Second World War took place on September 17, 1944. It was a bold and potentially decisive attempt to seize a crucial bridge over the river Rhine and speed the allied forces into a collapsing Germany. The allied commanders hoped this daring thrust would bring the European war to a rapid end. By the time of the Arnhem drop into Holland, the allies were already advancing rapidly, but if the strategic bridge could be captured before it was destroyed by the retreating Germans, the end of the war would conceivably come very much sooner. To coincide with the allied attack at Arnhem, the Dutch government in exile in London urged the Dutch population to resist the German occupation with any means at their disposal. A rail strike was called in an attempt to hamper German movement of munitions and personnel.

The events associated with this airdrop were depicted in the movie *A Bridge Too Far*. If you have seen the film or read one of the many books written about this brave attempt to shorten the wartime suffering, you will know that the bridgehead could not be established. The gamble failed. The occupying Germans responded savagely by restricting the supply of food to the western part of Holland. To make matters worse, the winter of 1944–1945 was exceedingly cold. Starvation was rampant throughout the winter since liberation by the allies did not come until early May 1945.

What the movie and books won't tell you is that the failed attack drastically affected more than the health and lives of the Dutch already born at that time and who were forced to live for months on starvation rations. The poor diets of women who were pregnant during the Dutch Hunger Winter also affected the lifetime health of at least one generation of people then unborn. The effects may still be with us fifty years later, since studies in animals show that the effects of poor maternal nutrition may be passed across several generations.

Before the imposition of the restrictions on transport of food by the Germans, the average Dutch person's wartime food intake was about 1,500 calories a day. By the end of 1944, this intake had fallen to around 750 calories a day. At the height of the very harsh winter, some people were only eating as few as 450 calories daily. Meals consisted of a few slices of bread, turnips and potatoes. Some people resorted to eating their famous Dutch flower bulbs. The Dutch government did everything possible to lessen the impact of the food shortage by setting up soup kitchens and arranging rationing. A black market existed, and people suffered differently according to their connections, wealth and local resources. In the countryside there were some limited food stores—at least at the beginning of the winter. People who lived in the cities were more seriously undernourished than those who lived in the countryside. Food shortages were worst in the city of Amsterdam. It is estimated that nearly 20,000 people died before the allied troops liberated the region in early May 1945.

Keeping alive through the *Hongerwinter* (as the Dutch call this period) required all the resources of body and mind that humans somehow summon up in times of adversity. As the very cold winter drew on, it was often all one could do to stay still and keep warm. People moved around as little as possible. On a visit to Holland in 1996, I spoke with one of the survivors, Mrs. Bakker. She delivered her baby, a daughter on May 2, 1945. The baby girl weighed 2,800 grams (6.16 pounds). Mrs. Bakker was fortunate to live in a rural area. Her family was hiding because they were Jews, and it was very dangerous for Jews to be outside their houses. When she did go outside, friends acted as lookouts to tell her if German soldiers were in the neighborhood. Generally, however, all she did was lie or sit in the same room, day after day. Movement requires the body to expend energy. If you are on starvation rations, unnecessary expenditures of energy lessen the chance of survival.

Although community efforts were made to provide pregnant women with as much food as possible, people were reluctant to make major exceptions to the limited rations available. There was not enough food to think of generations as yet unborn. Young pregnant

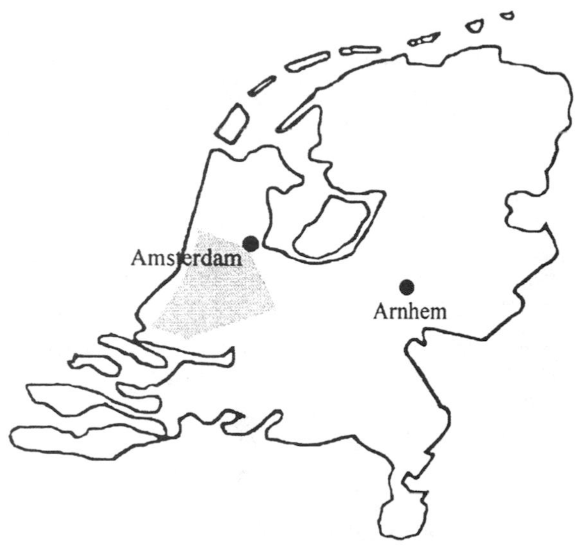

FIGURE 2.1

Map of Holland showing the site of the Arnhem airdrop of paratroopers and the area of Holland that the Nazis starved as a punishment.

women were not completely neglected. They were given more ration tickets for vegetables and potatoes, but their families often made them share the extra food among their brothers and sisters. It is easier to see the needs of young children standing before you than to be concerned with the special requirements of the unborn baby in the womb. Mrs. Bakker recalled that mothers and fathers were more concerned to feed the children who had already been born than the children as yet unborn. Mrs. Bakker was the third of fifteen children in a farming community, so she said they were relatively well off, though the situation became progressively worse. There was also the physical and mental stress to cope with. Being both short of food and pregnant, she found it hard to walk any distance. However, she knew throughout her pregnancy that when she went into labor, she would need to walk to Amsterdam where she was to deliver her baby at the Wilhelmina Hospital. Because of the impossibility of transport

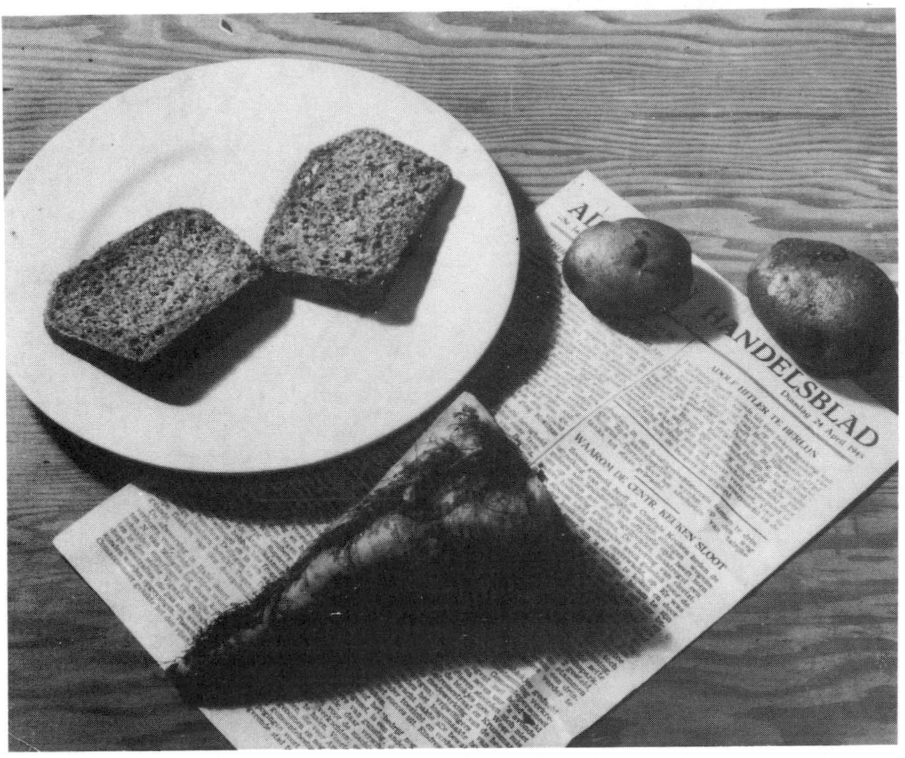

FIGURE 2.2

A typical meal for an adult during the Dutch Hunger Winter of Nazi occupation, September 1944 to May 1945.

and her reluctance to be seen outside the house, she could not visit her doctor. As a result, she had very little prenatal care. Newborn babies and young children suffered especially badly. Young children need calories to grow and develop their immune systems. The grossly underfed children were very vulnerable to infection. During this cold winter combined with pitiful nutrition it is not surprising that diphtheria and other childhood diseases killed large numbers of children.

The Effect on Pregnancy of Wartime Starvation in Holland

The period of starvation rations ceased early in May 1945 and the war ended soon after. In addition to the immediate provision of food after the war, medical aid was a top priority for Holland. Physicians from the United States and England were sent to survey medical needs. Clement Smith from Harvard Medical School, one of the founders of modern pediatrics, was among the first to witness the nutritional effects of the famine on the babies born during and after the period of starvation. He immediately saw an opportunity to obtain information that would help resolve important questions on how poor maternal nutrition affects the development of the fetus before birth. Clement Smith had available to him pregnancy records and newborn birthweights from the Dutch National School of Midwives at Rotterdam and from a major hospital in The Hague. He worked fast. Within a year, on May 2, 1946, he presented his first talk on the effects of the famine on the babies born during the Hunger Winter and immediately afterward. The effects on birthweight of the babies were dramatic.

Clement Smith's first paper was entitled "Effects of Maternal Undernutrition upon the Newborn Infant in Holland (1944–1945)." The second paper was given a more striking title: "The Effect of Wartime Starvation in Holland upon Pregnancy and Its Product." Some extracts from the first of these two papers highlight the importance of the problem and point to the difficulties faced by epidemiological studies.

Clement Smith understood the problem of proving cause and effect from epidemiologic data. When food is plentiful, underfeeding and malnutrition during pregnancy are due to personal emotional and psychological decisions the mother makes that result in poor eating habits. Consequences to the baby under such conditions may be due to the personal problems that led the mother to refuse to eat rather than the lack of nutrients. Clearly, in the famine situation, the mothers had not ceased to eat because of some psychological problem; the nutritional deprivation had been forced upon them. Smith set out to describe exactly *what* had happened as a result of

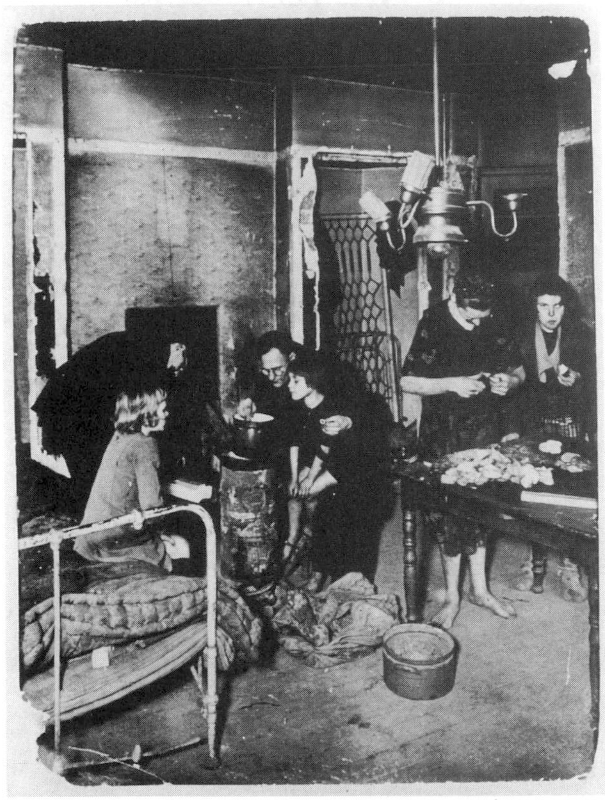

FIGURE 2.3

A Dutch family huddled around the stove in the Dutch Hunger Winter.

starvation in the hope that the data would help to show *how* nutritional deprivation harms the growing baby. Here was an opportunity to gain the firm information required to answer the *why, when, where and who* as well. Fifty years later, data from the Dutch *Hongerwinter* continue to provide an opportunity to evaluate the consequences of poor nutrition in pregnancy in a human setting.

Clement Smith wrote, "The great difficulty [in establishing a cause-and-effect relationship between maternal nutrition and the development of the baby] is to construct experimental situations producing incontrovertible proof that undesirable results of human

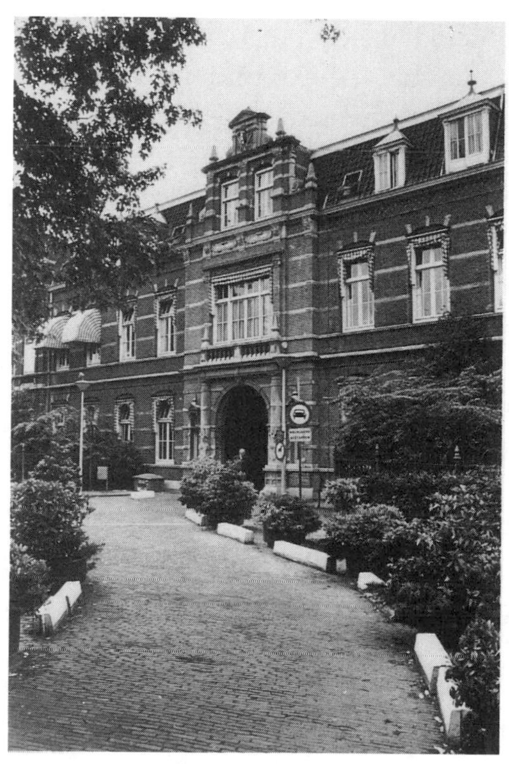

FIGURE 2.4

Wilhelmina Gasthuis, Obstetric Hospital in Amsterdam.

pregnancy, either maternal or fetal, are direct consequences of maternal dietary factors. The substance of this difficulty is stated by the proposition that women who eat poor diets may well be suboptimal individuals in various other ways, as in heredity, environment, and past history of disease . . . we still need proof that the infant's condition is the *result* [Clement Smith's emphasis] of the mother's diet. Or, if maternal malnutrition cannot be shown to be the sole cause of the fetal subnormality, we should like to know the relative degree of its influence."

The amount of food available varied at different times of the winter. Some women were already pregnant when food was first restricted. Others became pregnant at varying times during the winter. As a result, the period of fetal development affected by the poor nutrition differed in each pregnant woman. Since different fetal organs grow and mature at different times in pregnancy, the Hunger Winter data can throw light on the different unwanted poor outcomes that result from malnutrition at the various stages of fetal development. For example, the fetal kidneys are developing very rapidly around the middle of pregnancy and are likely to be damaged when undernutrition occurs during that time. Thus, knowing *when* the challenge of poor nutrition is experienced by the fetus will provide information on which of the fetal body systems are likely to be most affected. To gain information on the *how*, the mechanisms by which malnutrition adversely impacts development, it will be necessary to look at more epidemiological studies and conduct carefully controlled experiments in animals. In animal studies, it is possible for investigators to alter carefully chosen portions of the diet (for example, the amount of protein taken in by the mother can be altered independently of the amount of carbohydrate or the total calories) and observe how the pregnant animal and her fetus respond. The *who* in the story is each individual, since we all respond slightly differently to changes in the world around us, and the characteristic and idiosyncratic responses of each individual must always be taken into account.

Clement Smith continues, "There are at least four ways of securing data which may help to clarify these relationships. The simplest, though obviously suitable for animal investigation only, is the calculated restriction of maternal intake during pregnancy. . . . A second method is that of accurate analyses of diets voluntarily consumed by pregnant women, with later comparison of the maternal nutritional status with the outcome of the pregnancy. . . . A definite drawback is again that a group of conditions unfavorable to the pregnancy or the fetus may be present along with improper food habits. . . . A third procedure . . . employs the directed dietary improvement of an experimental group of women, whose pregnancies are then contrasted with those of a control group not so manipulated. This, if large enough numbers are employed, complete objectivity maintained, and *the two groups exactly comparable in all aspects except the nutritional* [Clement Smith's emphasis], would perhaps be the most informative procedure . . . the ideal program for such a procedure would select the two groups at the very onset of pregnancy, if not before." [So Clement Smith was aware of the *when*.]

"A fourth plan is that of observing the effects of widespread nutritional inadequacy due to war or other calamity affecting an entire populace. This type of study takes advantage of a period of starvation as an unhappy but nevertheless potentially serviceable human experiment somewhat like those conducted with animals in the first type listed above. Statistics from the pre- and post-starvation periods furnish the only possible controls."

It must be pointed out that the best investigations in biological science will always investigate what are called contemporaneous control subjects. Control individuals are studied at exactly the same time as the affected subjects. It is important that controls in any study are exposed to exactly the same conditions as the experimental study group *except* the one factor under study, in this case dietary factors that may affect the pregnancy.

This need for contemporaneous controls to enable evaluation of information from human studies is no small and insignificant point. The problem of obtaining contemporaneous controls is one of the major reasons why animal studies will always be necessary to understand how the body as a whole works. Most studies that evaluate the effects of the Dutch Hunger Winter on fetal development and lifelong consequences compare the pregnancies that occurred before or immediately after the period of starvation as controls with the pregnancies that occurred during the time of starvation as the experimental group. Throughout the whole duration of the wartime period, food was scarce, but the amount and quality of the food available was constantly changing. Several factors would make women who were pregnant before or after the Hunger Winter less-than-perfect controls for the pregnancies during the Hunger Winter.

The diets available before pregnancy began were unlikely to have been the same for a woman who started her pregnancy in December 1943 and completed it before the Hunger Winter and a woman who started her pregnancy in December 1944 following three months of ever-increasing shortage of food. The wide-ranging differences in maternal preparation for pregnancy is even more stark if we try to compare a woman who became pregnant in September 1944 and one who became pregnant in March 1945. The second woman would have suffered the worst ravages of food restriction for six months before her pregnancy even started. In addition, the critical first two months of her baby's development would take place at the height of the food shortage. Finally, the mental and physical stress on each pregnant woman varied greatly at different periods of the war as well as in different parts of the country. We should not underestimate the stress on a pregnant woman that comes from having to hide her husband or other loved ones under the floorboards each day, living in fear from minute to minute that the hiding place will be discovered or disclosed by a collaborator.

Consequences of the Hunger Winter for the Baby

Within a year after the end of the war, Clement Smith was able to conclude that maternal undernutrition had resulted in a significant drop in the birthweight of babies and a smaller but still significant decrease in the babies' length. This smaller effect on length than weight may reflect the fact that weight measures growth in all three dimensions, whereas height, or length, measures only growth in one dimension. Length is predominantly determined by the growth of the bones, particularly the spinal column and the long limb bones.

Nutritional restriction has varying effects on different tissues: muscle, fat, liver, skin, kidney, heart, gut and, of course, the nervous system. Thus, looking at effects of undernutrition on the baby's weight effectively adds up all the effects. The critical period at which each tissue grows and the degree to which each organ suffers depends on *when* the restriction occurs.

The *where* and *who* of each pregnancy will depend upon each individual mother's health both before and after she became pregnant. For all babies developing in the uterus, the health of their mothers is the single most important factor in the environment. A mother's weight and her health before pregnancy critically influence the development of her baby. If a woman is underweight and malnourished even before she becomes pregnant, the fetus will not get a good start.

The *when* of the adverse effects of the Hunger Winter is also clear. Clement Smith commented on the fact that babies who passed the last third of their preparation for birth during the Hunger Winter suffered worst. This finding should not be surprising. Most of the baby's growth occurs during the final weeks of pregnancy. As a result, this is the time that the growing baby makes the biggest overall demands on the mother.

Normally, a woman will gain about 25 pounds in weight during pregnancy. During the Hunger Winter, some pregnant women gained as little as 4.4 pounds. As a consequence, growth of their babies in the womb was markedly slowed. It is remarkable that the babies continued to grow in the womb at all. Since even the lowest group of birthweights of babies born during the Hunger Winter were around 4.8 pounds, which was greater than the woman's total increase in weight during pregnancy, it is clear that pregnant mothers must have cannibalized some of their own tissues to grow their baby. What then happened to the babies of women who were already pregnant or became pregnant during the Hunger Winter? How was their life before birth affected?

A woman who became pregnant on September 1, 1944, would have given birth soon after the time of the liberation by the advancing allied armies in May 1945. The majority of her pregnancy would have exactly coincided with the period of starvation. As we have seen, the availability of calories worsened continuously through this period. In addition, the demands on the pregnant woman's own body would have been impacted more severely when the winter weather was at its worst, during the second half of her pregnancy.

Women who gave birth in late 1944 were only exposed to the really severe food restriction at the end of their pregnancy. In contrast, the fetuses of women who became pregnant at the beginning of March 1945 would have been exposed to the famine during only the early weeks of pregnancy. Pregnancies that started between September 1 and March 1, 1945, would have resulted in exposure of the fetus to severe malnutrition in the womb for varying periods of between three and nine months, depending on exactly when the pregnancy began. So babies born in Holland from the beginning of September 1944 to the end of 1945 would have differed greatly in the critical periods of development in the womb during which they were severely undernourished. For convenience, we can break down the different patterns of exposure into three groups: babies who were undernourished in the womb for the whole pregnancy, just the first third, or just the final third.

Measurements of overall body weight at birth, the baby's length and head circumference all show that suboptimal nutrition during the last third of fetal life has the greatest impact on overall growth in size. This conclusion shows through from comparisons of these three measurements in babies who were only exposed to the famine during the first three months of development in the womb and babies who were exposed for the final three months only. However, the greatest effects were always seen in the babies who were deprived throughout the full period of their development. Their heads were the smallest of the three groups, they were the shortest and they weighed the least.

Study of the different effects of starvation restricted to the first or last thirds of pregnancy has yielded some fascinating results. The babies who only suffered in the last third of pregnancy had weight, length and head size less than babies born before the famine began or who spent their whole gestation after the famine finished. In remarkable contrast, babies who were only exposed to nutritional challenge when they were in the first third of pregnancy had larger head sizes, weighed more and were longer than controls. This remarkable observation of seemingly stimulated fetal growth if the period of nutritional restriction is only in the first third of pregnancy will be of no surprise to ranchers and sheep farmers. They have known for years that the best way to grow a large fetal lamb is to restrict the pregnant ewe's feed in the first third of pregnancy and then to provide a good diet for the rest of the pregnancy. Immediately after the war, the allies rushed food to Holland, rapidly converting the greatly restricted maternal diet to one of plenty. Thus, for those women who had only suffered restriction for a few months, the nutritional history of their babies was very similar to the program that farmers use to increase lamb weight.

There are some potentially very important biological processes that may account for this remarkable, somewhat counterintuitive observation. One would have thought the pregnancy that begins with poor nutrition, even if things then get better, would result in a small baby. However, there is a very rational explanation. In early pregnancy, the placenta is growing fast while the fetus is still a small ball of cells spending time sorting out the different cell types needed for all the various organs. At this time, the fetus is not growing substantially in overall mass but instead spends these early weeks growing a placenta. This is a clever strategy. First the baby grows the placenta she or he will completely depend upon to provide the good nutrition necessary to grow fast in the second half of pregnancy. Then, with a good placenta in place, the baby can start the process of growing quickly. If there is a shortage of nutrition in early pregnancy, the baby grows a bigger placenta to try to compensate for the shortage. If, for some reason, the mother's nutrition improves, the larger placenta will be available to produce an even larger-than-normal baby. It is as if a fetus that is poorly nourished early in pregnancy sends signals to the placenta to say that the adverse conditions under which he is developing will require more placental growth, more cells, more action to extract the necessary nutrients from the mother's blood. Professor Jeffrey Robinson in Adelaide, Australia, and his research team have kept pregnant sheep on a restricted diet in early pregnancy and then allowed them unlimited access to feed for the rest of the pregnancy. This dietary regimen led to large placentas and large lambs compared with ewes who were allowed to eat as they wanted throughout pregnancy. The biological processes occurring throughout pregnancy are complex and truly marvelous. They have to be, the survival of the species depends on them.

In all of our considerations about fetal growth, we should remember that size is not everything. It is quality that is required: a good brain, a sound heart, firm bones and functional kidneys. Given the correct environment, the baby intuitively gets this right. The baby's first task in development is to focus on the quality and distribution of different cell types to their correct destinations in the body. After that has been successfully accomplished, the body grows. Fortunately, when we attend to the rules of our biology, pregnancy is usually normal.

Because of the unique nature of the information available from the Dutch Hunger Winter, several groups throughout the world are currently analyzing the data in very great detail. In one ongoing follow-up study based at the Academic Medical Center in Amsterdam, Dr. Janna Koppe and her colleagues have noted that the death rate of babies in the first year of life was ten times higher during the Hunger Winter and immediately after than the death rate before the war. This high death rate suggests that the babies whose development in the womb occurred during the Hunger Winter were less healthy as a result of the suboptimal conditions they experienced in the womb. We shall see in chapter 3 how these early deaths in infancy can shed light on long-term problems.

Immediately after liberation, everything possible was done by the allies to improve the supply of food, and by September 1945, the average food intake in Holland had risen to just over 2,000 calories. The recommended dietary intake for women during pregnancy is around 2,500 calories. In addition to the prenatal deprivation these babies had suffered, many were now exposed to the consequences of poor or nonexistent breast-feeding. Surprisingly, some women were still able to breast-feed. Mrs. Bakker told me that she was able to breast-feed without any apparent problems, yet another tribute to the marvelous resilience of our human biology.

In addition to the lack of exactly contemporaneous controls, the Dutch Hunger Winter study has a second major limitation. Clement Smith and others such as Hugh Sinclair from Oxford University in England, working immediately after the war, used only records of babies born in hospitals. In human epidemiologic studies, selection of subjects solely on the basis of the availability of records or for other reasons of convenience may greatly influence whether the findings are applicable to all pregnancies. When a selected population is studied, the observations may only relate to that specific population under study.

Long-Term Effects on Health: The Unseen Victims of War, Those as Yet Unborn

One observation of the long-term consequences of the Dutch Hunger Winter is especially startling and central to the view that prenatal life programs important aspects of our health. Women whose own birthweight was low as a result of malnutrition when they were themselves developing as fetuses during the Dutch Hunger Winter have smaller babies when they themselves become pregnant. A very simple explanation is that the same processes that restricted the growth of other organs in her body during development will almost certainly have restricted the growth of her own developing uterus. When she reaches reproductive years, the available space in her uterus for her own growing babies will be less. There are several mechanisms whereby the mother may constrain the growth of her fetus. We will consider some of these mechanisms in chapter 5. The ability of a pregnant woman to restrain the growth of her baby is a very good strategy. If a small woman is carrying a baby with a high genetic potential for growth, she will need to constrain the growth of that fetus so that the baby can eventually pass through her pelvis. Before the days of cesarean sections, this maternal restraint on fetal growth would have been literally vital to small women since maternal death invariably occurred when the mother failed to deliver a large baby.

At forty-five years of age, women who were born at the end of the Hunger Winter and hence experienced the maximum negative effects are still lighter than women who experienced shorter durations of exposure to malnutrition during their own fetal development. Lifelong effects on obesity have also been shown in male children of the Hunger Winter. When 300,000 male military recruits who were fetuses during the famine were examined at nineteen years of age, the effects on their body shape and degree of obesity differed according to their stage of fetal development during which they were deprived. If nutritional restriction occurred during the last third of their life in

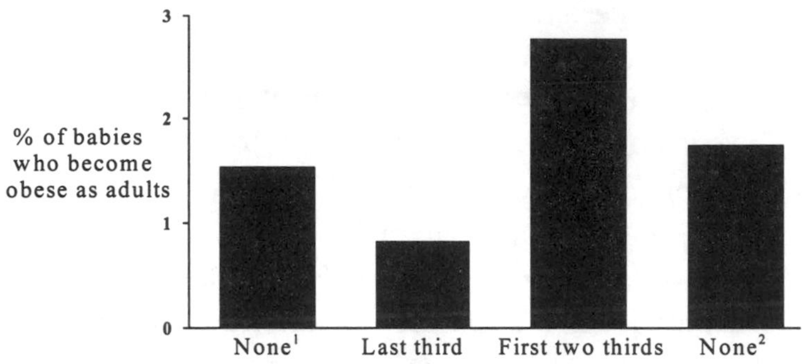

FIGURE 2.5

Portion of pregnancy during which the baby was exposed to low nutrition in the womb and the likelihood that the baby will be obese when s/he grows up. [1]Babies born before the Dutch Hunger Winter. [2]Babies born after the Dutch Hunger Winter.

the womb or in the first months after birth, the recruits were less likely to be obese in later life. In contrast, if they had been deprived during the first half of pregnancy, the men were more likely to be obese. The research group who undertook this study concluded that the centers in the brain of the developing fetus that regulate appetite may have been differently affected by food restriction early in pregnancy compared with late pregnancy. Studies in developing rats have shown that restriction of calories in the period of suckling produces a rat with smaller amounts of fatty tissue. Much of the development that occurs in late pregnancy in human babies occurs immediately after birth in the rat pup. There may be some similarities between the leaner humans whose nutrition was restricted late in their fetal life and the rat pups who were restricted during suckling.

In earlier generations, war and the mind-set of a society seemingly continually engaged in preparation for war had another harmful effect on children as yet unborn that we shall see in a different context later. Available food was given preferentially to the fighting men. If it was not freely given to the soldiers, they often took it forcibly.

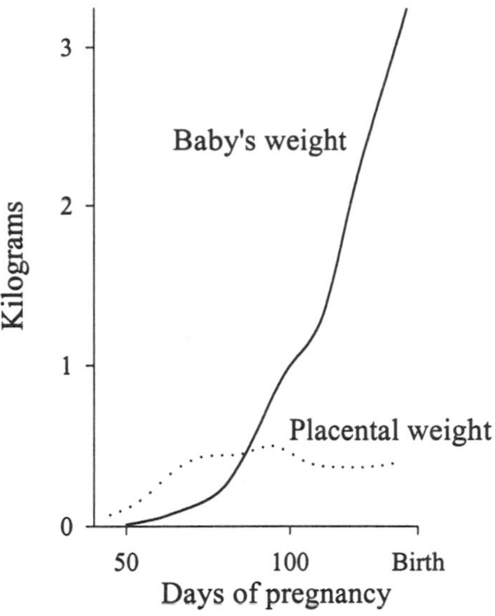

FIGURE 2.6

Diagram to show that the placenta in sheep grows early in pregnancy, before the fetal lamb begins to grow. The placenta also grows early in human pregnancy.

Pregnant women as well as growing girls who were biologically preparing their bodies for pregnancy were low on the totem pole for available food. These young girls were therefore not allowed the best opportunity for their bodies to be physically ready for motherhood. In this way, wars ravaged future generations by physiological processes that are only now beginning to be understood. It has always been clear that those who start wars visit destruction on more than one generation. However, postwar reparations have so far not considered the health consequences for future generations affected by intrauterine programming.

It is an interesting thought that many Dutch citizens in their early fifties likely have a continuing and previously undeclared case against the Nazi occupation. The lifetime health of these children of the Dutch Hunger Winter was adversely impacted by the period of starvation they experienced during life before birth. The consequences of the war have permanently altered the lives of babies who were in the womb at the time of the war. Cause and consequence

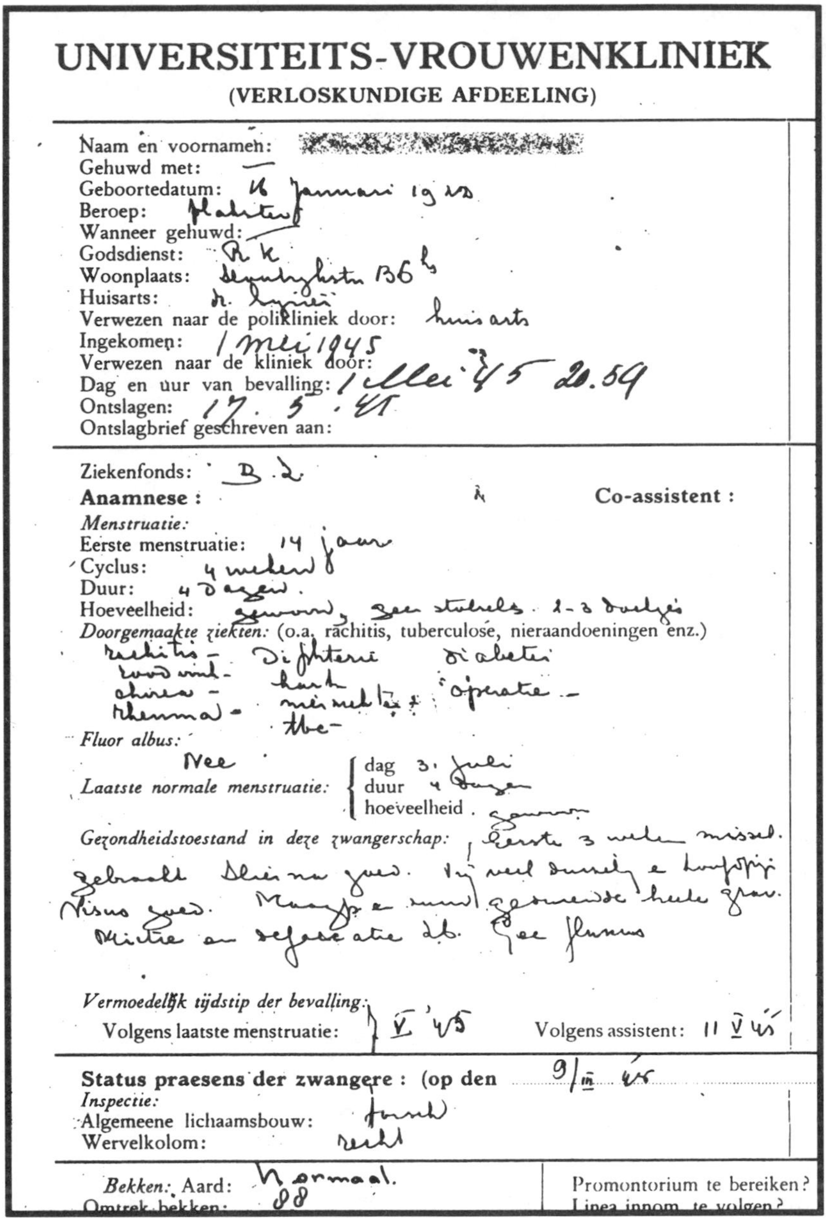

UNIVERSITEITS-VROUWENKLINIEK

(VERLOSKUNDIGE AFDEELING)

Naam en voornamen: [illegible]
Gehuwd met: —
Geboortedatum: 16 Januari 1918
Beroep: [illegible]
Wanneer gehuwd: —
Godsdienst: R.K.
Woonplaats: [illegible] 136
Huisarts: Dr. [illegible]
Verwezen naar de polikliniek door: huisarts
Ingekomen: 1 Mei 1945
Verwezen naar de kliniek door:
Dag en uur van bevalling: 1 Mei '45 20.59
Ontslagen: 17. 5. '45
Ontslagbrief geschreven aan:

Ziekenfonds: B. 2.
Anamnese : **Co-assistent :**
Menstruatie:
Eerste menstruatie: 14 jaar
Cyclus: 4 weken
Duur: 4 dagen.
Hoeveelheid: gewoon, geen stolsels. 1-2 doekjes
Doorgemaakte ziekten: (o.a. rachitis, tuberculose, nieraandoeningen enz.)
rachitis – Difterie diabetes
[illegible] – hart
chorea – [illegible] – operatie –
rheuma – tbc –
Fluor albus:
Nee
Laatste normale menstruatie: dag 3. Juli; duur 4 dagen; hoeveelheid . gewoon
Gezondheidstoestand in deze zwangerschap: Eerste 3 weken missel. [illegible] gebracht [illegible] goed. [illegible] hoofdpijn. Visus goed. Maag [illegible] hele [illegible]. Mictie en defaecatie [illegible]. Geen fluxus

Vermoedelijk tijdstip der bevalling:
Volgens laatste menstruatie: V '45 Volgens assistent: 11 V '45

Status praesens der zwangere : (op den 9/III '45
Inspectie:
Algemeene lichaamsbouw: [illegible]
Wervelkolom: recht

Bekken: Aard: Normaal. Promontorium te bereiken?
Omtrek bekken: 88 Linea innom. te volgen?

FIGURE 2.7

Obstetric records of a Dutch woman who was pregnant during the Hunger Winter.

are as clear as if these babies were physically disabled by injuries sustained in the war, the loss of a limb or an eye. Their children also have a case. Given current knowledge, it is difficult to evaluate the

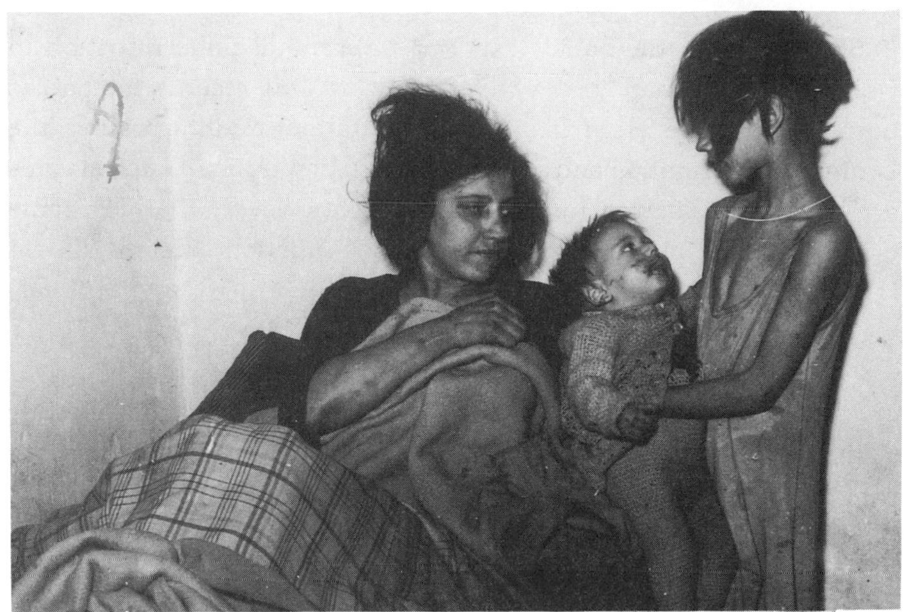

FIGURE 2.8

During the Hunger Winter it was important to look after the growing children and to keep warm. The children suffer the most long-term health consequences of war and famine because they do not grow properly—before or after birth.

extent of effects on future generations of poor prenatal nutrition and stress caused by wars. In a more modern context, the shortages of food that have resulted from Saddam Hussein's adventures in the Middle East, the late General Aidid's power struggles in Somalia, the racial struggles in Rawanda and the conflict in Bosnia will have repercussions on the health of thousands of children long after these of these aspiring warriors have been forgotten. An immortality of sorts, I suppose.

The concept of prenatal programming affecting health is so important that we must seek all the data we can find from unfortunate human experiences of deprivation. The Dutch Hunger Winter story does have a related Second World War parallel, the siege of Leningrad. Leningrad was blockaded for 872 days. Almost a million of its 2.4 million population died. At the siege's height, dietary intake was down to 300 calories, mostly bread and no protein. Birthweight fell by more than 500 grams (1.1 pounds), in contrast to 250 grams

(0.55 pounds) in the babies exposed to prenatal undernutrition in Holland. Unfortunately, the lack of birthweight records for babies born during, the siege is a great limitation in interpreting the Leningrad information and shows yet again how difficult such studies are to perform in the human situation. However, there is some evidence of problems with blood vessel function later in life in individuals born around the time of the siege.

Male Babies: The Weaker Sex

The number of baby boys born in any period is usually greater than the number of baby girls. The reason for this difference in birth rate between sexes is not known, but since the death rate in men is higher at all stages in life, even in the absence of wars, birth of a larger number of male children obviously has value in a society that until recently was relatively monogamous and in which the species depends on the production of large numbers of children. In Holland, 53 percent of pregnancies around the time of, but not including any part of, the Hunger Winter resulted in male offspring. In pregnancies in which any part occurred during the Hunger Winter, only 49 percent resulted in the birth of boys. Statistical analysis of these data show that they were unlikely to have occurred by chance.

Why should there be a fall in the proportion of boys being born as a result of pregnancies occurring at a time of very severe food restriction? Boys are normally heavier than girls at birth. They grow faster in the womb. Fetuses are most vulnerable to the challenges of suboptimal conditions when they are growing fast. It is therefore likely that the investment that male fetuses put into developing more muscle and forging ahead in their fetal growth make them much more vulnerable should conditions in the uterus be less than desirable.

The Continuing Search for More Evidence of Programming

The Dutch have always been excellent record keepers. Since Holland is a relatively small, highly educated society living in a compact area with good communication, it will be possible to obtain much more important information on the Hunger Winter's effect. It is relatively simple to track down those adults who formed the group of fetuses developing in the womb during the Hunger Winter. Once these individuals are located, they generally understand the importance of the investigations that are needed. Researchers at the Academic Medical Center in Amsterdam have found that the children of the Dutch Hunger Winter, now in their early fifties, are very willing to undergo the tests necessary to determine the consequences of the challenges of their fetal life.

The small survivors of one of the final acts of barbarity of a devilish military regime will help to throw light on how our bodies are affected when they cannot develop optimally according to the program given to us by our parents. It is now clear that periods of prenatal starvation alter blood pressure in later life, increase the likelihood of becoming diabetic, modify fertility and affect the performance of the brain. The story of the Dutch Hunger Winter starts us on a fascinating trail. Our journey will lead through Hertfordshire and Preston in England, Mysore in India and Beijing (previously known as Peking) in China to a story that is of fundamental importance to health everywhere. This worldwide story will show that when it comes to our health, getting things right at the beginning is the most important thing that we can do. Understanding this story is the key to better health for our children and their children.

THREE

DETECTIVE STORIES

The story always old and always new . . .
But the facts are facts and flinch not.

Robert Browning, *The Ring and the Book*

New ideas in science are always built on old ideas. The most innovative new ideas are often rejected when they first appear since they confront accepted dogma. Dr. David Barker and his Research Unit at the University of Southampton in England have been the leading proponents of the idea that human health is programmed as a result of prenatal experience. They observed that towns in Britain with a high incidence of death from coronary heart disease had experienced a similar high incidence of death of babies around the time of birth early in this century. David Barker concluded that suboptimal living conditions to which pregnant women in these towns were exposed led both to a high incidence of death of babies in late pregnancy and early newborn life and an increased risk of death from heart disease fifty years later in those babies who survived.

The innovative feature of these studies was the way they highlighted the critical importance of life before birth in determining lifetime health and disease. Prior to the reports by Barker and his colleagues, the emphasis was on the importance of the early months and years of life after birth. Lifetime health requires a favorable set of conditions throughout life: good nutrition, lack of stress, adequate exercise and avoidance of poor environmental conditions. However, a poor beginning in the womb increases an individual's susceptibility to disease for a lifetime.

The British Medical Research Council Epidemiology Group has followed these early clues—at times with trials and tribulations—through several areas of England and then into Europe, India and China. They have been joined in their quest for the prenatal origins of health and disease by other groups in the United States, Scandinavia and Europe.

New Ideas: Always Old, Always New

New ideas have always been around, in some form or another. Newton said, "If I have seen further than others it is only because I stand on the shoulders of giants." To obtain inspiration for his own work, Bach apparently walked two hundred miles to hear Buxtehude play the organ. Ecclesiastes tells us that "there is no new thing under the sun." Even an idea as revolutionary as the detailed, three-dimensional chemical structure of the DNA double helix was dependent on an earlier seemingly unimportant observation on the basic chemical composition of DNA. Where and when does a new idea originate? Always from a related, earlier, simpler, less detailed idea. It is seeing the significance of little hidden connections and clues that is the stroke of genius.

The generation of new ideas and the proof of their validity are two separate but related activities. Both events are of fundamental importance to progress. However, if there is any truth in the view that ideas have been around for a long time, then the major credit for changing the way we think about the world around us must surely go to those who roll up their sleeves and assemble the facts required to prove the validity of the new idea, not those who claim to have thought of it first. The arena of human accomplishment is full of authors, playwrights, inventors and scientists who claim they were the first with a particularly good idea. We need to ask who had the

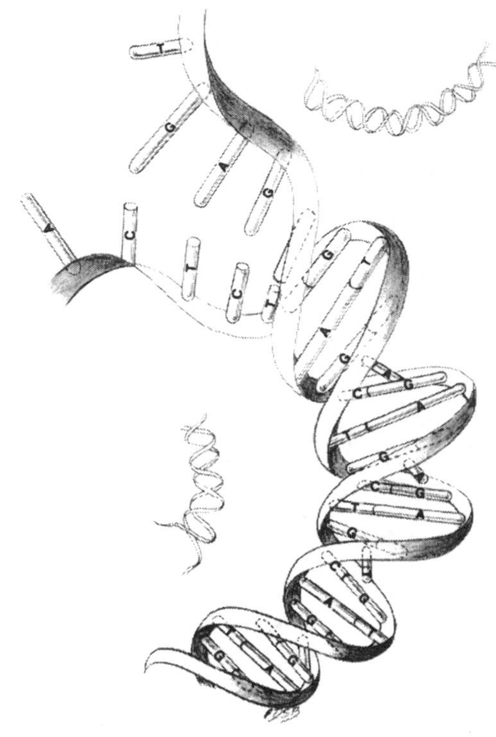

FIGURE 3.1

The double helix structure of DNA—the fundamental three-dimensional structure of the genes.

energy and creativity to do the work that convinced trained skeptics, the peers in their discipline, that the new idea is in large measure true. By the very nature of their training, scientific researchers must always be skeptical of new ideas until they are proven beyond doubt. The credit for progress should surely go to those who relentlessly pursue the goal of changing the mind-set of the entrenched establishment. Before any new notion is accepted, the establishment in the particular field of intellectual pursuit must be satisfied that the idea fits with currently accepted, well proven dogma that has stood the test of time and scrutiny. If the new idea doesn't fit, then the onus of proving where entrenched, conventional wisdom is incorrect will surely lie with the innovator of the new idea.

The What, Why, When, Where, How and Who—Again

There have been many contributors to the rapidly evolving research field on the prenatal programming of adult health and disease. Many investigators have provided information to answer the *what, why, when, where, how* and *who.* Modern biomedical science is divided into multiple specialities, each of them expanding at an exponential rate and dizzily spinning off new subdisciplines. The subdisciplines have their own jargons. It is very hard to be an expert in more than one area of human biology. It is difficult enough to have a firm grasp of the past history, modern technologies and recent discoveries in one's specific chosen subdiscipline and the areas immediately around it. The interaction between disciplines such as molecular biology and the study of hormones and how they regulate the cardiovascular system is what makes attempts to integrate the function of the whole human body so challenging and exciting. Each of us is not a separate brain, heart, lung, kidney and gut stuck together like some collage or inanimate jigsaw puzzle. Our various organ systems interact in very complex ways. Initially, the study of programming requires the reductionist analysis of the individual body systems to understand the rules by which they work. Having taken the pieces apart, the next step is the synthesis of disparate pieces of experimental knowledge to obtain a clear understanding of how the individual systems interact to make up each unique human being.

When it comes to piecing together the programming story as it relates to the origins of heart disease, it is clear that David Barker is due a very large portion of the credit. He is also due the credit of having recruited a most outstanding group of colleagues who travel all over the world in search of the evidence. Members of the group at the Medical Research Council's Epidemiology Unit at Southampton University on the south coast of England are the leading scientific truffle hounds of the programming story.

The Medical Research Council Epidemiology Unit at Southampton, England

Sitting in David Barker's corner office of a squat, unimposing building on the grounds of Southampton Hospital is a very relaxing affair. At least it is most of the time, since David Barker is a gregarious character in his late fifties. But do not let his quiet voice fool you into thinking that he is a tolerant man when it comes to scientific sloppiness or a reluctance to critically justify, substantiate and refine an idea. Educated at one of the major British public schools, Oundle, and then at the world-famous Guy's Hospital in London, David Barker continues to practice day-to-day emergency medicine while at the same time directing the Epidemiology Unit. One day a week, he takes charge of emergency admissions at the Southampton Hospital. The day I visited, he was struggling to understand the clinical problem of a middle-aged man who came to the hospital because his breasts were enlarging. This rare condition, called gynecomastia, can occur very suddenly in adult men. It is due to hormone imbalance and may be caused by a variety of conditions. So, in addition to his work on the lifelong effects of undernutrition before birth on high blood pressure and chronic heart disease in later life, Dr. Barker is a practicing general physician. He clearly enjoys the human contact with his patients as a counterbalance to the less personal computerized manipulation of health statistics in his chosen field of epidemiology. He spends much of his life immersed in the details of birthweight, calculations of newborn babies' growth rates and analyses of causes of death in Great Britain, India, China and other locations throughout the world.

To be a pioneer in any area of human endeavor, it is necessary to be at least a little focused. Many of the real geniuses and innovators—musicians, painters, authors, scientists—were totally obsessed with their chosen field. It is always interesting to know how individual researchers became fixated on particular areas of science or any other intellectual field. How did David Barker's thinking on the association between life before birth and the quality of health throughout life develop?

Fortunately, the power of computer databases allows us to go back to the start of the career of individual scientists and search their publication records. In the early papers of the scientific pioneers we can find fascinating hints of the subjects that will later come to dominate their careers. In 1966, David Barker published a paper entitled "Low Intelligence; Its Relation to Length of Gestation and Rate of Foetal Growth" in the *British Journal of Preventative and Social Medicine*, one of the world's leading epidemiology journals. The paper contains fascinating indications of the thoughts that would come to dominate David Barker's work twenty years later. He began this early paper by stating that more information was necessary in three areas relating low intelligence to birthweight: first, low birthweight was known to be associated with mental subnormality, but the significance of this connection remained unknown; second, high birthweight had been reported to occur more frequently in association with subnormality, but the evidence was inconclusive; third, prolonged pregnancy had been suggested as a cause of brain damage and consequent intellectual impairment, but no data on this issue appeared to have been published at that time

In search of data to prove or disprove these associations, David Barker first sought a suitable human population to study. He would repeatedly search for study populations in his later work on the interplay of nutrition during fetal development and lifelong health and disease. In his first major paper, the young physician observed 606 subnormal children from a population of 73,687 single births. Large numbers of subjects are needed because it is extremely difficult to identify and separate the multitude of factors, both genetic and environmental, that determine intelligence. Objective analysis in any area of knowledge requires that a researcher puts firm numbers to the phenomenon under study. Issues only become clearer when firm quantification can be obtained. Even with firm numbers, it is sometimes difficult to convince skeptics. The numbers must be reproducible and statistically significant. To show any association between birthweight and intelligence requires quantification of intelligence. Putting firm numbers to mental characteristics has always proven difficult. Brain function cannot be satisfactorily quantified unless widely accepted, objective measures are available for impartial observers to focus upon and compare between studies. The absence of such measures is the major cause of the current debate on the use of IQ testing to substantiate a genetic basis for intelligence as conducted by Hernstein and Murray in their controversial book, *The Bell Curve.* A numerically acceptable apportioning of the relative contributions of nature and nurture to mental performance is an area that moves slowly as we await breakthroughs in our understanding of how the nervous system develops and works.

Despite these problems in resolving the finer points relating intelligence (or some measure of it) to prenatal life, David Barker's concluding remarks in his early paper provide fascinating premonitions of his later work. He concludes, "Low intelligence is associated with both a *slower rate of intrauterine growth* [my emphasis] and a higher incidence of birth before 38 weeks than are found in the population." So already the idea of associating growth rate before birth and quality of function after birth is beginning to surface in his thinking.

David Barker's next major paper published in the *British Medical Journal* was titled, "Obstetric Complications and School Performance." Again, it is easy to see how obstetric and developmental themes were jockeying for attention in his mind. When one sits in David Barker's office, occasionally one will see his eyes glaze over. At times like this his wife, Jan Barker, will say, "He's fallen to thinking." All researchers should spend more time thinking, especially if they can come up with revolutionary new ideas as David Barker has.

CLUES IN OLD MAPS

Throughout most of the nineteenth century, there has been a North-South divide in the quality of health enjoyed by the population in England. In 1984, an atlas showing how death from selected diseases varied in different parts of England and Wales was published by the Medical Research Council. David Barker was one of the editors. David Barker and his colleague, Clive Osmond, were startled

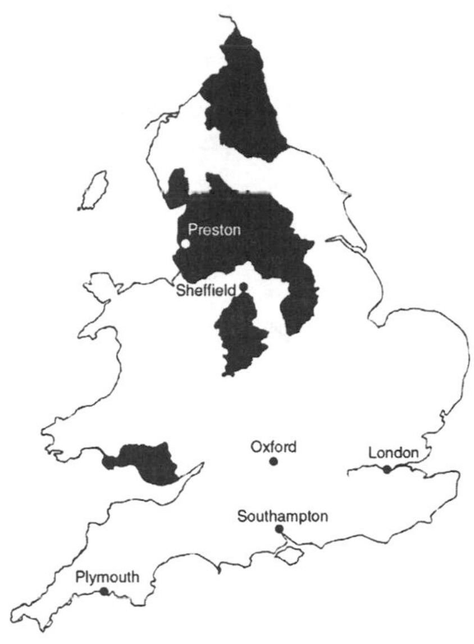

FIGURE 3.2

The dark areas show the areas of England and Wales in which infant mortality in 1901–1910 and death from coronary artery disease in men aged 35 to 74 during 1959–1978 were high. Note that these regions are the poorer industrial areas, not affluent London.

by the similarity of the regions of the country with a high incidence of heart disease among men aged 35 to 74 years during 1968–1978 and the distribution of areas with high rates of infant mortality in the early part of this century. Both heart disease in men in the 1970s and infant mortality earlier this century were highest in the industrial areas in England and Wales.

At the time David Barker and Clive Osmond were studying these maps, heart disease was considered a disease of affluence. Experts in the field considered lifestyle, smoking, diets high in animal fats and stress as the major causes of heart disease. The medical profession and nutrition experts have generally followed the view that heart disease is caused by too much good living and too little exercise. If this view is true, then coronary artery disease should be less common, not more, in the poorer areas of England and Wales. Barker and Osmond developed an innovative explanation for this apparent paradox. They reasoned that babies who were less well-prepared during fetal development were more prone to suffer from heart disease in later life. Of course, the same babies who died in infancy, contributing to the high infant death rates in the industrial areas of England and Wales at the turn of the century, could not themselves have suffered from coronary heart disease in later life. What was so striking was the indication that babies who managed to escape the high death rates were more likely to suffer from heart disease in later life.

Problems Before Birth or in Infancy

These ideas were not completely new. At the time David Barker was musing over the similarities in the maps of England, several important studies had already been published that related infant mortality to later coronary artery disease. Infant mortality is defined as the number of deaths that occur during the first year of life. In 1964, Geoffrey Rose showed that brothers and sisters of patients who eventually suffer from coronary heart disease were twice as likely to die in infancy. In 1977, A. Forsdahl in Norway pointed out that heart disease in different counties in Norway was well correlated with infant mortality rates. Both of these eminent physicians thought the important connection was between postnatal life and heart disease. Finnish studies also appeared around this time that showed a similar relationship of heart disease to childhood conditions. Even earlier, in 1946, Dr. Barnett Woolf, an anthropologist, published a paper entitled "Studies on Infant Mortality. Part II. Social Aetiology of Stillbirths and Infant Deaths in County Boroughs of England and Wales" in the *British Journal of Social Medicine.* This substantial paper of over fifty pages covered an enormous terrain. In addition to highlighting methodological problems that beset the collection and analysis of human data, affected as it is by a multitude of different factors such as social class, overcrowding, poverty, family size, infection and maternal employment or lack of it, Woolf concluded that improving maternal nutrition would likely prove more significant in preventing infant mortality than changes in housing. It would pay us all to give some attention to that conclusion today.

Many of the critical factors in the living conditions in which we grow up also influenced our mother's health during pregnancy. Thus, these environmental factors affect our early lives twice. They determine our mother's health and our home in the womb, programming our lifelong health. Then these same conditions in the environment continue to work on our own health during our own lives. Significant environmental factors include social class, size of family, poverty, environmental pollution or its absence and, of course, nutrition. If a mother is poorly fed while she is pregnant, it is likely that the child of that pregnancy will be poorly fed while growing. These adverse factors are also likely to be present at other stages of an individual's life, and we need to determine which stages are the most critical. Is poor nutrition before birth more important than poor nutrition after birth? Or are they both equally important?

The big breakthrough came when David Barker and his colleagues realized that throughout England, the area-by-area correlation of death rates of newborn babies in the first month of life with heart disease later in life was even closer than the correlation of death rates in the first year of life with the later incidence of heart disease in these same areas. They began to focus attention on the critical importance of fetal life in distinction to early childhood. They demonstrated that variability in death rates from coronary artery disease in England and Wales correlated best with death rates in the month after birth, better than any correlation with death rates in later childhood.

TROUBLE WITH THE ESTABLISHMENT

The progress of scientific knowledge depends on the ability of the scientific community to accept ideas that run counter to the perceived, conventional wisdom. Just as happens in any well-established bureaucracy, the scientific establishment often has trouble assimilating new ideas. The purpose of scientific training is to sharpen the wish to question everything. Training as a scientist makes you desperately hungry for evidence, for firm proof, to support new ideas. Preferably, proof should come from several sources and different methodological approaches. Ideas are fine, but they are only the first step. Ideas need proof before acceptance. Scientific researchers are trained to suspend judgment until strong evidence is obtained to show that an observation is reproducible in different laboratories and by competing research groups. Ideas will not be accepted until firm reproducible experiments show that new concepts have general validity. This reluctance to accept change is particularly true in relation to big, new ideas that totally revolutionize thinking. The idea that the origins of heart disease and other conditions later in life are programmed by conditions the fetus experiences in the womb is a very big idea. David Barker recalls that the younger epidemiologists were quicker than the establishment to accept an association of coronary heart disease in later life with the quality of fetal development. In retrospect, David Barker probably expected trouble from the establishment. He certainly met with it.

The Hunt Is Up: Old Records in Unexpected Places

As these connections took root in his mind, the time had come to search for birth records that might explore further the connection between prenatal development, especially birthweight, and adult disease. In 1985, David Barker found 500 birth records from the beginning of the twentieth century in the town of Plymouth in the southwest corner of England. The port of Plymouth is famous for Sir Francis Drake and his preparations to defeat the Spanish Armada. Drake's preparations were arduous and lengthy. David Barker's course was to prove equally so.

Barker was prevented from using these records because access was restricted under a 100-year rule of confidentiality of patient information. Then, in 1986, he discovered sets of complete birth records in six villages in Hertfordshire, a county just a few miles north of London. Again, his request to study the records was refused for similar confidentiality reasons. On this occasion, however, David Barker had a personal connection. He was able to tell the medical officer in the Hertfordshire records department that during the Second World War, he and his family had been evacuated to Hertfordshire to avoid the German bombing raids. It so happened that his own sister's birth records were in the very database his research group wanted.

David Barker was told that he could have the Hertfordshire birth records if he could find a safe place in which to store them. That very day, he telephoned the vice-chancellor of Southampton University to ask if the university could ensure this requirement while the Research Unit explored them. With speed that surprises anyone knowledgeable about university bureaucracy, he was told to promise the Hertfordshire authorities that the University of Southampton would house the records under complete security. Indeed, to convince the medical officer in Hertfordshire, David Barker was told to inform him that the records would be housed in the same location as the archives of the Duke of Wellington. The first set of birth records David Barker studied traveled to a safe haven alongside records of the Battle of Waterloo.

Finding the first set of records from six Hertfordshire villages proved to be the turning point. It soon became apparent that the whole county of Hertfordshire possessed similar detailed birth records. From 1911 onward, midwives visited every woman who had given birth in the county. They recorded the birthweight, the way the baby was fed, any illnesses and, very importantly as we shall see, the baby's weight at one year of life. A unique strength of this record of all the births in Hertfordshire is the fact that the records were not from a selected population but were a complete record of all the children born throughout the county.

Armed with the knowledge that it was possible to obtain the type of detailed birth records he would need, David Barker felt the time had come to hire a researcher to help him find and sort the information. He hired a young woman historian recently graduated from Oxford University who played a key role in exploiting the Hertfordshire records. But there was another stroke of luck in her appointment. She was the first woman from her school at Preston in the north of England to gain a place to study at Oxford University. On one vacation from her search for birth records, she visited her family in her hometown. She decided to visit her local hospital to search for further records. Her impulse was amply rewarded. There in the records room of Sharoe Green Hospital, Preston, she found the birth records from the delivery room on every baby born between 1934 and 1943. The value of these records lay in the fact that a multitude of measurements had been made on the babies at birth. The babies had been measured in such detail that David Barker says that he could have used the recorded measurements to make sketches of the individual babies in their cribs.

Each record at Sharoe Green contained one piece of unusual information that would open up new lines of enquiry of critical importance to future analysis. The babies' birth records contained the weight of the placenta. In the 1930s it was, unfortunately, very rare to weigh the placenta. The placenta contains much information about the baby's stay in the uterus. One day in the not far distant future the placenta may be used as the baby's prenatal diary. There is one further small item of human interest in the Sharoe Green records. Many attempts had been made to destroy them to create more space. Mrs. Freda Foden, the person in charge of the records, insisted they be kept because of the intrinsic beauty of the old handwritten ledgers as well as her perceived opinion of their historical medical value. She was now about to be proved right with regard to the clinical value of the records. The Hertfordshire records were uniquely valuable because they represented a whole unselected population of births over thirty-four years. In contrast, although the Preston records represented a selected population of hospital deliveries, they had their own special value because they contained information on the size of the placenta.

Then a third set of records then came to light. In an old boiler house at the Jessop Hospital in Sheffield, Yorkshire, the Medical Research Council researchers found a complete set of equally beautifully bound ledgers that contained details of every birth at Jessop Hospital dating back to 1907. The strength of the Sheffield records lies in the even greater details they contained of the babies' birth proportions, including length, abdominal and chest circumference.

Find the Man or Woman Who Was the Child

David Barker's goal was to use these records to determine whether babies who showed signs of impaired growth in the womb had health complications later in life. He was especially interested in heart disease. These excellent records would be of little use if the babies whose details were recorded in Hertfordshire, Preston and Sheffield could not be traced into their adult life. Barker reasoned that if these babies, now adults well into the second half of their life, could be traced, then it would be possible to correlate their birthweights and other measurements, such as the size of their abdomen at birth or the weight of their placenta, with the health they had enjoyed throughout life, the illnesses they had suffered and even, in many cases, the cause of death. Finding the adults whose birth details were recorded in these ledgers would enable the now-grown baby to visit the hospital for a rather belated postnatal checkup. At these visits, blood could be obtained for laboratory evaluation of the functions of various organs such as the liver or the pancreas. The current function of these grown organs could then be related to the size of the baby at birth many years previously.

Medical epidemiologists and detectives have much in common. I have this mental image of David Barker in a trench coat, standing by a lamppost on a dimly lit city sidewalk waiting for a sixty-five year-old man or woman who had been born at Sharoe Green Hospital to come home from an evening out at the pub or theater. There is a small notepad in his hand. When that little boy or girl born in Sharoe Green Hospital, now grown, comes home, she or he will be stopped and questioned. "Would you please come down to the hospital for an interview and a few tests?" Very soon they will be volunteering to step on the scales, have their blood pressure taken, their urine analyzed for glucose in case they have become diabetic and work out on the treadmill to test the ability of their hearts to respond to exercise.

Although epidemiologists have developed a far more comfortable lifestyle than the private eye, both epidemiologists and detectives need to track down the evidence "along the mean streets" as Raymond Chandler would say. The next step for the Medical Research Council investigators was to obtain records from the National Health Service

Central Register, which is kept in what once was the magnificent ballroom of a large and opulent holiday hotel on the northwest coast of England. This registry contains the health records of all patients who have had medical treatment under the British National Health Service. The records contain information on each individual's visits to the doctor, blood pressure measurements and the health problems that have afflicted the person throughout life. Tracing men is of course easier than women because many women change their names on marriage. Much of this hard detective work in the United Kingdom is now completed, and the details of the lifetime health of many of the Hertfordshire, Sharoe Green and Jessop Hospital babies are now safely entered on the computers of the Medical Research Council Epidemiology Unit.

Publish and Be Damned

Epidemiologists and detectives have other activities in common. First they must collect data. Then they must organize, correlate and interpret it. Both detectives and epidemiologists must identify and prove connections that satisfy not only themselves but also a jury of their peers. In the case of the detective, the evidence produced must stand before a jury in a court of law. For scientists, the jury is other investigators in their own field of knowledge who know the problem equally well but may be taking a different route to resolve it. To gain the attention of other scientists and try to persuade them to accept new ideas, a researcher writes a paper that presents the ideas and the experimental data that support it.

When a researcher submits a paper to a journal, the editor of the journal will ask two or three experts to review and evaluate it. The reviewers are asked to comment on the originality of the study, the validity of the methods and the statistical soundness of the conclusions. They then recommend to the editor whether the paper contains material that is both novel and sound enough to merit publication. Editors cannot be specialists in all the fields covered by their journal. Most important, editors cannot have firsthand experience of all the latest methods the various investigators use. For these and many other reasons, editors are very dependent on the reviewer's opinions. It is a good idea to have three reviewers so that in the event of a disagreement, the vote will be two to one. Once published,. the information is in the public domain for everyone, scientist and lay person, to review and evaluate.

Early on in their analysis of the Preston data, David Barker and his colleagues obtained the important clue that babies with large placentas were more likely to have raised blood pressure in later life. It seems initially to be paradoxical that babies with a large placenta should be less healthy in later life. However, this apparent paradox becomes easier to understand when we recall that sheep fetuses that are undernourished in early pregnancy grow a larger placenta. So a placenta that is large in relation to the size of the baby may well indicate that the conditions were not optimal in the uterus and the baby tried to compensate by growing a larger placenta.

When David Barker submitted his initial paper to his first choice among the major medical journals, the editor thought so poorly of it that he refused to even send the paper out for review. When editors reject papers in this fashion, it is usually because they do not consider the findings of enough interest, think the methods unsound or feel that the new, revolutionary idea is just plain wrong, too absurd to risk the journal's reputation. Undaunted, David Barker battled on. He did the only thing he could do. He submitted the paper elsewhere, to the *British Medical Journal.* It was accepted and published. An initial rejection was also the fate of his second paper, which showed that fetal and infant growth were related to the way in which individuals control the amount of glucose in their blood.

The reasons for these initial rejections of the two groundbreaking papers are unclear. As any new idea comes forward in science, there is a brief period of silence from the scientific community as the ideas are digested. Then people take sides. At the time David Barker submitted his original papers, some reviews had been published attacking the notion of the childhood origins of adult disease, and established researchers expressed caution about epidemiological studies because of the potential confounding influence of lifestyle and social class factors among the mothers. They also questioned the selection of subjects for study. Each of these potential criticisms is important. All epidemiologic work suffers from an inability to control the multitude of factors that may act on a particular individual. In order to control potential confounds, clinical research and data from animal studies must always be sought to confirm epidemiological connections. David Barker himself repeatedly calls for animal studies to verify the *why* and *how* of the epidemiologic findings.

Global Laws Applicable in Europe, India and Asia

Like all pioneers, David Barker was not prepared to wait around while people decided whether his ideas were right or wrong. He just determined to find more and more epidemiologic evidence until the whole story would be too strong to discount. Luck was on his side again. In 1989, he visited Belgium to teach an epidemiology course. At this course David Barker met Dr. Srinath Reddy from the All India Medical Institute in Delhi who invited him to visit India. The following year, he and his colleague, Dr. Caroline Fall, took up the invitation. Caroline Fall had lived many years in India with her father who had been a young officer in an Indian Army Regiment. As a result, she speaks Hindi. Her godfather is a colonel in the Indian Army. All of these associations were to prove extremely helpful.

By this time, the major focus of the Medical Research Council Group in Southampton was directed at the effects of nutrition on fetal growth and the influence of suboptimal fetal growth on longterm health and disease—especially heart disease. Various areas of India where there had been problems in maternal nutrition in the past seemed to hold great opportunities for investigation of the relationship of maternal nutritional deprivation, fetal growth and long term health. The researchers would, however, need to repeat the complicated procedures of finding birth records and then trace the babies described in these records through later life as they had begun to do successfully in England.

In the hope that she could set up a study on the effects of poor nutrition in pregnancy, Caroline Fall wrote to all the mission hospitals in India. In the course of these enquiries, she unexpectedly found birth records in Mysore, Bangalore and near the Pakistani border at Amritsar. From these three sites, the Southampton group chose to focus on the babies born at Mysore. Their studies in India are only in their early stages, but they already indicate that the general rules on how our prenatal history affects our health throughout our lives apply not only to Europeans but also to Indians.

In 1986, David Barker went to China in an exchange program. Always on the lookout for new populations to study, David Barker took the opportunity to ask whether collections of Chinese birth records might be available to him. He reasoned that the case for a fundamental influence of these prenatal biological mechanisms on lifelong health would be strengthened if similar relationships could be shown in China as well as Britain and India. He was not successful. Still looking, he returned to China in 1988. Again, he was unsuccessful. A few years later, Queen Elizabeth made an official visit to China. This time, David Barker's luck broke. Accompanying the Queen was Sir Norman Blacklock, a urologist who was introduced to Dr. Wu Jie Ping, Mao Tse-tung's personal doctor. Shortly thereafter, Sir Norman Blacklock arranged for Dr. Wu Jie Ping to make a visit to the Medical Research Council Unit at Southampton. David Barker told Dr. Wu Jie Ping about his wish to find birth records in China.

The Peking Union Medical College has an impeccable Western pedigree. It was founded by the London Missionary Society in the nineteenth century. The hospital was bought from the London Missionary Society by the Rockefeller Foundation in 1917. Miraculously hospital records had been preserved through the Japanese occupation of Peking. They had even been kept intact when the Rockefeller Foundation was thrown out of China by Mao Tse-tung. Perhaps most surprisingly, the records had survived the anti-intellectual onslaught by Red Guards and the cultural revolution. These Chinese records hold great promise. They are written in English and are extraordinarily detailed. The Chinese records of babies born at Peking Medical Union College Hospital contain even more information than those in Hertfordshire, Preston and Sheffield. In some records, the baby's head was measured in at least six different directions.

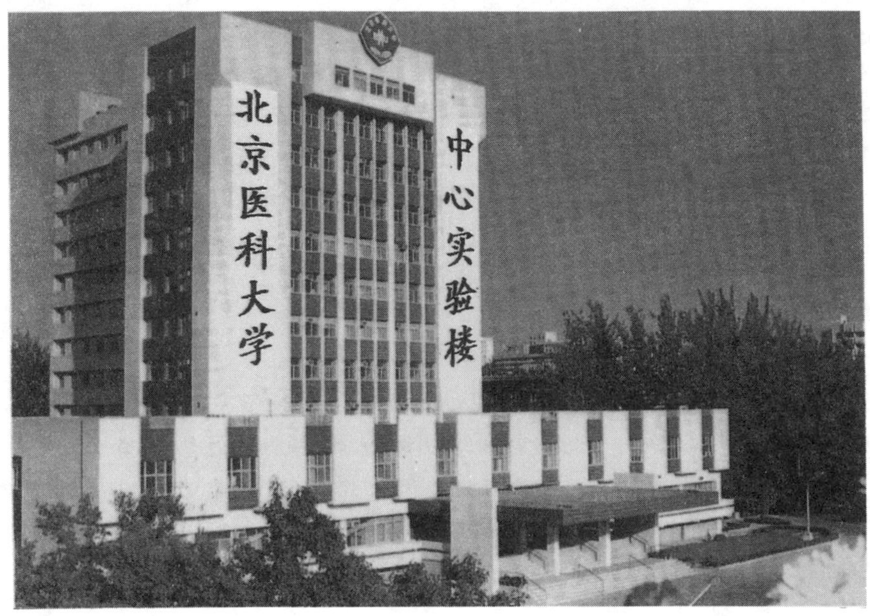

FIGURE 3.3

Beijing Medical College.

For David Barker and his colleagues, it is not yet time to rest. The worldwide journey still goes on. Taken together with the remarkable finding that the growth-retarded daughters of the Dutch Hunger Winter had a higher likelihood of having growth-retarded babies themselves, the epidemiological data from China and India has been an enormous stimulus to thought and research. Together, epidemiology, clinical research and laboratory experimentation constitute a triad of approaches to the unraveling of the prenatal origins of health and disease. Throughout the rest of this book we will pursue this triad through our considerations of how fetal development programs our lifetime health and susceptibility to disease.

FOUR

TRANSGENERATIONAL ORIGINS OF HEALTH AND DISEASE: DISEASE FIGHTS FORWARD

Visit the sins of the fathers [and mothers] upon the children unto the third and fourth generation.

Book of Common Prayer

Diabetes is one of the major diseases of Western civilization, occurring in epidemic proportions in some areas of the world. There are two different types of diabetes. The less common but rapidly progressing form that generally starts early in life is thought to be caused by genetic factors. In contrast, recent research indicates that environmental, rather than genetic, factors play a key role in the second, later-onset form of diabetes. In both forms of diabetes, the function of the pancreas is abnormal. Animal studies show that feeding a low-protein diet to the mother during pregnancy can decrease the size of the fetal pancreas and result in a higher incidence of diabetes in later life. Female offspring of diabetic mothers have a greater tendency to become diabetic when they themselves become pregnant.

When a diabetic mother cannot keep her own glucose in the normal range, her fetus is exposed to the excess of sugar that builds up in the mother's blood. As a result of the high levels in the mother's blood, excessive amounts of sugar pass across the placenta to the fetus. This abnormally high exposure of the fetus to sugar stresses the developing fetal pancreas, producing eventual long-term problems including a higher incidence of diabetes in later life. This tendency can be passed across several generations. These observations of the transgenerational passage of diabetic tendencies in animals have been made independently in the United States and Europe. So, just as we saw with the small babies of mothers who were themselves growth-retarded following the Dutch Hunger Winter, unwanted consequences of an unfavorable environment in the womb can be passed across generations.

The interaction of nature and nurture that will affect our whole lives is also played out in the womb. The baby's development is not solely regulated by the genes inherited from the parents. The idea of transgenerational passage of nongenetically determined conditions is a fascinating and fundamental piece of our biology. It is difficult to dismiss these findings as inapplicable to our own human species when we consider the multitude of similarities in the various developmental processes that occur before birth in many different animal species.

THE FETUS OF THE DIABETIC MOTHER

Diabetes is a cash flow disease that occurs because specialized cells in the pancreas, known as beta cells, cannot produce enough insulin to keep the levels of glucose in the blood within normal limits. Glucose is the main fuel burned by most cells in the body to provide their energy supply. Insulin regulates the flow of glucose (cash to expend) into muscle and fat cells so that they have enough fuel to burn to carry out their normal functions. By performing this function, insulin is an important regulator of availability of sustenance to cells. Without glucose, all cells have great trouble keeping their production lines going. However, not all cells in the body depend on insulin to help them take up glucose from the blood. One important exception is the brain. Most cells of the nervous system can get their glucose without the help of insulin. In diabetes, there is not enough insulin circulating in the blood. As a result, working muscle and fat cells rapidly get short of glucose. These cells must now start to burn up their own internal fat and protein. They have to resort to cannibalizing important components of their own structural framework. It is as if a building started to consume the fundamental steel girders from which it is itself constructed. This is the reason young diabetics whose pancreas fails completely lose a lot of weight in a short time even though they eat voraciously. Nerve cells do not need insulin to extract their glucose from the blood. As a result, when diabetes strikes, the brain can go on functioning relatively normally until the side effects of the lack of insulin begin to build up. This is one of the few fortunate aspects of the disease.

In addition to regulating the flow of glucose into cells, insulin also stimulates the uptake of amino acids. It is now generally accepted that insulin is a major growth-promoting factor during development. Amino acids are the bricks from which we build the structural proteins that make up every cell in the body. Studies conducted by Dr. Abigail Fowden at Cambridge University in England on developing fetal sheep show that, in the womb, insulin is probably the major factor regulating growth. If we look at growth as a factory production line with good, healthy cells as the product, then insulin plays a major role in providing both the energy (the glucose) as well as some of the major raw materials (amino acids) to keep the production line going.

The second result of any deficiency in insulin production is that the concentration of glucose builds up in the blood. There is plenty of glucose in the blood in diabetes, but because of the lack of insulin, glucose cannot get into the cells where it is needed. Insulin is necessary for glucose to go into the muscle and fat cells. For this reason, diabetes is sometimes called "starvation in the midst of plenty."

If the mother's diabetes is not well controlled by diet or insulin, the fetus faces major problems. In uncontrolled maternal diabetes, the blood glucose level is high and there is an abnormal mix of nutrients, particularly the amino acid building blocks, in her blood. As a result, there is an abnormally large amount of glucose going across the placenta to the fetus. The mix of amino acids that go across the placenta is also abnormal. A tendency to diabetes during pregnancy is a very widespread problem. For each pregnant woman who has been diagnosed as a diabetic before she is pregnant, there are ten times as many women whose body metabolism has lesser but still significant problems with the correct use and distribution of glucose during pregnancy. This condition of impaired glucose control in pregnancy has been called *pregnancy diabetes* because of the sudden appearance during pregnancy of glucose in the mother's urine and high levels of glucose in the blood of otherwise seemingly healthy women. Before they became pregnant, these women had no problems with handling sugar in their bodies. During pregnancy, the placenta, fetus and the changed circulating hormones in the mother's blood alter the way her body handles and burns different fuels. Pregnancy diabetes generally resolves and is no longer a problem after the baby is born. However, the likelihood that a woman will become diabetic later in life is increased if the changes in her pregnancy led to pregnancy diabetes. When pregnancy diabetes occurs, it is a signal that something may be wrong with how the mother uses her glucose.

The amount of many nutrients—not just glucose—circulating in the blood of the pregnant diabetic may be abnormal. The actual pattern of nutrients that are affected will vary from woman to woman. Thus there is a very wide variety of environments in which the baby of the diabetic mother can develop in respect to the availability of glucose, protein, fat, vitamins and other important nutrients in the mother's blood. The mother is the baby's quartermaster, and the mother's blood is the baby's supply depot. When essential materials are missing from the depot, there is no way the baby can obtain a supply. Alternatively, if the developing baby is forced to take too much of some nutrient—glucose in this case—the baby's developing body may be exposed problems of excess.

What does this all mean for the woman who develops pregnancy diabetes? The importance of understanding the effects of pregnancy diabetes is clearly shown by recent advances in management. Most specialists who treat diabetic women in pregnancy are convinced that when a diabetic woman is carefully checked out and supervised throughout her pregnancy, the risk that she will lose her baby before birth is not significantly greater than the risk for a woman who does not have diabetes. If a woman with diabetes or a tendency to diabetes

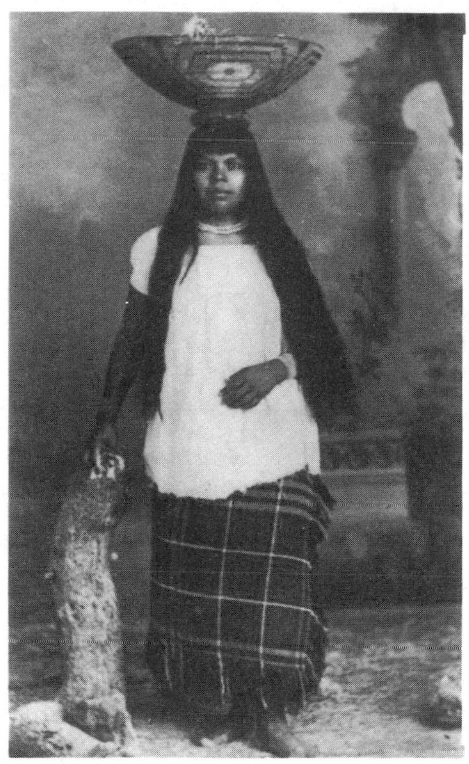

FIGURE 4.1

A Pima woman in traditional dress.

wishes to become pregnant, it is extremely important that the proper steps be taken to ensure that the diabetes is well under control, even before the pregnancy begins. Overall, between 1 and 3 percent of women show some abnormality of glucose function during pregnancy, but some ethnic groups such as the Pima Indians of the Sonoran Desert in New Mexico and northern Mexico have a much higher likelihood of showing signs of diabetes during pregnancy than others.

Clinicians and researchers who deal with diabetes on a day- to-day basis talk of an epidemic of diabetes that is currently occurring throughout the Western world. This epidemic cannot be accounted for solely by a gene for diabetes, since the rise has been too rapid to

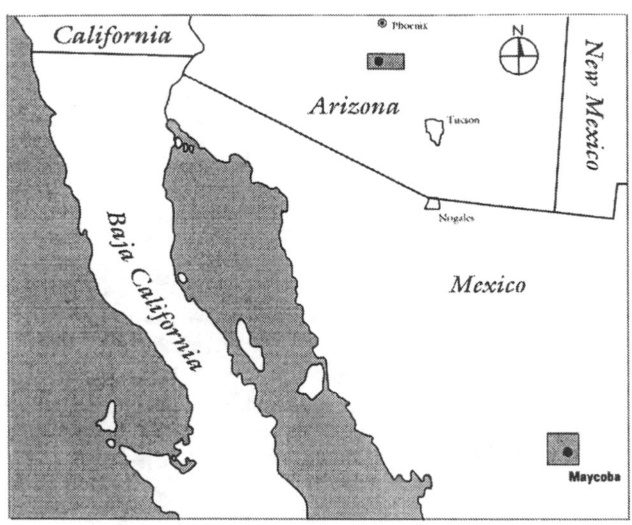

FIGURE 4.2

Map of Southwest United States and northern Mexico, showing where the Pima Indians live.

be accounted for by a change in the gene pool. This explosion of diabetes is occurring preferentially throughout developed—in distinction to developing—world communities. It is likely that the rise in the incidence of diabetes results from a mismatch between the world some babies, especially those who are nutritionally deprived, prepare for in the womb and the world of overabundance they eventually experience throughout their lives. This explosion of diabetes has to be explained, at least in part, by a conflict between environment and lifestyles: a poor environment before birth and a plentiful one after birth.

A Low Protein Diet During Pregnancy **Damages the Fetal Pancreas in Rats**

Dr. Joseph Hoet and his colleagues at Leuven in Belgium have shown that when the amount of protein eaten by a pregnant rat during pregnancy is decreased by just over half, there is a significant reduction in the number of insulin-secreting cells in the pancreas of the fetal pups that mother is carrying. Interestingly, there is a also a reduction in the number of blood vessels that develop in the pancreas. As we saw in the fourth of our list of ten principles of programming, reduction in the number of blood vessels that form is very bad news for a developing organ. Reduced blood supply is one of the fundamental principles by which programming can become permanent. Developing fetal tissues need a very good blood supply to get off to the right start. It has been shown that a brief period of twenty-one days of poor nutrition immediately after birth also results in impaired development of the pancreas and a tendency to diabetes when the rat pups grow up.

The clinical biochemistry group at Cambridge University directed by Dr. Nicholas Hales has gone a long way toward describing the specific cell problems that are caused by the short period of undernutrition during early development. They showed that protein deficiency in fetal life alters the proportions of different cell types in the liver. The cells around the blood vessels that bring glucose and other nutrients to the liver are good at producing glucose and passing it out into the blood in times of shortage. Protein deficiency during development permanently increases the activity of cells in this area of the liver while decreasing the activity of the cells in other areas of the liver that take up glucose and store it. Thus there is a greater tendency for the liver of the fetus that has become used to glucose deficiency in the womb to put out rather than store glucose. This is a good adaptation to times of shortage. It is not good, however, if after birth, food is available in abundance.

The Cambridge University group has also shown that a low-protein diet before birth will decrease the activity of the fetal pancreatic cells that monitor the amount of glucose circulating in the blood. When this happens, glucose in the blood has to build up to higher levels before enough insulin is produced by the pancreas in an attempt to bring the sugar down to normal amounts.

Transgenerational Effects: Influences on Insulin Production

Low-protein diets during development result in permanent unwanted changes in the liver and pancreas of individual rats. Two groups of researchers, one on either side of the Atlantic, have conducted studies in pregnant laboratory rats that have been made diabetic experimentally. These diabetic rats have pups with a higher likelihood of becoming diabetic than the offspring of nondiabetic pregnant rats. We should note right from the start that this is an environmental effect. The rats in the studies I am about to describe were not diabetic for any genetic reason. They were made diabetic experimentally. These remarkable observations are strengthened by the fact that similar experiments with essentially the same results have been conducted both in Europe and the United States. Both sets of researchers have shown that the daughters of untreated diabetic pregnant rats themselves have a higher tendency to pregnancy- induced diabetes. As a result, this programming may go on for several generations, passing from daughters to granddaughters and onward down families. There is transgenerational passage of disease by mechanisms that are not genetic. A detailed look at these fascinating and informative experimental studies will also help you to decide just how firm is the overall concept that our health throughout life is programmed in the womb.

We have seen that a single injection of male hormones given to a female rat at a critical time in her development permanently programs the function of areas of the brain that control her reproductive cycles. We should then ask the question: Are there also periods in development when regulation of nutrition is similarly programmed? Studies in rats show that if blood sugar levels are high in the mother's blood during pregnancy, some factor—probably high glucose concentrations in the fetal rat's blood during development—can modify pancreatic insulin function permanently.

Among the Pima Indians, the risk of individuals becoming diabetic is more likely if their maternal grandmother suffered from diabetes than if their maternal grandfather was a diabetic. Transgenerational effects due to abnormal glucose tolerance when the grandmother was a fetus or the mother was a fetus may influence these differences in the incidence of diabetes in the offspring. It is epidemiologic evidence like this that fits with the concept that environmental causes are just as likely as classical genetic factors to lie at the root of some forms of diabetes.

To gain significant insights into the interactions that govern the function of insulin in mother and fetus as well as the transport of glucose and amino acids across the placenta between mother and fetus, we must turn to animal studies. Human fetal tissue obtained following spontaneous abortion is not particularly suitable for these studies since it is always likely to show the signs of the abnormality that caused the abortion. In addition, it is impossible to study transgenerational effects in humans if the first generation has not survived. So we must start with the most commonly studied experimental species, the laboratory rat. We will eventually return to the human condition: to Pima Indians, to McDonald's fast foods and lack of school playing fields, to couch potatoes and computer junkies. But first to the rat.

Pregnancy in the rat lasts twenty-one days. The baby rat is born in a very immature state. At birth, the rat pup's eyes are not yet open. During their very short stay in the womb, fetal rats must develop the ability to perform the many tasks necessary to live an independent life in the challenging outside world. After birth, rat pups must control their own body temperature. Their mother did that for them when they were in the womb. Newborn rat pups must feed when they are hungry in order to get more glucose, protein and fat into their growing bodies. In the womb, these fuels and building blocks came directly across the placenta from the maternal supply depot. Before birth, they did not need to do anything actively to obtain food. Now, after birth, they must be able to take in and digest the glucose and to pack it away into cells. Glucose is needed by all the cells of the body so that they can function efficiently. To pack the glucose into the cells, newborn rats need to be able to secrete insulin from their pancreas. Fortunately, producing insulin is not something they have to learn all of a sudden. While in the womb, rat pups secreted insulin to push amino acids into cells to help them grow. The pups learned to produce and secrete insulin while in the womb, so at least that function is ready at birth. But after birth, glucose will no longer be as steadily available as it was during fetal life, coming as a continuous stream across the placenta from their mother. Admittedly, there were blips, ups and downs, as the mother rat's glucose rose and fell when she ate, but the supply line from the depot was fairly constant and assured. After birth, the rat pups will need to secrete more insulin when the level of glucose in their blood is high and secrete less insulin when glucose availability is low. Newborn pups, like adults, must keep the amount of glucose in their blood at fairly stable levels.

STUDIES IN BELGIUM IN THE ANCIENT CITY OF LEUVEN

Because the level of glucose and amino acids are often altered in the blood of the pregnant women in his clinic, Dr. Andre Van Assche and his colleagues in Leuven, Belgium, are interested in the way these changes may affect the development of the baby. It has been known for many years that the newborn babies of diabetic mothers are less able to control their own blood sugar levels immediately after birth. These babies also show deficiencies in the development of other vital systems such as the lung. As a result, newborn offspring of diabetic mothers whose glucose and insulin have not been well controlled during pregnancy are more likely to have breathing troubles when they are born.

In order to find out how the fetal pancreas forms, Andre Van Assche and his colleagues, Drs. Hoet, Aerts and Holemans, have spent countless hours dissecting out the pancreases of fetal rats at different stages of development. This is no mean feat. A pile of pancreases from one hundred newborn rats would fit easily on a teaspoon. One of the fundamental needs of research is to understand and carefully describe the normal before we can begin to tell how things go wrong in disease states. The Belgian investigators are skilled at preparing thin tissue sections so that they can study this minute organ under the microscope. They stain the microscope sections with various dyes so that they can distinguish the different types of cells and observe the changes that occur at the critical stages of fetal life. They are experts at knowing the detailed appearance of the normal fetal rat pancreas. Under the microscope, insulin-secreting cells can be seen at about eighteen days of fetal life in the normal fetal rat pancreas. Their numbers and maturity of appearance increase rapidly just before birth.

The Belgian researchers wanted to compare the insulin-producing cells in the pancreases in the fetuses of normal, healthy pregnant rats with the pancreases of fetal rats whose mothers were diabetic. Pregnant rats can be made diabetic by giving the mother a single injection of a drug, streptozotocin. This drug rapidly and relatively selectively destroys the insulin-producing cells of the pancreas. If streptozotocin is injected into pregnant rats on the very first day of pregnancy, most will rapidly become diabetic. It should be noted that when the drug is given, it damages only the mother's pancreas. Since the fetal pancreas has not yet developed at this early stage of pregnancy, the fetal pancreas is not harmed by the drug. The degree of damage to the mother's pancreas can be varied according to the amount of drug she received. As a result, the degree to which the drug makes her insulin-deficient and the level to which her glucose rises will also vary. This variability in response is not a shortcoming that makes the interpretation of the study difficult. In fact, the range of responses allows researchers to relate the various grades of severity of the diabetes in the mother to the extent of the effects produced in the fetus.

The placenta, acting as the fetal gut, transfers glucose to the fetus. The concentration of glucose in the fetal blood is directly related to the glucose concentration in the mother's blood. In this regard, as in so many others, the fetus is captive to the mother's physiology. I have referred to the mother’s role as that of a quartermaster. Another somewhat unappealing analogy for the relationship of mother to fetus is that the mother is the baby's jailer. So that you don’t consider the metaphor too severe, she is a good jailer in at least one respect. She shares her food, both good and bad, with the prisoner. The baby can only obtain more glucose when the mother eats more food. Glucose passes across the placenta all the time, but it is only when the mother’s blood glucose and nutrient concentrations rise that the amount of glucose and other nutrients going from mother to baby increase markedly.

If the mother's glucose level is really high, as it could well be in human pregnancy when the mother is a diabetic who receives no insulin treatment, fetal glucose levels are also high. As a result, the fetal pancreas is forced into greater and greater action. The immature, developing fetal pancreas is ill-prepared for such hard work. If the challenge is too great, eventually, the fetal pancreas can no longer cope. The fetal insulin-secreting beta cells begin to show signs of exhaustion. They have been responding as best they can to secrete enough insulin to pack away the abnormally high amounts of glucose coming across the placenta from the mother, but the insult has been more than they were designed to deal with at this stage in their development. The challenge of the high blood glucose is too much, especially if sustained day after day, as may well be the case in the untreated diabetic. The microscopical findings of exhaustion of the insulin secreting beta cells observed in the human fetal pancreas obtained from dead babies of poorly controlled diabetic mothers are very similar to those seen in the fetuses of diabetic rats. If the amount of glucose coming across the placenta from the mother is continuously more than it should be, the fetal pancreas eventually gets worn out, exhausted, as a result of the abnormally high workload.

If the mother is short of insulin, the concentrations of glucose and amino acids in her blood will be high. More of these compounds will be available for the placenta to transport to the fetus. As long as the fetal pancreas can respond by secreting more insulin, the fetus will be able to pack away these extra building materials in growing cells. Fetuses of diabetic mothers are often overweight, and their bodies are composed of more and larger cells than normal. Just as with small, growth-retarded babies, this overgrowth scenario may have unwanted consequences later in life.

It is of interest that when insulin is secreted in greater amounts by the fetus of the diabetic mother rat, more receptors to insulin appear on the developing cells of the fetal organs. Hormones like insulin exert their action on cells through their specific receptors. So the effects of insulin are further enhanced in the developing rat fetus whose mother is an untreated diabetic as a result of the increase in insulin receptors. This phenomenon in which a hormone actually causes an increase in the number of receptors on its target cells is called *up regulation.* The opposite effect, where an increase in the hormone level decreases the number of receptors, is called *down regulation.* Up and down regulation, if permanent, can potentially alter the level of activity of the system in many ways. Later on, we will see that permanent down regulation changes can occur in the number of receptors in some regions of the brain that monitor the amount of stress steroids circulating in the blood of rats who were exposed to excessive amounts of these steroids while they were fetuses. This alteration in receptor numbers leads to permanent resetting of the level of activity of the brain's stress axis. Long-term programming of health may in some measure reflect permanent changes in receptors caused by up or down regulation. In this way, an individual's regulating mechanism for a particular function can be reset.

When baby rats born to diabetic mothers grow up, they are more likely to have troubles with their pancreas. By one hundred days of life, which is well past puberty and into midlife for a rat, the pups whose mothers were diabetic during their pregnancy often have higher levels of insulin in their blood than normal rats would need at any particular level of glucose. It seems that in these rats, prenatal exposure to high glucose levels results in development of resistance of the cells in the body to insulin. This form of insulin resistance is similar to the more common form of diabetes, the noninsulin-dependent diabetes in humans.

Van Assche and his colleagues were careful to show that the abnormal handling of glucose by the second generation, the offspring of diabetic rats, was due to prenatal problems rather than events that take place after birth. To find out how much of the problem could have been due to the mother's milk, they fostered rat pups of diabetic mothers onto normal mothers. They also did the reverse study, fostering pups of normal mothers onto diabetic mothers. From the results of these investigations, they were able to show with confidence that the glucose handling and pancreatic problems in the offspring of diabetic rats was caused by something they were exposed to in the womb of their diabetic mother before birth rather than any consequences of the mother's diabetes after birth during the suckling and weaning periods. However, the Belgian researchers did show that feeding by a diabetic mother results in a delay of growth in the pups. So there are long-term problems if the diabetes is not controlled, both before and after birth.

What happens when the female rats born to diabetic mothers become pregnant? When they become pregnant, they have more glucose in their blood and lower insulin levels than normal pregnant rats. They have a picture similar to human pregnancy diabetes. During pregnancy, the insulin-secreting cells in the pancreas of these second-generation pregnant offspring of diabetic mothers look very inactive compared with normal pregnant rats when studied under the microscope. The consequences of being the fetuses of diabetic rats are about to play out again and pass across the generations. One begins to think that similar mechanisms may explain the very high incidence of diabetes passing across generations as in the Pima Indians where the maternal side of the family has more influence on an individual's tendency to diabetes than the father's side.

Let us recap the story so far. A first generation of rats that were made diabetic at the beginning of pregnancy had high blood glucose levels throughout pregnancy. This high maternal blood glucose resulted in more glucose passing across the placenta to their fetuses, producing high fetal blood glucose. The elevated glucose in the fetal blood overstimulated the fetal pancreas, and the cells that secrete insulin grew and divided at a greater than normal rate. When the challenge to the fetal pancreas was moderate, the pancreas enlarged but did not collapse under the strain. When the maternal blood glucose was wildly out of control and as a result the fetal glucose was very high, the fetal ability to secrete insulin was exhausted under the excessive, unusual and constant challenge. The constant need to secrete more and more insulin to bring the very high blood glucose levels back to normal was eventually too much for the developing pancreas. It became exhausted by the effort to keep up with the large amounts of glucose coming across the placenta from the diabetic mother. Just as with the pups of rats fed a low-protein diet by Dr.

Hoet, second-generation fetal rats whose mothers (the first generation) were diabetic had fewer blood vessels in their pancreas than second-generation rat pups whose mother were not diabetic.

Since the second-generation mothers have a decreased ability to secrete insulin, like their own mothers, they also will have a tendency to become diabetic when confronted with the challenge of pregnancy, exposing their own pups, the third generation, to high levels of glucose during prenatal development. So it comes as no surprise that when these third-generation fetuses reached adulthood, they, too, demonstrated abnormal responses to a glucose tolerance test, having a decreased ability to secrete insulin in response to the glucose. Since the increased tendency to diabetes occurs in successive generations of pregnant mothers, there is no reason for it to stop passing across generations until the maternal diabetes is controlled during pregnancy. When this is done, the fetal pancreas will not be excessively challenged during development. That's the good news. Understanding how programming works will help us to prevent its adverse, unwanted effects.

What influence does the father have on this nongene-dependent, transgenerational passage of the tendency to diabetes? In one study, Van Assche and Aerts examined the ability of rats at eighty days of age (early adult life) to handle a glucose load. They found that rats born to second-generation diabetic mothers showed abnormality in their ability to use glucose regardless of whether the father was a normal rat or a second-generation diabetic rat. In contrast, rats born to normal mothers and second-generation diabetic fathers had normal responses to glucose similar to the response in rat pups born to a normal mother and normal father. This observation is very similar to the findings in Pima Indians referred to above, in which the tendency to the noninsulin-dependent form of diabetes is passed down through diabetic mothers and grandmothers, not fathers and grandfathers.

STUDIES IN THE UNITED STATES IN PROVIDENCE, RHODE ISLAND

This story of the nongenetic transfer of diabetic tendency across generations has also been shown by Dr. William Oh and his colleagues from Brown University in the United States. The only difference of note in how they conducted their study is that they made the mother rats diabetic by injecting them with the beta cell- killing drug streptozotocin on day five of pregnancy. You will recall that Van Assche gave the injection on day one in the studies from Leuven. In the Providence study, pregnant rats were allowed to deliver, and their offspring were studied at eighty days of age when they showed a decreased ability to keep their blood glucose levels down when challenged with a glucose load. By breeding the daughters of the original diabetic rats, the problems with the pancreas and insulin secretion was shown to be present in the third generation, just as in the Belgian study. These third-generation pups were larger, and both males and females had more body fat than pups of the third generation from nondiabetic mothers—the controls.

Transgenerational biological endowment can be either harmful or beneficial, depending on how we as a species use or abuse it. We can choose to help successive generations have a better home in the womb or allow problems to pass down generations, unchanged. As we learn more about transgenerational passage of both health and disease, the knowledge gained will be available to help us determine how to alter many of our political, economic and personal behaviors. The consequences of ignoring these prenatal antecedents, these fundamental causes of good health as well as disease, are clearly more intractable and long-lasting than previously considered; they may not be easily amendable to the quick fix.

I am reminded of Macbeth's comment on seeing the ghost of his rival, Banquo. In the first scene of the play, Macbeth and Banquo are returning from a famous victory. They are greeted by three witches who predict that Macbeth will become king, but Banquo, although he will never be king himself, will be the father of a long line of kings. Macbeth will not pass on his lineage transgenerationally, but Banquo will. Macbeth seeks to frustrate this prediction by arranging Banquo's murder. Assassination successfully completed, later in the play, Macbeth sits down to feast with his wife and nobles. Suddenly, he sees the ghost of Banquo, followed by Banquo's son and many, many other kings, all descendants of Banquo. The dead Banquo clearly will pass on his linage across multiple generations. Macbeth rages in horror, "What, will the line run on until the crack of doom?"

We may well ask, "Will the consequences of prenatal suboptimal development run on until the crack of doom?" It need not be so if we understand how these adverse outcomes occur and take the necessary steps prospectively to prevent them. The bad effects can be reversed. That's the good news. The bad news is that it may take a few generations. In chapter 9, we will see that it takes at least three generations of normal nutrition to recuperate some of the consequences of feeding low-protein diets to twelve generations of rats. At present, no one knows the speed at which these different bad effects can be washed out of the human system. It is important to find out how good health can be recuperated. It is clear that unwanted transgenerational effects don't just fade away at the first attempt to put them right.

FIVE

GROWTH IN THE WOMB. SIZE IS NOT EVERYTHING

When I have pluck'd the rose,
I cannot give it vital growth again,
It needs must whither.

William Shakespeare, *Othello*

A good start is critical for almost everything we do in life. It is particularly true for how we grow before birth. The available space in the womb and the quality of the placenta are key determinants of growth before birth. The environment in which we grow in the womb has a greater effect on whether we reach our full growth potential than our genes. The placenta completes most of its growth early in pregnancy. Normal growth of the placenta is vital to everything that happens later. The placenta and the umbilical cord are the only pipeline from mother to fetus. Everything the baby needs has to pass this way, as does everything the baby wishes to dispose of.

The placenta contains a detailed record of what happened as we grew in the womb. It is in essence a diary of our life before birth. Advances in molecular biology will soon make it possible to decode the language in which this placental diary is written. Throughout pregnancy, there is a two-way conversation between the fetus and the placenta; hormones pass backward and forward, regulating growth and development.

Teenage pregnancy has many disadvantages, including one major biological problem that helps us to understand how the baby grows under suboptimal conditions. Mothers who themselves are still growing compete with their baby and the placenta for nutrients. After all, growing mothers have to grow their own cells.

At a critical stage in development, cells have to make a fundamental decision either to go on dividing to produce more cells or to specialize to perform a particular function. Fetal cells are most vulnerable when they are growing and dividing fast. Since different fetal organs— heart, brain, liver—are growing at differing rates at various stages of fetal life, the long-term results of fetal compromise may be very different according to the precise time when the fetus is challenged by unfavorable circumstances. Size is not everything. However, it is important that all growing babies in the womb get the opportunity to grow all the important components of their bodies in the optimal fashion. The challenge of developing under adverse circumstances may program an individual for problems later in life. The problems may be general or restricted to specific organs such as the heart, brain or pancreas.

The body shape of growth-retarded babies varies according to whether the unfavorable conditions in the womb occurred during early pregnancy or late pregnancy. Adverse conditions early in pregnancy produce symmetrical growth retardation where the whole body is affected. The overall number of cells in all parts of the body is reduced. Unfavorable conditions in late pregnancy produce asymmetrical effects since different organs are affected to a varying extent according to their rate of growth at the time of the insult. In some forms of growth retardation, it is possible for the baby to catch up at a later stage of life. However, studies in rats have shown that such catching up may be associated with a decreased life span. So, as always, prevention of growth problems during fetal life is better than to attempt cure later in life.

Cancer is caused by unrestricted growth and division of cells. The precise reason why cells suddenly begin to divide in an uncontrolled fashion varies in different body organs. There is good evidence that adverse programming of the ovary, breast and prostate gland during fetal development can increase the risk of cancer of these tissues in later life.

Room in the Womb Constrains Growth

Since the vast majority of cells are born and do their early growing before birth, it is not surprising that the events before birth are so important. In addition, it is easy to see how, if something goes wrong in one of the early stages, the problem is retained or even multiplied as damaged or improperly constructed cells continue to divide. If the deprived cells are administrative, regulatory cells, they may give out the wrong instructions or even the right instructions at the wrong times, later in life. Thus, perpetuation of errors made during growth and development resulting from adverse conditions in the womb has the potential to be carried on for the rest of life. As I have said before, we pass more developmental milestones during life before birth than we do after birth.

We all need space in life, preferably quality space. This need for space applies to our prenatal development, too. The overall health of the mother, her nutrition, the proper function of her heart and her blood system, even her own prenatal history (shown so well in the transgenerational effects of the Dutch Hunger Winter), are major regulators of prenatal growth and development of her baby. Analysis of the factors that determine weight at birth of large numbers of children who are related by birth to varying degrees has shown that 62 percent of the variation in birthweight between children is determined by the environment in the uterus in which they developed. The remaining variation in the size of babies at birth is split roughly equally between factors in the mother's and the father's genes. Thus, from the point of view of general growth, nurture is certainly quantitatively more important than nature. As in all other matters, whether each fetus reaches her or his growth potential depends on the extent to which the environment in the womb allows this potential to develop in full. All the experimental evidence shows that the environment in the mother's uterus acts as a powerful constraint to

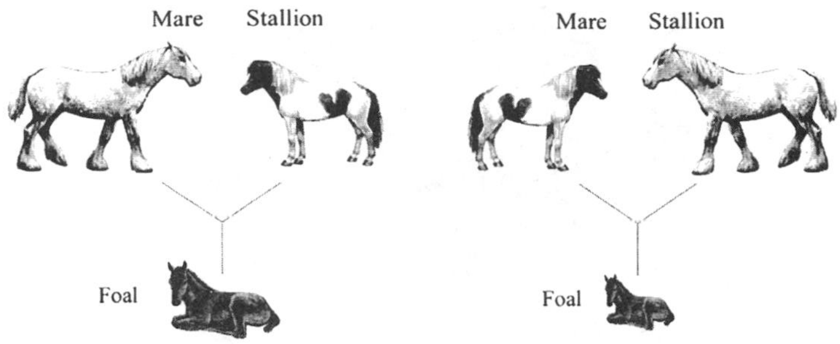

FIGURE 5.1

Difference in the size of the foal that results from crossing Shire horses and Shetland ponies.

growth during life before birth, controlling the degree to which the fetus reaches his or her maximum potential size.

The first scientific demonstration of the constraints the mother places on the ability of the fetus to grow in the womb was given by John Hammond, a pioneer in the field of animal science. In the 1930s, he performed a pioneering—and often quoted—controlled breeding study. Hammond crossed small Shetland ponies with large Shire horses. When the mother was a Shetland mare and the father a Shire stallion, the foal was smaller than when the mother was a Shire mare and the father a Shetland stallion. This classic experiment indicated but did not prove that the environment the mother provides before birth is crucial to the amount of growth the fetus can accomplish within the womb.

Embryo Transfer Studies

Because of its design, the Hammond study is not conclusive proof that the maternal environment is critical to the development of the fetus. Since these were natural matings, the genetic make up was different between the two crosses Hammond used in his study. The genetic makeup of the foal growing in the Shetland mother came from a Shire father and a Shetland mother. In contrast, the foal growing in the Shire mother had a Shetland father. Thus, the two situations

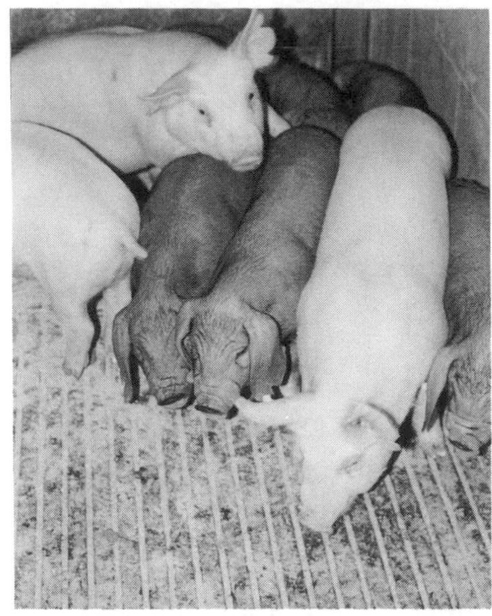

FIGURE 5.2

Small dark-skinned Meshian and large light-skinned Yorkshire pigs.

differ not just in one but in two factors: the maternal environment and the genetic composition of the fetus. The constitution of the embryo is not the same in the two cases. This means we cannot say with complete confidence that the differences in growth are due to the environments of the Shetland and the Shire uterus. We must reserve judgment because in the Hammond study, the differences may be due at least in part to the genetic makeup of the embryos.

To answer the specific question of how the quality of the uterine environment provided by the mother affects the growth of the baby, Dr. Stephen Ford at Iowa State University has used the more modern approach of embryo transfer. Stephen Ford studied the growth and development of identical embryos transferred between two strains of pigs, the small Meshian pig from China and the large American Yorkshire pig. These two strains of pig are very different in size and temperament. It is possible to transfer embryos that have both a Yorkshire mother and father to either surrogate Meshian or Yorkshire sows. When this is done, the genes that make up the embryos are kept constant; only the environment of the surrogate womb is different.

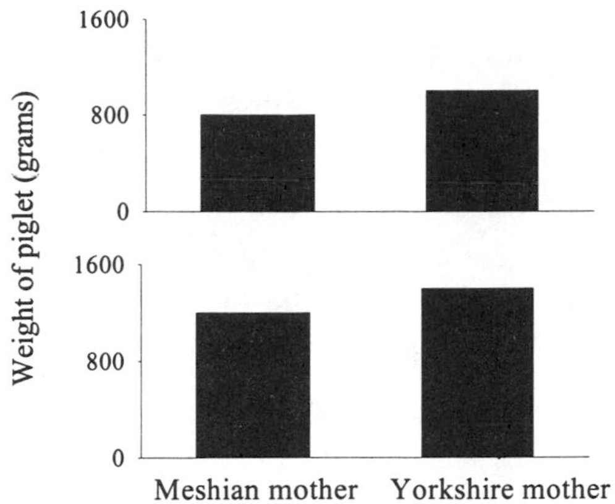

FIGURE 5.3

Weight of piglet just before birth when Meshian (top panel) and Yorkshire embryos (bottom panel) are transplanted to Meshian or Yorkshire mothers.

Stephen Ford weighed the fetuses growing in the two different uterine habitats, either the Yorkshire or the Meshian uterus, four days before they would normally have been born. The two groups differed very clearly in weight. At the very end of pregnancy, the largest fetuses were the Yorkshire-Yorkshire fetuses (those whose parents were both Yorkshires) developing in a surrogate Yorkshire mother. Fetuses with the same Yorkshire-Yorkshire parentage growing in a Meshian mother were much smaller. From this comparison, we may conclude that the environment in the Meshian uterus does not allow the pure Yorkshire fetuses to grow to the full size of which they are capable when they are developing in a Yorkshire uterus. This embryo transfer approach to the question of whether the mother controls the rate of growth of her babies provides much firmer data than the Hammond approach because the genetic material in the two groups studied by Steve Ford was the same. In both of these groups, the fetuses were all Yorkshire and had the same genetic background, both mother and father. The only difference was the environment provided in which to grow, either a Yorkshire or a Meshian uterus.

To clinch the point, Dr. Ford undertook the reverse embryo transfer. He transplanted embryos whose parents were both Meshian pigs to either surrogate Meshian or Yorkshire mothers. The results were as expected. Piglets whose parentage was pure Meshian grew faster in the uterus of a Yorkshire sow than in a Meshian sow's uterus. As in the previous embryo transfer study, the findings show that the larger Yorkshire uterus again allows more growth. Other information in Dr. Ford's elegant study shows clearly that the genetic makeup of the fetus does also play a critical role in how fast the fetus grows. The Yorkshire piglets grow larger in either the Yorkshire sow or the Meshian sow when compared with fetuses with both Meshian parents. We can conclude with some certainty that the genetic growth potential of the Yorkshire breed is greater than the Meshian.

Time and time again, as we analyze these and other data, we must remember that size is not everything. We must always consider quality as even more important than quantity. From the point of view of human health, it is our ability to function in a complex world and resistance to disease that each of us needs to develop optimally.

To understand the origins of health and disease, we need to ask searching questions about the importance of the quality of growth before birth to long-term health. We need to know in particular the conditions that are optimal for brain growth. Optimal brain development is fundamental to good health through life. The rate of brain growth changes at different times of pregnancy. There are spurts in brain growth rate that occur at different times for the various specialized regions of the brain. We need to know the conditions that encourage the correct rates of growth. We need to know if there is a price to pay later in life for growing too large or too small. Evidence from human epidemiologic studies certainly shows that being born either smaller or larger than the size your genetic program would produce under normal conditions is not good for your health in later life. It is the correct balance of growth between different organs growing at the right time in relation to each other that appears to be the key to a long and healthy life.

RULE NUMBER ONE: GROW A GOOD PLACENTA

In Steve Ford's embryo transfer study, there are four different groups: Meshian fetuses growing in either Meshian or Yorkshire mothers, and Yorkshire fetuses growing in either Meshian or Yorkshire mothers. Close inspection of the placentas of both types of fetuses (Meshian and Yorkshire) in the four situations shows that the maternal environment also plays an important role in allowing the baby's genes to express themselves. The early development of the placenta is faster when the piglet is growing in the Yorkshire uterus, regardless of the genetic makeup of the fetus. Thus, the placenta of Yorkshire-Yorkshire cross fetuses grows faster when growing in the uterus of a Yorkshire than in a Meshian sow. Similarly, the placentas of the Meshian-Meshian crosses grow faster in the Yorkshire sow than in the Meshian. So there is something in the environment of the Yorkshire sow's body that makes the placenta grow faster early in pregnancy.

The first third of pregnancy can be considered a time for the placenta to grow rather than the fetus. It is important that the mother and fetus work together to grow a good placenta in this first third of their combined prenatal effort. It is a combined effort, both mother and fetus play critical interactive roles in determining how well the placenta forms. Steve Ford's current hunch, supported by good preliminary experimental data, is that the Yorkshire mother or her developing embryo produce more estrogen early in pregnancy than the Meshian sow. Estrogen plays a critical role in regulating blood flow to the uterus and developing fetus. Thus, it is highly likely that the Yorkshire placenta provides a better start to fetal life by boosting the early growth of the fetus.

We have already seen that in the early days of pregnancy many critical phases of the baby's development are riding on the rapid and effective development of the placenta. If the placenta does not perform well, then the baby is at a great disadvantage and growth and development will be impaired throughout pregnancy, and this impaired prenatal growth can have consequences throughout life. Just as we know that the newborn child is dependent on a good start in life, so is the developing embryo. Parents and teachers know that the early stages of a child's education are critical to everything that follows. If a child does not learn to read, she can't learn much else. If a good placenta does not form, normal growth and development are impossible. The priority given to protecting the growing placenta early in pregnancy is very similar to the priority given to protecting the brain later in fetal life. It is intriguing to think that at one stage of life, the placenta is more important than the brain.

The hormones and nutritional factors that regulate placental growth have received all too little research attention. It appears to be difficult to persuade even research scientists that there are certain times in pregnancy when the placenta is more important than the fetus. So it is understandable why the general public is not all that interested in this fascinating structure. However, in some cultures the placenta does hold a higher place in people's esteem. The ancient pharaohs paraded their placenta before them on ceremonial occasions. In the Andes and other parts of the world, the placenta is often buried at the corner of a new house, symbolizing the foundation on which everything is built. The placenta is a fetal diary; in it is written information on many of the important happenings throughout the pregnancy. The diary entries are encoded in changes in the cell structure and the exact mix of genes that have been switched on and off by the prevailing conditions in the womb. The time may yet come when a small piece of every baby's placenta is frozen away at birth to measure the activity of specific genes. Another piece will be stored in ways that allow special microscopical examination. Then, in later life, it will be possible to consult our individual prenatal diaries. The story written in the placenta will assist in treatment of diseases in later life and clearly will have medico-legal implications.

TEENAGE PREGNANCY: GROWING MOTHERS COMPETE WITH THEIR GROWING BABIES

There is an optimum biological time for a woman to be pregnant from the viewpoint of her physical response to the needs of pregnancy. Although obstetricians and reproductive scientists would strongly debate the best age range from the point of view of the fetus, a woman's biology is probably at its peak reproductive efficiency between the age of twenty and thirty. The exact age span that is optimum will differ from woman to woman according to her physique, her own developmental history and her general state of health. One thing, however, is certain; teenage pregnancy, especially in the early teen years, is not an optimal scenario for either fetus or mother. The demands of pregnancy on the maternal circulation and food resources are very significant. When growing at the maximum rate at around thirty-two to thirty-four weeks of pregnancy, normal human babies are increasing their weight by nearly 250 grams (over half a pound) a week. It is not optimal for a woman to be pregnant at a time when her own body is still maturing and building her own tissues. The demands of the baby at this time will inevitably lead to suboptimal development of both mother and baby. It is not in the best interests of either mother or baby for a woman's body to grow a baby before she herself is fully grown. The information from the daughters of the Dutch Hunger Winter shows that suboptimal growth when a woman is herself a fetus can adversely impact growth and function of her own children, and so on across generations. Fetal growth is certainly not going to reach its full potential in the majority of teenage pregnancies.

Some elegant recent studies in pregnant sheep have clearly demonstrated the problems of fetal growth in mothers who have not yet completed their own growth. Dr. Jacqueline Wallace and her colleagues in Aberdeen, Scotland, have studied young ewes who received transplanted embryos before they would normally have become pregnant. At the age at which the ewes were made pregnant, they were still growing fast—they were essentially teenagers. Dr. Wallace's interest was to discover how rapid growth of the young mother would affect the growing lamb in the womb. She wanted to know just how the cells of the growing mother would compete with the cells in her baby growing in her womb. So she allowed one group of young pregnant ewes to eat just as much as they wanted and to grow as rapidly as they could. To provide a comparison, she fed a second group with just enough food to grow normally. You've probably guessed. Somewhat counterintuitively, the rapidly growing, well-fed ewes had smaller babies. It is as if, when nutrients are

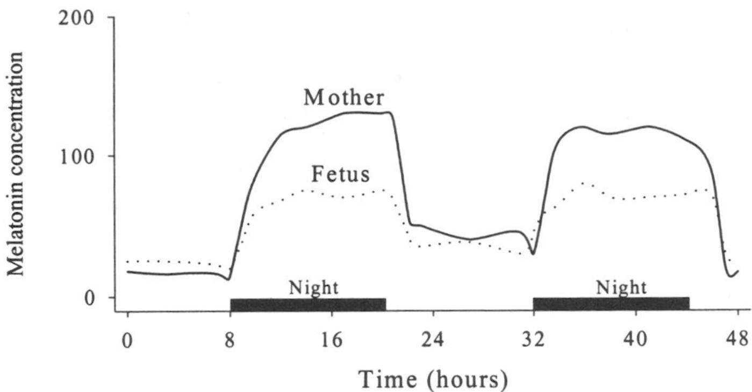

FIGURE 5.4

The rhythms of the hormone melatonin in the blood are very similar. The melatonin in fetal lamb blood comes across the placenta from the mother.

unlimited, the young mothers grow as fast as they can, ignoring the needs of their babies in the womb. These are exciting and important observations that need further exploration.

The Umbilical Cord: Information Superhighway and Fetal Supply Pipeline

Throughout pregnancy there is a two way conversation between the fetus and the placenta. The communication is not by messages that flash along nerves. There are no nerve fibers running through the umbilical cord to carry messages from placenta to fetus and fetus to placenta. The words in this dialogue are a wide variety of hormone molecules of different shapes: prostaglandins, peptides and many steroids. Sometimes, the mother may get in on the act by sending her own messages across the placenta. Melatonin is a maternal message that allows the mother to tell her baby the time of day in the world outside. Melatonin helps to drive our day and night rhythms. It is a hormone secreted by the pineal gland, a collection of nerve cells that sits on the top of our brains. These cells receive instructions from a very special group of cells in the hypothalamus that serve as our daily, or circadian, clock. During the hours of darkness, the pineal gland secretes the hormone melatonin. So, during the nighttime hours, the level of melatonin in our blood increases. Since melatonin can cross the placenta very easily, as the melatonin level rises in the mother's blood, it will also rise in the baby's blood. The rise and fall in melatonin in the baby's blood tells the fetus whether it is day or night out there.

The placenta produces a large number of hormones that help to control the activities of the developing baby. As we have seen, the baby also plays a critical role in regulating the growth and function of the placenta, especially early in development. In a very general way, the amount of blood the baby's heart pumps to the placenta is crucial to the normal growth of the placenta. It is now clear that there are also many very special signals that regulate placental growth. These signals enable the baby, in times of need, to increase the growth and function of the placenta. The prioritization of placental growth may even take place sometimes at the expense of growth of the baby. Signals from baby to the placenta play a key role in the ability of the placenta to grow to compensate for adverse conditions. A better understanding of how the placenta functions will make it possible in the future to use hormones and other growth factors to reverse inadequate placental growth and prevent the lifelong health problems associated with low birthweight.

Growth and Specialization: Two Competing Processes

At all stages during prenatal life, cells have to make a fundamental choice: to grow or to specialize. Growth and specialization during prenatal life are two important but competing processes. The cellular processes that govern the production of more cells differ from the processes that prepare cells to perform their unique functions. At some stage during fetal development, each cell comes to a point at which it must decide whether to continue to divide so that the baby's body can grow or to specialize for a specific function so that the baby is more biologically versatile after birth. This is the developing cell's dilemma. When to divide, when to specialize? Each cell in the developing fetus has to make this choice at some time in its life history. The agony of decision does not go on forever. Eventually, the decision is made. It is of great consequence to the body that each developing cell makes the right decision at precisely the right time. Normal prenatal development requires a finely tuned and regulated balance between growth and specialization. Once the decision is made, some cells—for example, nerve cells—will never divide again. They have become just too specialized to change their ways.

At some stages of fetal life, the body benefits when cells divide to produce more cells. At other times in development, it is more advantageous to the developing fetus if a particular cell begins to specialize, to perform a specific function, on behalf of all the cells in the body. In the early phases of development, the cells that will eventually comprise each organ in the body divide repeatedly to provide adequate numbers of cells for each organ to perform its specific functions throughout life. If the decision to differentiate rather than divide is made too early, an organ will end up with too few cells and thus be unequal to the challenges of later life. Inadequate numbers of cells will result in small organs. A good example of suboptimal growth is the depleted muscle mass of poorly nourished children. It is also important that the correct proportions of different types of cells are present within an organ. When there are too many cells of one type or too few cells of another, the critical balance between different cell types will be permanently changed.

One area that currently is receiving extensive attention is the growth of blood vessels. If too few blood vessels are present in a developing organ, there will be less ability to change the blood flow to that organ at times of need in later life. You will recall that the fetal rat pancreas exposed to inadequate nutrition before birth starts life after birth with an impaired blood supply.

The steroid stress hormones produced by the adrenal glands inhibit growth and cell division. This function is quite appropriate since at times of real danger, there are more important things to do than grow. Cortisol is the major steroid stress hormone in humans. In the fetus, cortisol plays an important role in instructing cells to specialize and stop growing. Perhaps the most important example of this action is cortisol's role in the regulation of production of surface tension lowering molecules in the developing lung. Without these molecules, collectively called surfactant, it is impossible to keep the lungs distended with air. In late fetal life, cortisol matures this function but at the price that it slows lung growth. This function of cortisol was elegantly worked out in fetal sheep by Dr. Graham Liggins from Auckland, New Zealand. For this work he was knighted by Queen Elizabeth. He received his knighthood at the same time as General Schwarzkopf. It is not often that researchers receive as much attention as warriors.

In chapters 6, 7 and 9 we will see how too much cortisol crossing the placenta from the mother to the fetus can adversely impact the development of fetal circulation, the fetal liver and the fetal brain. The long-term harmful effects of cortisol on the program of development of the fetus probably occur as the result of cells responding to cortisol's instruction to differentiate before they have finished growing and dividing.

Cells Are Most Vulnerable When Growing Fast

Growth is a demanding business for cells. Cells are most vulnerable when they are dividing rapidly. Growing cells have much greater energy and structural needs than cells that have completed their growing and settled down contentedly to perform their appointed function. Growing cells need more oxygen, amino acids, vitamins and glucose than those that are not trying to expand their activities.

Although most cells do have a small store of glucose and other necessities to stay alive, there is one vital necessity cells cannot store: oxygen. As a result, oxygen deprivation is fatal if it continues for more than a few minutes. It has been said jokingly that humans can only live without oxygen for a few minutes although they can live without water for days, without food for weeks and without ideas for a lifetime. It is the vulnerability to lack of oxygen that exposes all cells in the developing fetus to problems if the long pipeline to the outside air is interrupted for an appreciable length of time. Unfortunately, the fetal oxygen supply line can be impaired by inadequate performance of a number of organs: the maternal lungs, the maternal heart, the uterine blood vessels, the placenta, the fetal blood system and the fetal heart.

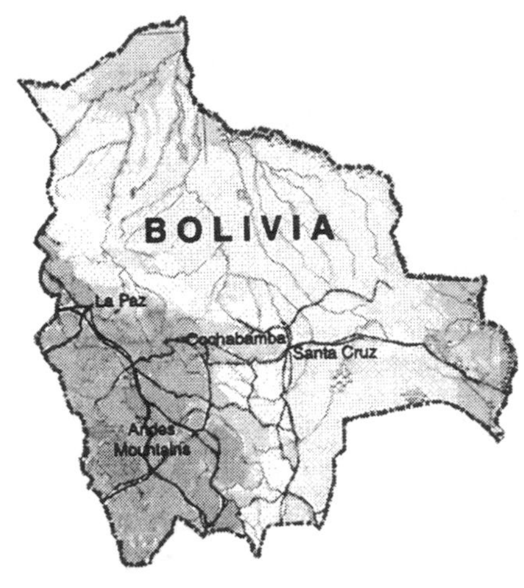

FIGURE 5.5

La Paz, the capital of Bolivia, and Cochabamba are in the Andes Mountains. Santa Cruz is at a lower altitude.

The effects of oxygen deficiency in pregnancy on fetal growth and newborn health have been studied in both pregnant sheep and llamas. The llama living in the altiplano in the Andes has adapted over the centuries to breathing air that is short of oxygen. When a llama living at high altitudes becomes pregnant, the transfer of oxygen to her fetus is a greater challenge than if she were living at sea level. In human pregnancy, the problems of oxygen delivery to the fetus at high altitudes are seen at their most pronounced in areas such as Colorado, the Himalayas and the Andes. Babies are not only smaller at birth in these high-altitude areas, but they are also more prone to die in the first year of life. By comparing infant death rates in different cities in Bolivia, Dr. Dino Giussani at Cambridge University has shown that both nutrition and oxygen availability appear to play a role in the health of the newborn baby in the first year of life. He compared Andean cities at similar altitudes but with very different socioeconomic conditions (La Paz, the capital of Bolivia, with Cochabamba) or cities with similar socioeconomic conditions but

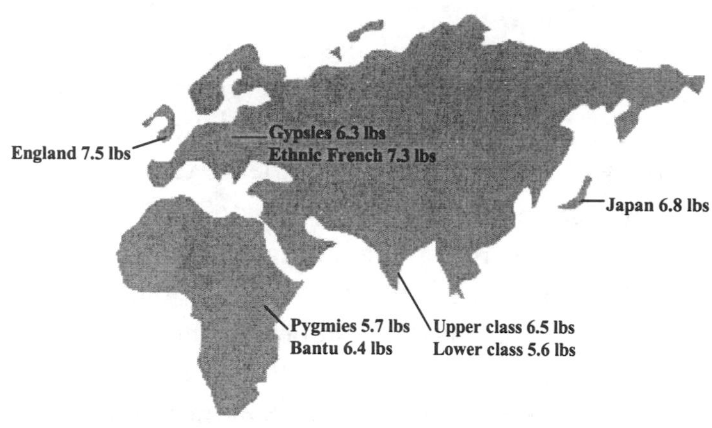

FIGURE 5.6

Average birthweights in different parts of the world.

at different altitudes (La Paz and Santa Cruz). The infant mortality rate is higher in Cochabamba than La Paz, showing, as we might expect, that socioeconomic conditions play a role in death in the first year of life. However, despite being the capital city of the country, infant mortality is higher in La Paz than in Santa Cruz, showing that altitude is also an important factor.

The Importance of the Fetal Pancreas in Regulating Growth

The pancreas is a fascinating and important organ. Firmly attached to the back wall of the abdomen, it lies snuggled in a curve of the small intestine into which it secretes a number of digestive enzymes that play a critical role in breaking down all the major classes of food components: fats, carbohydrates and proteins. In addition to its digestive functions, the pancreas secretes several hormones directly into the bloodstream. The best known of these hormones, and in many ways the most important, is insulin. Insulin instructs most cells in the body on how and when they should take up, use and store both glucose and amino acids. Glucose is the major fuel burned by the body to provide energy. By altering the rate at which glucose is made available to cells, insulin plays a major role in regulating the level of the body's activities. Since insulin also regulates how cells in the body take up amino acids, the building blocks from which proteins are made and growth is accomplished, insulin plays the role of both the supplier of the building materials and the workforce. Together, these activities determine how fast and to what extent cells and tissues grow. It is not, therefore, surprising that insulin plays a key role in regulating the growth of the fetus.

Very skillful and elegant studies by Abigail Fowden, the late Dr. Marian Silver and the late Dr. Robert Comline at Cambridge University in England have highlighted the precise and critical role of the fetal pancreas in regulating the growth of the fetus. When Abigail Fowden and her colleagues surgically removed the pancreas from fetal sheep about two-thirds of the way through fetal life, the fetuses virtually stopped growing. After the fetal pancreas had been removed, the uptake of glucose and amino acids from the mother and overall growth slowed dramatically. The same marked slowing in growth occurred if the fetal pancreas was destroyed by injecting the fetus with streptozotocin to target and kill the pancreatic cells that produce insulin. Infusion of insulin to the fetus reversed the effect of removal of the pancreas.

In contrast to the marked effect on fetal growth of removal of the fetal pancreas, removal of the fetal pituitary, thereby removing the source of any fetal growth hormone as well as the hormone that regulates the thyroid gland (thyroid stimulating hormone), has very little effect on fetal growth. While unimportant before birth, growth hormone and thyroxine are very important after birth. Newborn babies and infants who lack growth hormone and thyroid hormones have markedly stunted postnatal growth patterns. This difference in the action of these growth promoting hormones shows that growth in the fetus is regulated in a very different way than that of the newborn and infant. In the newborn and infant, growth hormone plays the key role; in the fetus, insulin is the major growth promoter. So, yet again we see that the fetus lives by its own special biological laws.

Different Body Forms in Growth-Retarded Babies: Symmetrical and Asymmetrical Growth Retardation

When considering the reasons why a particular baby is small, we must make the distinction between babies who are constitutionally small—genetically small, in other words—and babies who are small because before birth they developed in a prenatal environment that did not allow them to reach their full potential. The precise stage of development before birth at which growth impairment occurs has very different effects on the baby's body shape and the size of individual organs. When growth is restricted early in pregnancy, there is a reduction in the total number of cells throughout the baby's body. Everything about the baby is smaller. In this type of growth retardation, the baby is considered as being *symmetrically* growth retarded. Following significant early insult, growth will occur at a slower overall rate, and the baby's body remains uniformly small.

A different body form emerges when the baby's growth is restricted later in pregnancy. By the second half of pregnancy, the fetus has developed clever responses to compensate for inadequate nutrition or oxygen supply. Function of the fetal heart and blood vessels are now well under the control of the fetal brain. In chapter 1, I described how blood is channeled preferentially to the most important organ of all, the fetal brain, at times of oxygen or nutrient deficiency. This regional redistribution occurs at the expense of organs that are less vital to survival. There are several organs the baby does not need to use to their fullest while in the uterus: the skin (the baby does not yet need skin either as a protective barrier against the outside world or as an organ to help regulate body temperature by sweating), the bones (antigravity support of the body will only become important after birth), the gut (the baby isn't eating food yet), the kidneys (waste products are removed across the placenta) and the liver (liver functions such as excreting cholesterol are not critical until after birth). As a result, during nutritional or oxygen deprivation late in pregnancy, blood is redirected toward the arteries supplying the head and brain and away from these less vital organs. The result is an irregular decrease in growth. To preserve the brain, growth at the front end of the body is less impaired than at the tail end. Affected babies are *asymmetrically* growth retarded. Their body form is relatively long and thin for their overall weight. The measurement of head circumference is relatively well maintained, while abdominal circumference is decreased. So, in asymmetrically growth-retarded babies, the ratio of head circumference to abdominal circumference is increased compared with babies who have grown to their full genetic potential. Since different organs are growing at different rates at various times of fetal development, the organs most affected at any particular period of asymmetrical retardation will be those that are growing fastest at that time.

Catch up Growth: It May or May Not Be Possible to Make up for Early Growth Problems

Even when symmetrically growth-retarded babies are fed adequately after birth, they may not be able to catch up to the optimum weight and size that nature intended. Because symmetrically growth-retarded babies have fewer cells in their bodies, they will always be small. They will never reach the full size (especially height) that their genetic potential could have produced under favorable conditions. As we shall see later, attempts to stimulate catch-up in growth-retarded rodents shortens their individual life span. Thus, the consequences of the mother impeding early cell division of her baby by excessive intake of alcohol or drugs of abuse or even pronounced maternal undernutrition are likely to be a permanent part of an affected offspring's life. Where prenatal problems lead to major functional impairment, the family and society will have to shoulder the consequences for a long time and the cost may well exceed the cost of prevention. Strong evidence suggests that some of the costs may also be multigenerational.

In order to make the connection between prenatal growth retardation and long-term disease, it is necessary to remember that the human body functions as the sum total of its individual parts. Each one of these parts is specialized to perform specific tasks. It is easy to understand how an adult with a decreased number of liver cells will be less well adapted in later life to handle excessive cholesterol intake from our hamburger patty munching and popcorn popping diets. A small pancreas that contains fewer insulin-secreting cells will be less able to cope with the challenge of sugar-coated donuts and repeated candy snacks. Human epidemiologic studies show that growth-retarded babies are more likely to become diabetic later in life. Starting life with fewer insulin-secreting cells in the pancreas does not help an individual avoid diabetes. To fully appreciate the consequences of adverse prenatal conditions, we must see both the wood and the trees of this argument. The trees are the individuals organs: the liver, lung, brain, kidney, pancreas and gut. It is necessary to understand how each of these critical organs responds to an adverse prenatal environment. A clear knowledge of the significance of the individual trees will provide a better understanding of normal function and development of the whole individual, the wood. The big picture is our general health, yours, mine, and our children's health, for a lifetime.

When growth impairment occurs after the correct number of cells in the body has been established, growth slows as a result of the deprivation, but when normal nutrition is resumed, there is a good chance that the body can catch up to its full potential. In this case, catch-up is possible because the body has the correct number of cells. There is evidence that cells that were deprived at one stage and then given the materials that permit catch-up may never be completely returned to their normal state. We should beware of thinking that catch-up growth returns affected babies to their full potential. It would be much better to prevent the problem of suboptimal prenatal development than to try to correct it. The old adages our parents taught us, such as "a stitch in time saves nine" and "prevention is better than cure" are often considered clichés. Clichés or not, the rules of biology are incontrovertible, inescapable, and unforgiving, rail as we may against them. Prevention is better than cure in biology—always.

The reduction in the number of cells in an organ that occurs during periods of suboptimal growth includes a reduction in the number of blood vessels that grow into the smaller organ. This reduction in blood vessel number may be one of the most fundamental ways in which suboptimal conditions at critical periods of life adversely program an individual. The absence of an adequate blood supply fundamentally impairs that organ's ability to increase its workload at times of challenge. Correct and adequate function of all organs depends not only on the specialized enzyme- or hormone-producing cells they contain but also on the blood supply that brings oxygen, nutrients and instructional molecules, such as other controlling hormones and growth factors, to the growing organ. Normal function both before and after birth also depends on the nerves that enter the developing organs to alter function at times of changing need. There is evidence that exposure to alcohol during the first weeks of embryonic life will decrease the number of nerve fibers in the optic nerve and permanently impair vision. Supporting structures around the organ are also critical to its normal development. For example, normal development of the lung depends on correct development of the chest cage. Unless the muscle of the diaphragm and the ribs and muscles of the chest wall develop properly, the baby's lungs will not develop to their maximum capacity. If the correct arrangement of all the vital functional components of critical systems is not achieved in an orderly fashion during fetal life, it is understandable how the individual can be programmed for health problems later in life.

Nutritional deprivation in the period before and immediately after birth markedly alters life span in male rats. Prenatal nutritional deprivation shortens the life of rats, whereas postnatal deprivation can increase longevity. What is more remarkable is that when rats who are growth retarded as a result of poor nutrition before birth are fed well immediately after birth to encourage catch-up, they have a reduced life span. This observation is both fascinating and extremely worrying. It shows how little we know about the consequences of growth retardation and what to do to improve the outcome of babies who are growth retarded.

Cell Death Is as Important to Normal Development as Cell Growth

Many cells don't make it to birth but are programmed to die during development. Cell death is an important part of normal growth during development in the womb. This apparent paradox may seem surprising, but from the very earliest stages of embryonic development, some cells are dying, their roles completed. The dead cells make way for other cells to take over their location and supersede their function. This programmed death of cells is not random and does not occur because of adverse conditions. Cell death is a vital part of the overall genetic blueprint. The programmed death of cells is called *apoptosis*. Apoptosis is a natural process and should be distinguished from the traumatic premature death, or necrosis, of cells that results from oxygen lack, nutrient deficiency or damage to vital cell machinery by toxic chemicals. Under the microscope, cell death due to apoptosis looks very different from cell death due to necrosis.

During apoptosis, specialized genes are switched on to bring about the cell's own destruction in a carefully programmed way. During programmed cell death, these suicidal genes get to work within the cell and instruct the cell to produce enzymes that cut up the cell's DNA, making it impossible for that cell to carry out its vital functions. The cell destroys its own blueprint for life, its own intracellular recipe for how to get things done. In contrast, death by necrosis is not due to a self-determined set of intracellular processes that result in failure of the cell to continue living. Necrosis of cells is due to some unwanted influence in the cell's environment. Apoptosis can be seen as ritual suicide, while necrosis is essentially murder by outside influences. Cells undergoing apoptosis may die because they have received instructions from other cells to terminate their own existence. In this scenario, these administrator cells have apparently passed a sentence of redundancy on the doomed cells. The regulation of the switch in cell function that brings about apoptosis is poorly understood. Learning more about this regulatory switch that starts apoptosis and the mechanisms that control it may well improve our understanding of cancer.

Death of cells by apoptosis at precisely programmed stages of fetal development is critical for the remodeling of tissues to perform new functions after birth. The intestine is a good example. The lining cells of the intestine have no digestive function before birth. After birth, digestion and absorption of food is critical to the newborn baby's survival. In the first few days of newborn life, the digestive tract undergoes marked changes in the lining cells that produce the enzymes that digest food. Remodeling also makes it possible for the body to perform old functions under new conditions. For example, after birth, the large arteries in the body are subjected to a sudden increase in pressure compared with the pressure in the vessels before birth. The walls of these arteries have to be remodeled to withstand this change. During these growth and remodeling phases, many cells come to the programmed end of their useful lives. One major reason apoptosis occurs is to allow other cells with different characteristics and capabilities to move in and take over space and hence change the form and function of the tissue or organ. As a result of death by apoptosis of one cell type with a specific function, other cells already in an organ will be left to carry on their functions unopposed. The changes in form and function that accompany the remodeling of tissues as they develop and grow have very important long-term consequences.

Prenatal Growth Is Important for Lifetime Health

The concept that unfavorable conditions in the environment to which the fetus is exposed during prenatal life may permanently alter the functional capabilities of the baby can be very clearly demonstrated if we look at the effects of iodine deficiency during fetal life. In certain mountainous areas of the world, the drinking water does not contain enough iodine. Iodine is an essential component of the hormone thyroxine. Thyroxine plays a critical role in the function of nearly every cell in the body. Under the influence of thyroxine, the rate at which cells function speeds up.

If thyroxine availability is insufficient in adult life, cells gradually slow down their level of function. The slowdown often occurs over many years, and may be almost imperceptible to people who see the affected person on a daily basis. The almost imperceptible development of the effects of low thyroid activity can be illustrated by the apocryphal story of the blacksmith who was the prize pitcher of the local baseball team. Year after year, he would dismiss visiting teams with hardly a hit, so fast was his fast ball, so cunning his curve and slider. But then, almost imperceptibly, his dominance began to fade. One year he lost a game or two. The next year he lost a few more. Then, over the next two or three years, his record slowly deteriorated until he was no longer the same force to be reckoned with, even though he was still young. Eventually, the blacksmith sought medical advice and was diagnosed as suffering from a deficiency of thyroxine production by his thyroid gland. Thyroxine deficiency had slowed him down, gradually ruining his statistics. Once his physician had realized this, thyroxine treatment had him again retiring opponents one after the other without a hit.

As with many features of fetal life, the effects of iodine deficiency during development have the potential to be much more damaging than iodine deficiency that starts during adult life because unless recognized and treated immediately after birth, the deficits that occur before birth are irreversible. When the fetus is short of thyroxine as a result of iodine deficiency, many tissues, especially brain and bone, do not develop properly. If the iodine deficiency continues during the early years of life, the baby will begin to show the classical features of cretinism. Most of the abnormalities of cretinism can be prevented by giving the newborn baby supplementary thyroxine immediately after birth. However, some developmental deficiencies may persist. The window during which this treatment is capable of reversing the deficiency is only a matter of days. Because of the danger of permanent, irreversible damage, all babies in the developed world are screened at birth for iodine deficiency. If they need thyroxine, they are treated immediately. The long-term effects of thyroxine insufficiency during fetal life are good reminders of the two critical features of programming: the existence of critical windows of vulnerability and the permanence of many of the unwanted consequences of suboptimal conditions in our home in the womb.

Cancer: Another Word for Excessive Growth

Cancer is not a single disease. It is best considered as a process that occurs when cells suddenly begin uncontrolled growth. There are many forms of cancer. The origins of cancer must be sought tumor type by tumor type. There are certainly some underlying cellular processes by which cancer is caused, and the rapid advance in knowledge of how cells function is providing valuable information of the cell growth cycle. However, the cause of melanoma will certainly be different from smoking-induced lung cancer or leukemia or breast cancer. However, despite the differences, the basic problem in any form of cancer is that growth has become excessive.

Could cells be programmed in the womb to unnatural rates of division and a greater tendency to cancer later in life? Several recent epidemiological studies do suggest that prenatal programming can increase susceptibility to some forms of cancer. A study published from Harvard in 1997 reported findings from nurses that showed that prenatal influences may increase the risk of breast cancer. Over 2,000 nurses born between 1921 and 1965 were included in the report. Women who weighed around 5.5 pounds at birth had approximately half the risk of breast cancer compared with women who weighed just under nine pounds. The investigators allowed for the usual risk factors associated with breast cancer, especially a family history.

The processes responsible for the greater tendency to breast cancer in larger female babies is unknown. However, high levels of estrogen in the mother's blood may be involved. Estrogen plays a key role during pregnancy by regulating blood flow to the uterus. High uterine blood flow would deliver more nutrients to the fetus and is thus likely to be associated with an increased fetal growth rate. So the high birthweight of women at risk may just be a marker for exposure to a higher level of estrogen at critical times in development. Breast cancer can be induced in developing female rats by exposing them to cancer producing compounds during fetal development. It is also of interest that the lower birthweight of Asian women matches their lower incidence of breast cancer.

When searching for the mechanism that might result in prenatal determination of an increased risk of cancer, it is of interest that high birthweight has also been linked with other forms of cancer that are likely to be regulated by hormones. Thus, cancer of the prostate has also been linked to increased birthweight. In a related fashion, cancer of the ovary has been linked with rapid growth in early life and an early onset of menstruation, suggesting that the setting of the hormone controls that regulate female reproduction have been advanced and possibly are working at a higher level.

In summary, it is clear that prenatal growth is critical to health throughout life. It is important to focus on health rather than disease. We need to relentlessly pursue knowledge of what makes for healthy, optimal prenatal development. To do so, we must investigate unfavorable, suboptimal climates, but the ultimate goal must be a better understanding of what is necessary for a baby to grow to her or his full potential before birth and enjoy the best health possible throughout life.

SIX

PRENATAL SETTING OF STRESS LEVELS

Pain is inevitable, stress is optional.

Life after birth is full of challenging and stressful situations. Similarly, life before birth provides its own challenges to the developing fetus. Fortunately, we are equipped with tried-and-true mechanisms to respond to stressful conditions in the environment before, as well as after, birth. These stress responses enable us to maintain our biological integrity. So that we do not confuse the challenge and the response, the challenging situations in the world around us are best referred to as stressors. It is our bodies' responses that produce the stress within us.

The brain-pituitary-adrenal system is a major player in the body's stress responses. One of the secretions of the adrenal gland, the hormone cortisol, mobilizes reserves to respond to external and internal challenges. Cortisol also affects the performance of our heart and blood vessels. At all times of life, too much cortisol secreted by the adrenal gland is just as harmful as too little. Steroids endanger cells that are exposed to other challenges such as oxygen deficiency.

The hormone changes a mother uses to respond to protein deficiency during pregnancy are similar to those that occur in nonnutritional stress situations. When cortisol levels rise in a pregnant woman as a result of various stressors in her life, cortisol passes across the placenta to the fetus. Studies in sheep, rats and monkeys—as well as humans—show that the placenta does its best to protect the fetus by inactivating the cortisol as it crosses the placenta. However, this protection by the placenta is limited. If maternal cortisol crosses the placenta in excessive amounts, the level of activity of the fetal brain-pituitary-adrenal system can be reset for life.

Prenatal resetting of the baby's brain-pituitary-adrenal system may play a role in programming conditions such as chronic depression and other alterations of mood in later life. The fundamental bodily twenty-four-hour rhythms that govern life are also altered when the fetus is exposed to high adrenal steroid levels before birth. Environmental influences postnatally, particularly maternal behavior and exposure to infection, are also able to program the level of activity of the baby's brain-pituitary-adrenal system.

The possibility arises that mothers with high adrenal steroid levels during pregnancy will alter the setting of the pituitary adrenal system in their daughters and hence set up transgenerational transmission of the adrenal hyperactivity in a fashion similar to the nongenetic transgenerational passage of a tendency to diabetes that occurs in the diabetic rat.

THE BRAIN'S STRESS PATHWAY

Most people have their own idea of what they mean when they talk about stress. It is unfortunate that the word has two related but different meanings. It is used to describe the multitude of external and internal influences that exert unwanted and abnormal effects on our bodies. The same word is also used to describe the body's response to these powerful challenges to a quiet, undisturbed life.

Often, the external stresses that impact the body are normal environmental influences. What makes the situations stressful is the exposure to an excessive amount of conditions that are quite normal in a lesser degree. We all react adversely to too much heat, too much cold, too much food, too much noise. In order to understand how stress impacts our lives, we need to distinguish clearly the external events that happen to us (which I will call *stress stimuli*) from the responses that occur within our bodies (which I will call *stress responses*). It is when stress responses are exaggerated that they can be harmful to the body. The stress response can be an increase in blood pressure, nervousness, mood changes, abnormal eating behavior, or lack of sleep. It is the stress response or reaction, not the original stress stimuli, that can do damage to our life and even shorten it.

It is difficult to differentiate cause (the stress stimulus) from our bodies' response (stress response) if we use the word *stress* for both the external event and the internal one. A well-known medical dictionary defines stress as "the sum of the biological *reactions* to any adverse stimulus, physical, mental or emotional, internal or external, that tends to disturb the organism's homeostasis [a scientific term for balance or equilibrium]; should these compensating reactions be inadequate or inappropriate, they may lead to disorders." In this case, stress is the body's responses to exaggerated external or internal stressful influences that produce the disturbed bodily responses. Yet most people use the word *stress* to refer to the external influences themselves. We talk of being under the stress of a death in the family, the loss of our job or failing an exam. None of these stress stimuli take place within our bodies. However, any marked stress stimulus does tend to produce a stress response within the body. Because of the confusion, the same medical dictionary goes on to carefully cover itself by saying, "The term [stress] is also used to refer to the stimuli that elicit the reactions." I will use the term *stress stimulus* to describe the event acting on the body and to distinguish it from the *stress response*, the body's attempt to cope with the stress stimulus. This is a very necessary distinction, since the bodies of different individuals clearly have different stress responses to the same stress stimuli. Evidence is accumulating that these stress responses are programmed in large measure by prenatal events.

Stress responses are the mechanisms that evolution has provided to enable us to escape from danger or to cope with the challenge provided by the stress stimulus. The danger may be a predator in whose presence we should mobilize all available resources to flee or fight to ensure our survival. In a situation where flight is necessary for survival and our muscles must carry us away as fast as they can, we mobilize fat. Fat is an excellent source of fuel that can be mobilized rapidly. At the same time, glucose is discharged into the blood from the liver stores. The beating of our heart is geared up a notch to pump more blood around the body, to provide more oxygen to the muscles (to fight or flee) and to the brain. These responses served our ancestors well in the primitive jungle. Unfortunately, our current lifestyles do not generally result in such a physical response to the stress. Now, instead of responding to the stress stimulus by running away and burning up the glucose and fat that our bodies mobilize expressly for that purpose, we stay in the same place, often fuming over the stressful situation but not dissipating our stress response in a burst of physical activity. The fat we have mobilized as a stress response hangs around and circulates in the blood and is redeposited, often not in the best of places.

Unfortunately, as in so many instances of modern life, our bodies respond and function inappropriately. In many ways, the biology of our bodies is no longer completely in tune with our surroundings. We have changed our environment faster than our bodies have changed their responses: the city in which we live is markedly different from the jungle and the prairie, but our biology is still firmly rooted in the past. It is not so easy to make rapid changes in biological responses that were vital to our survival in a different era.

The major system in the body that responds to stress stimuli is the brain-pituitary-adrenal system. A wide variety of sensory inputs to the brain, such as the sight of a predator, noise from the environment, or the acrid smells of a forest fire enter the brain via the eyes, ears and nose. These sensory stimuli produce changes in endocrine activity, energy usage and brain function via a very old part of the brain, the hypothalamus. Lying just beneath the hypothalamus at the base of the brain is the pituitary gland, a major regulator of our stress responses. As a result of its proximity to the brain, the pituitary can receive instructions directly and rapidly. The pituitary regulates the secretion of cortisol from the adrenal gland by itself secreting a hormone that travels around the bloodstream until it

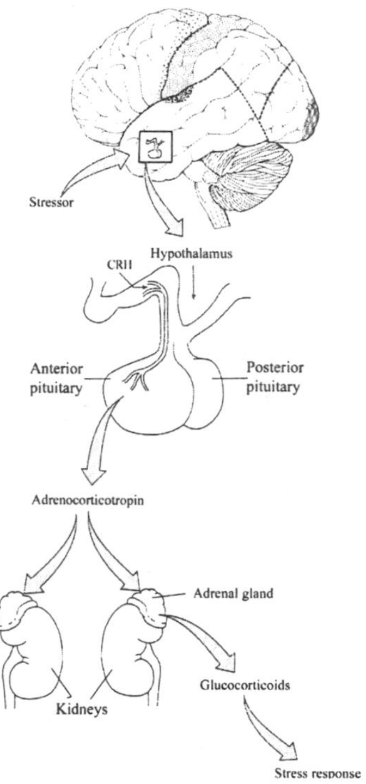

FIGURE 6.1

The pituitary-adrenal stress axis.

arrives at the adrenal gland. This hormone, adrenocorticotropin (ACTH for short) stimulates the adrenal gland to pour cortisol out into the blood. Once in the blood, cortisol has a multitude of actions. One of them is to act on the liver to release glucose, vital to rapid exercise; another is to release fat from the fat stores. The brain controls the amount of ACTH secreted by producing a hormone, corticotropin releasing hormone (CRH). CRH production is controlled within the hypothalamus in response to messages from many parts of the brain. One of the most important higher regulatory centers that controls the level of activity of this system is the hippocampus.

The Placenta Protects the Baby from Maternal Stress

Cortisol is a steroid hormone, one of a group of the glucocorticoid family of steroid hormones. The steroid group of hormones includes several hormones with a similar structure including the sex hormones estradiol and testosterone. Glucocorticoids have a wide range of actions in adults. They act on the brain, liver, fat tissues, blood vessels, kidneys and the immune system—almost every cell in the body in one way or another. Cortisol acts, like other steroids, by binding to a receptor on the cells whose actions it changes. After binding the cortisol molecule, the receptor carries the hormone molecule to the nucleus of the cell. Inside the nucleus, the complex formed by cortisol and the receptor attaches to the specific genes cortisol influences in response to the stressful situation. Cortisol then tells these selected genes to increase or decrease their activity. The usual effect is an increase or decrease of the production of critical enzymes. Enzymes regulate the rate at which various activities occur in a cell. They speed up or slow down the target cell's production line. In rats, the glucocorticoid produced is corticosterone, a steroid molecule very similar in structure to cortisol.

In the developing baby, Glucocorticoids play key roles in regulating the maturation of the lungs, liver, kidneys, immune system and many other body systems that will be critical for independent life in the world outside the womb. Fetuses need Glucocorticoids for normal maturation and produce most of their needs from their own adrenal glands. This is fortunate since the placenta has an enzyme that inactivates most of the mother's cortisol that tries to cross the placenta. Thus the fetus is protected from rapid increases in cortisol in the mother's blood when she responds to stress stimuli in her surroundings.

Unfortunately, the protection conferred by the placenta is not complete. If a pregnant rat is exposed to an excessive amount of stressful stimulation, her adrenal glands begin to secrete more and more corticosterone. In this situation, enough steroid may get through the placenta to produce permanent effects on the fetus. Small placentas or placentas that are not functioning properly may be deficient in the enzyme that destroys the corticosterone as it tries to pass from mother to fetus. As a result, more corticosterone than normal crosses the placenta from mother to fetus. Anything that interferes with the formation of a normal placenta early in pregnancy will potentially leave the baby at risk should the mother be exposed to stress later in pregnancy.

Unfortunately, many of the adverse, suboptimal factors in the mother's health that lead to inadequate growth of the placenta are also likely to be stressful stimuli. Babies of stressed mothers with poorly functioning placentas will be in double danger—danger from increased amounts of cortisol in mother's blood and as well as exposure to increased cortisol crossing from mother as a result of the decreased ability of the placenta to protect them by inactivating cortisol. In this type of situation, when the placental protective mechanisms against stress hormones are weakened, it will be even more critical to ensure that the mother is not stressed and the baby put at increased risk. The protective mechanisms that have evolved over the centuries are adequate for normal pregnancy. It is when the mother is subjected to an overwhelming set of adverse circumstances—poor nutrition, constant financial worry, physical abuse, drugs, alcohol, and other extreme circumstances—that the placental barrier may prove inadequate.

Several experimental studies with pregnant rats show that the fetus may pay a long-term price for exposure to excessive amounts of corticosterone during critical periods of development in the uterus. The best examples of this long-term price are the effects of excessive corticosterone exposure during fetal life on the developing brain. There are also pronounced effects of too much corticosterone on the developing heart and blood system. These effects on the brain and circulation in response to high levels of corticosterone coming across the placenta from the mother throughout pregnancy are certainly not beneficial for the individual when the quality of lifetime health is evaluated.

Steroids Endanger Cells, Enhancing Dangerous Responses to Other Stressful Stimuli

The level of activity of the brain-pituitary-adrenal system determines how much cortisol circulates in the blood at any time, both at rest and when we are responding to stressful situations. It is important that our bodies are not exposed to too much or too little cortisol for any extended time. Both too much and too little cortisol have adverse effects on our health. Too little cortisol results in weakness and inability to mobilize energy in times when we need a good stress response. Too much cortisol results in ulceration in the gut, weak bones, greater susceptibility to disease and death of nerve cells.

Too much cortisol in the blood is not by itself usually lethal to cells, but it does make them less able to survive risks. Cells exposed to high levels of cortisol cannot easily survive other risks such as low levels of oxygen or deficient supplies of energy. While the dangers of the combined effects of too much cortisol and various natural challenges are very real for adult animals, they are even more threatening for the fetus. If the placenta begins to fail in its task of transporting oxygen and glucose, fetuses respond by secreting more cortisol. Studies in sheep have shown that in the last fifth of pregnancy, the fetal lamb is very capable of secreting cortisol in response to a wide variety of stressful situations such as shortage of glucose or low oxygen in the blood. Both of these situations occur if the placenta is not functioning properly. A poorly functioning placenta will also allow more cortisol to pass from mother to fetus. The extra cortisol coming across the placenta from the mother will add its effect to the extra cortisol secreted by the fetus. Bad news for the fetus indeed. For cells already short of glucose and oxygen, exposure to high levels of cortisol from the mother in addition to increased production by the fetus's own adrenal gland constitutes a triple whammy. As a result, trouble may occur that will have continued repercussions throughout life. In the presence of too much cortisol, we are more susceptible to "the thousand heartaches and the natural shocks the flesh is heir to," as Hamlet might say.

The extra sensitivity to damaging stimuli following exposure to high cortisol levels has been termed *endangerment* by Dr. Robert Sapolsky from Stanford University and others working in the field of long-term effects of adrenal steroids on the brain. The causes and effects of endangerment have been extensively investigated in adult rats. Following excessively stressful situations, degenerative changes occur within as short a period as three weeks. Several studies in adult rats have shown that continual exposure to stressful conditions results in rapid aging and premature death. Excessive amounts of corticosterone circulating in the blood of rats has been associated particularly with accelerated aging of the hippocampus, the part of the brain that is responsible, among other things, for our memory stores. In contrast, if lifelong exposure to corticosterone is reduced, animals live longer and age more slowly. There is clearly a biological basis for the long life enjoyed by happy, relatively unambitious individuals who lead a relaxed life, taking things as they come. I am impressed by the longevity of many accomplished musicians. Vladimir Horowitz is an example, playing the piano so beautifully well into his eighties. Performing may have been an effort, a veritable tour de force, but these individuals find true joy and relaxation in what they do, though to those of us not wrapped up in the activity, it seems very stressful. Pain may be inevitable, but for some, it seems that stress is optional.

Each of Us Has a Different Response to Stress

We all know people who appear calm and collected under almost any circumstance. Stress certainly appears to be optional to them, or at least controllable to a level they can tolerate. Perhaps we can learn something from a bizarre and somewhat gruesome story I read in a British newspaper at the time of the fall of the shah of Iran. One of the shah's generals was interviewed by a western reporter the night before the general was to be executed by the new fundamentalist regime of Ayatollah Khomeini. The shah had flown off to the comfort of his several personal havens in the West, determined to avoid the same fate. Left behind were the less fortunate henchmen who had carried out his orders: the generals and other members of Savak, the shah's secret service.

The ayatollah had taken over. The generals and the leaders of Savak were rapidly rounded up and summarily sentenced to death. The reporter enquired about the general's views on the new developments, the changes in power. The general simply replied, "Things change, don't they?" If the general was stressed by his impending execution, he was not prepared to show it.

Few of us could exhibit this outward degree of calm. The world is mostly populated by more volatile people. Most humans have less equanimity and are more prone to stress responses of rage and fear. It is more common to come across people who have a very short fuse and high anxiety levels than the outwardly calm and collected general of my somewhat macabre story. We need to know the underlying mechanisms that lead stressed individuals to shoot other motorists on the freeway in road rage. It is important to discover the extent to which, and the mechanisms by which, the antecedents of aggression are laid down before birth. Another mood extreme is excessive anxiety. We all know people who always irrationally fear the worst. Another variant of the overanxious personality type is the brooding, quiet individual who says little but worries continuously. For them, the most pessimistic outcome is always the most likely. A friend of mine once coined the word *pessimal* as an opposite for *optimal.* We all know people who are unshakably convinced that, for them, the pessimal outcome will surely be the outcome that will happen in every situation.

Altered Stress Responses in Adult Life Following Prenatal Exposure to Stress Hormones Passing from the Mother Across the Placenta

What are the causes for these differences in mood and anxiety? Clearly, there are genetic influences. However, recent studies by several groups of researchers in a variety of laboratories throughout the world have shown that exposure to excessively stressful situations either by the mother prenatally or by the mother and newborn will permanently alter the level of activity of critical components of the stress axis in the offspring. The activity of the baby's stress axis will be programmed for life. This information comes from studies in both rats and monkeys.

In one study, pregnant rats were exposed to restraint stress each day during the last week of their twenty-one day pregnancy. The amount of corticosterone in the mother's blood was raised three times a day by placing her in a transparent plastic cylinder that restricted her movement. Being placed in the tube was a stress stimulus because she could not leave it and could not turn around. This stress stimulus was repeated three times a day between fourteen days of pregnancy and the day of delivery. The mother's adrenal glands were removed in a second group of pregnant rats so that she could not secrete corticosterone when she was exposed to the same stressful situation. Rats who were not placed in the restraint tube at all were studied for comparison.

To find out whether the stress responses of the fetuses in the womb were altered by exposure of their mothers to stress situations during pregnancy, the pups delivered by the mothers were allowed to grow up. At ninety days of age (when they are young adults) the investigators tested responses of the young rats to the same restraint stress that their mothers had been exposed to when pregnant. Young male rats whose mothers had intact adrenal glands and were thus able to secrete corticosterone when they were stressed during pregnancy had a greater response to their own stressful restraint experience than either young rats who had been born to mothers who had not been stressed or rats born to mothers who had not been able to respond to the stress of restraint because their adrenal glands had been removed. Something permanent had happened to the stress axis in the pups of the intact, stressed mothers. The remarkable fact was that there was a permanent increase in the stress response in the rat who had been a baby in the womb at the time of the mother's stress exposure.

How does the increase in the level of corticosterone in the mother's blood permanently alter fetal development? The level of ACTH secretion by the pituitary is controlled by the feedback of corticosterone that has already been secreted and is circulating in the blood. This is a typical negative feedback system like the thermostat in a home heating system. The higher the concentration of steroid already in the blood, the less activity in the axis. This makes sense. If a rat already has enough corticosterone circulating in the blood, it does not need to secrete any more for a while. But when is it enough? That depends on the level at which the feedback has been set.

In the study on the effect of maternal restraint stress during pregnancy, the number of corticosterone receptors was reduced in the brain of the pups delivered by mothers who had been stressed in the last week of pregnancy compared with rats born to mothers who were not stressed. This finding explains why the pups of the stressed mothers secrete more corticosterone in response to their own stressful experience later in life. A similar situation, if it exists in humans, might explain why the levels of cortisol circulating in the blood are chronically elevated above normal in some individuals with mood disorders. Individuals with damped feedback secrete more cortisol under stressful conditions than individuals with normal amounts of the receptors in the brain that monitor cortisol in the blood and set the level of the whole system.

There may be several other problems that lie in wait for the rats who were exposed to high levels of adrenal steroids while they were fetuses. Although there is little currently available evidence to prove a transgenerational effect of high steroid levels in the mother during pregnancy, we can immediately see some parallels with the transgenerational passage of diabetes described in chapter 4. Experimental studies have shown that rats who were exposed to high levels of corticosterone while they were fetuses have elevated blood pressure in later life. It is both fascinating and worrying that the developing cardiovascular system can be programmed for life in this way. In the next chapter, we will examine the link between maternal stress, increased exposure to adrenal steroids before birth and the programming of high blood pressure.

There are many reasons why maternal adrenal hormones may be abnormally high during pregnancy. These include mental stress, physical stress and nutritional stress. Feeding rats low-protein diets results in elevated plasma corticosterone levels in both mother and fetus. In this situation, some key enzymes that are regulated by adrenal steroids are increased in the placenta and fetal brain. In chapter 7, we will examine the effects of low-protein diet during pregnancy in programming blood pressure. It is clear that adrenal steroids may play a role in altering function of several key systems.

Altered Stress Responses in Adult Life Following Exposure to Stress Hormones in the Period Soon after Birth

The brain-pituitary-adrenal system is part of the body's rapid reaction force. Its purpose is to protect all the organs in our body against a variety of insults throughout our lives from the womb to the tomb. The highly variable responses of the system to different situations are made even more fascinating by the differences that can be demonstrated between individuals. There are differences in responses between the sexes as well as in the same individual at different times of reproductive and developmental life. In addition, it is clear that genetic influences are pervasive.

We have seen that prenatal exposure to Glucocorticoids alters the set point of a rat's adrenal stress response axis for life. In the 1950s, Seymour Levine was the first to show that early postnatal experience also programs the responsiveness of rats to stress in later life. Levine showed that early handling of rats, even for just a few days, permanently altered the animal's response to stress in later life. Since those classical early studies were conducted, an overwhelming body of evidence has built up to support the concept that early life experiences, especially maternal care, can alter the set point of the brain-pituitary-adrenal stress axis. Early handling will increase the number of receptors for adrenal steroids in the hippocampus of the rat. This is the opposite effect to the effect of increased steroids before life. As a result, the stress axis is set at a lower level. When newborn rat pups are handled and returned to the nest, the presence of odors on the pups stimulates their mother to lick and groom them more often. To show that maternal licking and grooming behavior is a key in programming, Dr. Michael Meaney and his colleagues compared the number of receptors in the hippocampus of rats whose mothers pay different amounts of attention to their pups. The more licking and grooming the mother performs, the lower the level of activity at which the stress axis in the pups is set for later life. It is fascinating that the effects of maternal licking and grooming can be reproduced by stroking the newborn rat with a paintbrush. There is much to learn, if humans are equally tactile individuals.

The observations made on the lifelong effects of increased maternal care are supported by the opposite situation, maternal deprivation in the newborn period. Dr. Charles Nemeroff at Emory University showed that isolation of rat pups from their mothers for six hours a day from day two to day twenty of newborn life resulted in increased steroid secretion in response to stress in later life. The human correlate would be that the more attention, love and care received in the days immediately after birth, the less stressed the individual will be in later life in any given environment. Of course, even someone with a stress axis set at a low level will respond vigorously to very stressful situations, so the differences are relative.

Depression, Mood Disorders and Developmental Setting of the Stress System

In order to see whether there are parallels between rats and other species, Dr. Nemeroff has studied the effects of maternal stress on young monkeys. Information from studies in nonhuman primates is essential to enable us to extrapolate to the human condition. Charles Nemeroff compared three groups of monkeys and their young babies. The young monkeys in the first group were reared in conditions in which there was plenty of good food available for their mothers. As a result, the mothers did not need to exert too much energy and mental effort in foraging. A second group of mothers had to work hard to find adequate food. This high-foraging group was working at gathering food all the time. A third maternal group had a constantly changing availability of food, a very insecure situation that is difficult to adjust to. The infants of the mothers who had constantly to change their behavior were highly stressed. Their mothers were obsessed with every aspect of the process of finding food. The babies became pathologically shy when put in mixed social groups. Measurement of hormones in the brain-pituitary-adrenal stress system showed that the levels were the same in the babies of the high- and low-foraging groups but were elevated in the variable foraging group.

The overall conclusions from maternal deprivation and maternal stress studies in the prenatal and postnatal period fits the concept that interactions between the mother's biology and the baby's biology both before and after delivery are important to normal growth and development. That seems a very trite statement. However, experimental studies are now exposing the specific mechanisms responsible in the brain and other organs. The developing brain responds to outside stimuli and reaches down within itself to modify function of specific nerve cells in its own structure. At the present time, it is uncertain which of these changes are compensatory, which are protective, and which are signs of damage. Some alterations may just represent a loss of the normal sequence of organization. Exactly which gene functions are permanently altered, and how, remains to be elucidated, but clearly there are changes in receptors in key areas that alter the set level of feedback.

Depression is one of the major causes of the 32,000 suicides that take place in the United States every year, the origins of depression are as important to society as the cause of automobile accidents. Certainly, the impact of psychiatric illness on the functions of individuals and families is enormous. There is considerable evidence that the level of setting of the brain-pituitary-adrenal system is abnormal in depressed individuals. Depressed patients have a higher cortisol concentration in their blood throughout the day and their daily rhythms of cortisol are blunted. When individuals get better either spontaneously or as a result of treatment, their plasma cortisol levels decrease. High blood cortisol may only be a marker of the state of depression, not necessarily the cause. However, we have seen that chronically elevated cortisol can damage the brain and lead to premature aging.

The rise and fall of cortisol production throughout the twenty-four-hour day is one of the most fundamental biological rhythms of our bodies. This twenty-four-hour rhythm represents the response of our brain's internal clock to the world around us. Deep within our brains, each of us has our own private timepiece. We each have an independent clock that cycles by itself. To show that our internal clock cycles continuously, even in the absence of clues about day and night from the outside world, researchers have spent months in caves or isolated laboratories where they had no clues on the existence of day and night. This deep-seated brain clock is called our circadian clock because it has a cycle of about one day.

Whether you are a morning or an evening person can greatly affect your character. Many people do not like to be sociable early in the morning. In the mornings, their personal internal clock makes them feel moody and withdrawn. The same people may well be the very life and soul of the party later in the day, transformed from who they are in the early hours. If you have a child, friend or spouse who is a true early bird, you are well advised to make allowances for their different rhythms. I am told that there is a regiment in the British army that recognizes this individual idiosyncrasy by giving soldiers the option to talk or remain silent at breakfast. In this regiment, if one prefers to be left alone until later in the day, one wears a hat at breakfast. People do not talk to someone who wears a hat at breakfast.

Our circadian rhythms are characteristic expressions of our relationship to the world around us. They are driven and organized by a multitude of outside clues. The major clue is the dark-light cycle. The alternating phases of darkness and daylight, moonlight, and sunlight as the world moves around the sun make sure that the whole of society keeps to somewhat the same routine. Although in a constant environment, you and I may have cycle lengths that differ by up to an hour, in real life our brain responds to the changing seasons, and our sleep-wakefulness cycle and our cortisol cycle track the outside world. Thus the inherent cycle length of our brain clock is overridden, and we can keep in tune with each other and the world about us. Since the combined daylight and nighttime periods of only two days in the year are precisely twenty-four hours long, we need to constantly adjust our body cycles as the days change. If we don't do this, we will have jet lag all the time.

Careful regulation of daily activities in relation to day and night can be a matter of life and death for animals in their natural habitat. If animals cannot adjust their activities to the constantly changing world around them, they might arrive at the watering hole at the same time as their predators rather than at other, safer times of the day. Having a freely adjustable clock that continuously changes allows us to make the necessary adjustment to the seasons. The sun sets four or five hours earlier in the winter than the summer. Between June 21 and December 21, our internal clocks make gradual bodily adjustments to this change in the world about us.

Levels of cortisol in the blood are highest early in the morning and decrease through the rest of the day only to rise again in the late hours of sleep. The basal levels of these rhythms and the extent of their rise and fall have an important role to play in our moods and behaviors. One study has shown that 60 to 65 percent of depressed patients have blunted cortisol rhythms. In addition, the average level of cortisol in their blood is elevated above the average for the whole population. If a patient suffers only intermittently from depression, the rhythms revert to a more normal form when depression is absent. It is important to look at the nature of these rhythms in greater detail.

Much more work needs to be done before these changes in steroid function in human depression can be linked to prenatal steroid exposure in the same way that similar changes have been demonstrated in rats and monkeys. In addition to needing knowledge on the mechanisms responsible for the increased steroid production, more information is needed on the consequences of this over activity on brain function and mood. It is abundantly clear that adrenal steroids, like anabolic sex steroids used by athletes to enhance their performance, are good for you at one level but very harmful in excessive quantities.

How does this new knowledge of programming of critical brain functions as a result of influences in early life play out in the context of nature and nurture, genetics and the environment? The structural framework of the brain is constructed like the rest of our bodies from a blueprint of genetic messages encoded in the germ cells. The division of the primitive cells that go to make the brain, their early journey around the brain as they move to their final resting place and their ability to respond to incoming signals by bursts of activity are all clearly properties that are coded for in the genes. In chapter 9, we will see that the genes carry the indispensable plans for the siring, wiring and firing of the brain. But as the rapidly progressing process of interactive serial changes during fetal development begins to gather pace, each event becomes dependent on the events that took place before. These prior changes help to create the environment in which subsequent changes occur. Every cell is dependent on local hormone concentrations, local cell-cell interactions and the availability of nutrients such as oxygen and glucose in the correct amounts. During fetal development, many of these critical ingredients are supplied entirely by the mother.

How do we incorporate this information on programming of brain function into concepts of free will and choice? How do these observations in rats and monkeys alter our views of individual responsibility? How do they help us to understand the consequences of our actions as human beings? A synthesis of the influences of nature and nurture in making us who we are is a deeply philosophical and ethical issue that only clearer information and a better understanding of available knowledge from behavioral biology and brain chemistry will provide. What is clear is that the prenatal and postnatal environments are major influences in the normal development of the brain. Did we really need to be told that? When a book that enjoyed as much popularity and acceptance as *The Bell Curve* can propose the extreme view that ability, especially the emotional and functional ability of the brain, is essentially determined by heredity and is not open to outside influence, we are forced to look hard at the evidence for genetic and environmental factors in programming intelligence and other brain functions. The studies I have described show that brain function and behavior are critically influenced, even permanently modified in major ways, by the environmental conditions that exist during development. How we think, reason and see are not just inherited characteristics. Brain function, behavior, mood, IQ and emotional stability are not solely a product of our genes. The way our brains function throughout life can be altered by the level of receptors that develop on critical brain cells as a result of pre- and postnatal environmental influences.

After birth, the body's stress responses to stressful situations may be processed differently by those who experienced a suboptimal intrauterine environment. Their mood and behavior may need a different type of education from those who have not experienced the same developmental history. This thesis has powerful support from both the epidemiological and the animal studies now coming to light.

One final word. If the tendency to diabetes can be passed on transgenerationally from mother to child, it is necessary to find out whether the resetting of the pituitary ACTH axis can be passed on across the generations through the daughters of mothers who themselves have an elevated level of adrenal steroid hormones in pregnancy. We had better pay attention to our biology, each and every one of us, if we wish to be better placed to determine how we can help our children and our children's children.

SEVEN

HEART DISEASE, OBESITY AND DIABETES

If you fail to prepare, you prepare to fail.

Heart disease and cancer are the two great killers of modern times. Over the last fifty years, research on the origins of heart disease has focused on four major factors that are thought to increase the incidence of heart disease: diet, smoking, exercise and a stressful lifestyle. New epidemiological, clinical and animal research studies have challenged these deeply ingrained notions. Together, these three approaches show that programming of our cardiovascular system by the environment in the womb in which we develop before birth may be the most important predisposing factor of all.

Suboptimal growth during fetal life and the early years of postnatal life raises the risk of high blood pressure and death from heart disease and stroke in later life. The harmful effects of poor prenatal development on blood pressure in adulthood can be observed as early as the first ten years of life. There are many determining factors, but the nutritional state of the mother during pregnancy appears to play a key role. This challenging concept of major prenatal causes of heart disease opens up important new areas of research that will guide prevention and treatment.

Nutritionally deprived fetuses slow their growth rate to match diminished resources that cross the placenta from the mother. This compensation by the fetus is a sensible adjustment to the suboptimal conditions in the uterus. A nutritionally deprived fetus who takes steps to lessen demands on the mother has been called a thrifty fetus. Thrifty fetuses learn to survive with less in the womb. Over the millenia of evolution, this thrifty approach has had survival value for human and animal fetuses born into an environment in which food supplies are restricted. In our modern era of conspicuous consumption, when they grow to be children and adults, thrifty fetuses are likely to be exposed to plentiful food supplies after mistakenly preparing their appetite and metabolic control mechanisms for a lifetime of thrift. When this mismatch happens, people tend to become obese and are more likely to suffer from diabetes. Babies who prepare in the womb for a thrifty existence after birth pay the price if they live a life of overconsumption in a situation in which food is plentiful. Prenatal adjustments that help the fetus cope with austerity before birth may be an incorrect and even fatal preparation for the food-laden riches of modern civilization after birth. This faulty preparation explains why the incidence of diabetes is higher in adults who had low birthweights and were thinner at birth.

Animal-based research studies have begun to clarify the mechanisms whereby suboptimal development before and immediately after birth leads to heart disease. In situations in which the fetus is short of oxygen or nutrients, the fetus protects the brain at the expense of other developing organs. Growth of the developing liver is particularly slowed. In addition, there may be an abnormal distribution throughout the liver of the mix of cell types that perform different functions. One of the major functions of the liver throughout our lives is to regulate the production and use of cholesterol and the factors that promote blood clotting. The liver also regulates the level of glucose that circulates in the blood. Abnormal liver development before birth can have lifetime consequences that result in high blood cholesterol levels leading to blocked-up arteries and an increased tendency to release glucose into the blood, thereby predisposing to diabetes. Both these situations will cause damage to blood vessels and increase the tendency to high blood pressure in adult life. Raised blood pressure is associated with an increased risk of death from cardiovascular disease in later life, both coronary heart disease and stroke.

Firm evidence for the linkage of heart disease to unfavorable conditions in the womb now comes from studies throughout the world, from Finland, India, the United States, South America, England and Sweden. What are the implications of these animal and epidemiological studies for human health? Should the knowledge that our cardiovascular health and diabetes are programmed in the womb lead to a feeling of fatalism, or can we take action to improve the future for ourselves and our children?

HEART DISEASE: THE GREAT SLAYER

"Forty million people in the United States suffer from diagnosed cardiovascular disease, and an even larger number don't yet know they have a heart problem. Sixty million people have high blood pressure. Eighty million people have elevated cholesterol levels. Over 1.5 million Americans have heart attacks every year. And for almost one third of them, having a heart attack was their first indication that they had a problem—clearly, not the best way to find out." So begins the first chapter of Dean Ornish's best-selling book, *Reversing Heart Disease.* This 631-page book is subtitled, *The Only System Scientifically Proven to Reverse Heart Disease Without Drugs or Surgery."* The understanding of the origins of heart disease and its relationship to our biology expressed in Ornish's book is a combination of the straitjacketed thinking of the medical community and the increasingly popular mix of biomedical science and unscientific New Age homilies. Recent human epidemiological research and related animal investigations, not mentioned anywhere in Ornish's book, indicate that, like research and treatment connected with cardiovascular disease, current efforts are essentially attempts to shut the stable door after the horse has bolted. However, Ornish's book has one overriding merit. It questions the value of the modern high-tech approach to treating heart disease and recommends a proactive preventive approach. With those sentiments I agree. We should try to focus away from high-tech drugs and surgical approaches. We spend far too much of our financial resources and mental energy on desperate efforts and heroic procedures to put right what we should avoid.

The ultimate way to deal with heart disease should be the avoidance of its root causes. The critical question in relation to the high incidence of heart disease in Western society is: What are the fundamental causes of heart disease? We need to identify the major causes and determine which, if any, are preventable.

It would be wrong to deny that our adult lifestyle plays a role in causing heart disease. Four major lifestyle issues merit attention: smoking, exercise, diet and stressful conditions in our lives. Smoking damages blood vessels. It also has a transgenerational effect. When young women take up smoking, they put their children as yet unborn at risk, even if they stop smoking when they are pregnant. Smoking damages all blood vessels, including those that will carry blood to the placenta during pregnancy. Decreased blood flow to the placenta will result in unfavorable conditions for the fetus. There is a growing trend in modern society for young people to take very little vigorous exercise as they pass increasingly sedentary lives in front of television and computer screens. Exercise improves the performance of our hearts, as well as making us feel better. In general, our exercise patterns are laid down during the early years of our lives. Much more effort needs to be made in helping children learn the habit of taking regular exercise for a lifetime. Dietary imbalance, especially the feeding frenzy on junk food, predisposes to heart disease. We can and should modify our eating patterns. Not a week passes without a new onslaught in the media about the rampant epidemic of obesity in the United States. We are told that anywhere between 40 and 60 percent of the population is overweight. Overarching all of the other considerations of this enormous health problem are the new ideas that the origins of both good cardiovascular health and heart disease are laid down in the womb. The recent evidence is compelling that unfavorable conditions in the womb increase the risk of developing high blood pressure, suffering from heart disease or having a stroke in later life. When should prevention start? Avoidance comes by taking measures earlier in life—in fact by paying attention to life before birth.

Epidemiological Studies That Link Heart Disease in Later Life to Prenatal Health

The history of the early epidemiologic ideas about programming of cardiovascular disease was examined in chapter 3. Excellent correlation was obtained between maps of the distribution of heart disease in the second half of the twentieth century to death of babies in the first month of life in the same regions of England half a century earlier. In these early observations, David Barker and his colleagues showed that death from heart disease was greatest in babies who were of low birthweight and who grew slowly over the first year of life. They traced nearly 8,000 baby boys born in the prosperous county of Hertfordshire just north of London between 1911 and 1930. Baby boys who weighed 18 pounds or less at one year of age had death rates from coronary artery disease later in life that were three times the death rate of babies who weighed 27 pounds or more. The group of people studied was generally poor, but most mothers had good diets during pregnancy. Over 90 percent of the babies were breast-fed, and analysis was restricted to the breast-fed babies to avoid the possible confounding effect of the different quality of nutrition in bottle-fed and breast-fed babies.

In another study linking low birthweight to cardiovascular disease, the body proportions of the babies at risk for coronary artery disease were very different from the babies at risk for stroke. One group of babies had a relatively normal head size but lowered birthweight. They showed no evidence that the placenta had tried to compensate for any lack of nutrients. This suggests that their growth was normal as they developed early in pregnancy when, as we have seen, there is a tendency for the placenta to try to compensate. However, later in pregnancy, when the demands on the mother are greater during the period of fastest fetal growth, it seems that their mothers were unable to supply these babies with enough nutrition. In contrast, babies at risk for coronary heart disease had smaller heads and were thin and short. Of particular interest was the finding that they had a higher placental to birthweight ratio, suggesting that there had been an attempt by the placenta to compensate by growing larger early in these pregnancies. The reason why these babies were growth retarded was less clear.

The researchers who made these observations include an interesting quote from the 1884 edition of the *Encyclopedia Britannica* connecting maternal socioeconomic conditions with placental growth: "The building of the placenta by the mother and the performance and function of that wonderful organ require certain favoring conditions.

These are certainly not to be found in factory labor." The investigators conclude their article with some historic comments and a remarkable conclusion. They suggest that the improvement of social conditions and maternal nutrition in the first part of this century has led to a decrease in the occurrence of stroke, which has fallen in the last fifty years. During this time, the incidence of coronary heart disease has risen and fallen. The differences in the pattern of incidence of these two forms of cardiovascular disease may provide clues to their cause and management. The researchers suggest that the form of growth retardation that leads to a higher incidence of stroke in later life is due to a failure of the placenta to grow to its full size, perhaps because the mother's uterus was reduced in size during her own development. Small birthweight is also more common in those who will eventually suffer from heart disease, but in these individuals, the cause does not seem to be a reduction in size of the placenta. Quite the opposite, there are indications that the placenta tried to compensate for some other mechanisms that resulted in less oxygen and nutrients getting to the fetus. In this second group of small babies, the size of the mother's uterus does not seem to be the problem. Instead, it is likely that, although the womb is adequate, there are now some adverse factors in the environment (perhaps smoking, junk food, and stress) that prevent the baby from growing to the full potential.

The adverse impact of suboptimal fetal development on cardiovascular health in later life is rapidly being shown to be a universal human biological characteristic applicable to all cultures and ethnic groups. A recent small study of adults at one hospital in Mysore in India found a strikingly similar result to the English report mentioned above. The incidence of cardiac disease in a relatively small group of adults studied in Mysore showed that babies who were small had the highest incidence of coronary artery disease. The effects were greatest if the mother was small and undernourished.

The association of low birthweight and high blood pressure in later life has been shown in countries all over the world. The research group at Harvard has studied both male and female health professionals. In one study on a group of women health professionals followed up from 1976 until 1997 they conclude, "Data provide strong evidence of an association between birthweight and adult coronary heart disease and stroke." The same group concluded from studies on males that "men with low birthweight were at significantly higher risk for hypertension [high blood pressure] . . . we conclude that early life exposures affecting birthweight may be important in the development of hypertension . . . in adults." Another study of 3,302 men born in Helsinki during 1924 to 1933 showed that those who had low weight at birth were at increased risk of developing heart disease. Like the people studied in Mysore, India, the effect was enhanced when the mothers were of small stature. A Swedish study concludes, "A failure to realize growth potential in utero . . . is associated with raised adult blood pressure." Similar conclusions have been drawn from a study in Chile. Bringing all these studies together, we have agreement from Finland, India, the United States, South America, England and Sweden.

The concept that intrauterine conditions program the development of the cardiovascular system has been called the *Barker hypothesis* after Dr. David Barker. All scientific discovery begins as a hypothesis when certain observations suggest a causal connection between two events such as the idea that the fetal brain sends out signals to start the birth process or that diabetes is due to a lack of insulin from the pancreas. The next stage is to undertake carefully controlled studies that change just one factor in the situation and see whether the system changes in a way that could be predicted by the hypothesis. Finding the predicted results does not prove the truth of the hypothesis, it just shows that the hypothesis is compatible with the observed facts. Technically, it is never possible to directly prove that a specific hypothesis is completely true. Even if the observations produced in clinical or laboratory research are compatible with a hypothesis, they may be the result of another similar but different mechanism that produces the same end result. It is impossible to say that there is definitely no other explanation. In contrast, if the observations do not support the hypothesis, we can conclude with certainty that the hypothesis is definitely *not* true. Because of this difficulty in proving that a process definitely works in a given way, experiments are always set up to reject the hypothesis. It may seem strange to someone not versed in the scientific method that researchers must design their experiments to reject the ideas they put forward. However, when experiment after experiment yield's information that is compatible with their proposed hypothesis, investigators can begin to be confident that the system works in the way they think it does.

There are many pieces of epidemiologic evidence that support the view that socioeconomic factors in early life play a key role in the origin of heart disease. One recent study showed a correlation between heart disease and the social class of the father. The father's social class is closely correlated with both the prenatal conditions and early life conditions in which a child develops. This study concludes with the statement, "Childhood socioeconomic status may be a persisting influence on ischemic heart disease risk in adult life." This and many other epidemiologic studies now point to important prenatal and childhood factors that predispose to heart disease in later life. While postnatal events have been considered important for many years, the new concept embodied in the Barker hypothesis is that preparation prenatally is probably even more critical than development after birth.

Critical Phases in Development of the Heart

Because the blood vessels are the waterways along which vital materials will be passed around the developing embryo, the anatomical beginnings of the blood system can be seen very early in embryonic life, at a time when the embryo is just a small ball of cells. At this stage of development, oxygen, glucose and other nutrients can reach every cell in the spherical embryo simply by diffusion. As the embryo grows, the distances become too great for diffusion alone to supply the embryo's needs. The blood distribution system develops to pass oxygen, energy-providing molecules and cell- building materials around the fetus. The embryo's heart and blood vessels begin to form by the fourth week in the womb. This very early start to development of the heart and blood vessels exposes the rapidly growing components of the blood system to any problems of lack of oxygen and nutrients that may be present. Every part of the developing blood system is extremely vulnerable to the insult of suboptimal conditions at critical times. Blood vessels are proliferating at a great rate in these early weeks. Cells are dividing rapidly as new arteries and veins branch off already-formed vessels. This exposes the whole system to the increased susceptibility to damage characteristic of rapidly growing cells.

Correct preparation of the blood vessels that will supply each organ of the body has a lifetime impact on the function of that organ. We have seen that problems with development of the blood supply to the developing pancreas may set the pancreas up to fail in later life. Failure of the pancreas to get enough blood to deal with the challenges of closely regulating the amount of glucose in the blood may lead to diabetes in later life. This is particularly likely if the poorly prepared pancreas is severely challenged by an abnormally high dietary intake of carbohydrates day after day, year after year, after birth. More potato chips anyone? The same considerations very likely apply to blood vessels all over the body, including the coronary arteries that grow into the heart muscle itself at early stages of development. These coronary blood vessels will prove vital later in life at times of increased demands on the heart. At such times, the heart must pump more blood to its own muscle cells to provide them with adequate oxygen and nourishment to perform the extra workload. It is vital to future cardiac health that an adequate number of those conducting channels for the blood to flow along are laid down correctly to start with. This is as true for the heart as for other organs. The wide-ranging harmful consequences of suboptimal development of the heart and blood vessels on organs such as the pancreas shows the functional interdependence of all the organs. What started off as a simple problem of too few blood vessels may end up as diabetes or heart disease in the adult forty years later. Remember, the heart beats 100,000 times a day, nearly a million times a week.

In addition to direct effects on the growth of blood vessels, some abnormal prenatal preparations for life after birth predispose to conditions that secondarily damage the cardiovascular system. Such indirect factors that may eventually give rise to heart disease are diabetes and obesity. However, as happens so often in life, when conditions are suboptimal and things go wrong, they go wrong in multiple ways. It is likely that the same poor diets during pregnancy that produce abnormal blood vessels in the pancreas also impair normal growth of the vessels in the brain and other parts of the body. As a result, if diabetes strikes in later life, the cardiovascular system is already in a worse position to cope.

When considering the consequences of suboptimal fetal nutrition, it is important to realize that the problem does not just involve malnutrition of the extreme starvation type that occurred during the Dutch Hunger Winter. Mild to moderate malnutrition may also play a part in programming the quality of health for a lifetime. The emphasis of current research on effects of maternal nutrition during pregnancy on fetal development is moving—as it should—from the effects of extremely abnormal diets to the consequences of marginal deficiency. It is important to obtain a clear idea of fetal needs throughout pregnancy and to evaluate how the mother can best provide them.

The Placental Connection

The quality and quantity of the diet a mother eats during pregnancy alters the size of her placenta. As we have already seen, fetal growth is regulated by the growth of the placenta. In general, the larger the placenta, the larger the baby. This is true unless the increase in placental size was an attempt by the baby to compensate for suboptimal conditions. Placental size is altered by the balance of different food—protein and carbohydrates, particularly—in the mother's diet.

The placenta also plays a critical role in transporting oxygen to the fetus. Fetuses that do not get enough oxygen make a dramatic choice. They preferentially distribute more of their blood to their brain and heart, depriving the liver, muscles and fat. At the same time, regulated by compensatory mechanisms that are not yet known, the placenta enlarges to help the baby get more oxygen. If a baby has a large placenta in relation to body size, that is a clear indication that something was amiss in the womb, and the fetus did not grow to his or her full potential. Concerns about a large placenta in relation to the size of the baby may seem somewhat counterintuitive. One would have thought that a relatively large placenta would have been good for the fetus. However, a placenta that is larger than it should have been is often a sign that precious resources were assigned to growing the placenta and not to fetal growth because of a scarcity of essential nutrients and oxygen.

The placenta acts as a protective barrier across which it is difficult for foreign molecules to pass to the fetus. The protection is provided by several mechanisms. First, the transport capabilities and diffusion resistance of the placenta do not allow large foreign molecules to pass from mother to fetus. In addition, there are enzymes in the placenta that inactivate many types of chemicals, both natural and synthetic, as they try to cross. We have seen in chapters 4 and 6 how the placenta inactivates the highly active adrenal hormone cortisol. If this conversion is impaired, maternal cortisol gains access to the fetal blood in greater than normal quantities. Studies were described in chapter 6 that showed that in this situation, cortisol itself alters the number of its own receptors in parts of the developing fetal brain. As a result, the activity of the brain-pituitary-adrenal system is altered permanently. This resetting of the stress controls is an important example of long-term programming that may be involved in depression and other mood alterations.

Administration of cortisol directly to fetal sheep or corticosterone (the equivalent steroid in rats) to pregnant rats produces high blood pressure. In fetal sheep it can be shown that the cortisol and related synthetic steroids actually cause constriction of some of the peripheral blood vessels, helping to raise the fetal blood pressure. Fetal rats and sheep exposed to excessive amounts of adrenal steroids during life before birth have raised blood pressure in adult life. Several studies have also shown that rats whose mothers ate a low-protein diet, during pregnancy develop high blood pressure in early adult life. When rats are fed a low-protein diet, they grow a small placenta. As a result, the ability of the placenta to stop corticosterone from crossing from mother to fetus is impaired. Consequently, the fetus is exposed to abnormally high amounts of corticosterone at critical times of development of the heart and blood vessels and the pups have high blood pressure when they grow up.

Corticosterone may play a major role in the programming of high blood pressure in the pups of pregnant rats fed a low-protein diet. These growth-retarded pups have the same type of asymmetric-growth retardation that is seen in the human babies who are of low birthweight and tend to have high blood pressure in later life. The investigations in rats have shown that the enzymes in several fetal as well as placental cells show clear effects of exposure to excessive levels of corticosterone. So the placenta performs a key function as a mechanism to protect the fetus against abnormally high amounts of cortisol. It is very important for a fetus to grow a good placenta. Even the early phases of pregnancy are very important in the origins of health and disease.

How You Set Your Blood Pressure

Critical functions of the body are regulated within a narrow optimal range by feedback loops that work in a way that is similar to the thermostat in a home hot water system. The mechanisms that control body temperature also work on the feedback principle. In the hot summer sun, you increase the activity of your sweat glands to lose heat. You also try to be as inactive as possible to decrease the amount of heat produced by your muscles. In contrast, when exposed to cold winter winds, you shut down the blood supply to the skin to decrease the amount of heat that can be lost because your skin is at a higher temperature than the world around you. These regulatory changes are controlled by nerve reflexes. The sense organs in the periphery tell the brain what the temperature is and the brain then sends out signals to the sweat glands and blood vessels, appropriately modifying their level of activity.

Regulation of blood pressure depends on feedback systems that oppose any tendency of the blood pressure to fall too low or rise too high. These feedback systems contain sensors that monitor the existing blood pressure and inform the brain of the present level. The information goes to central brain controller mechanisms for analysis. The brain then sends out instructions to make the changes necessary to keep the blood pressure within normal limits.

The sensors that measure blood pressure in the body are placed right at the center of the system in the large blood vessels that leave the heart, the aorta and the carotid arteries. At these locations, they are able to monitor the blood pressure at which the blood is provided to the brain (through the carotid arteries) and the heart (through the coronary arteries). This is a very appropriate place to measure blood pressure. When the blood pressure rises, nerve impulses flash up the nerves from the pressure sensors to specialized areas of the brain that control blood pressure. The brain evaluates the information that comes in via these special sensory nerves and integrates the information with many other pieces of information coming in from other areas involved in controlling the cardiovascular system. This integration is important because body temperature, the working of the kidneys and the pumping action of the lungs all greatly affect how much blood is available and how it is coursing around the body. If the pressure is too low, not enough blood will get to the tissues all over the body. If blood pressure is too high, there is the likelihood that the heart will fail to push enough blood out against the load (as when the heart muscle itself does not get enough blood and an angina attack occurs) or that a vessel will rupture (as in a stroke).

The human body's ability to regulate blood pressure within fine limits depends on the ability to increase or decrease the volume of blood pumped into the network of blood vessels as well as the degree of constriction of the vessels into which the blood is being pumped, the resistance of the system. The amount of blood pumped depends on both the force of each beat and the number of beats per minute. Thus there are many options and the whole system is fine-tuned to need, minute by minute. For example, blood pressure falls when you are sleeping. This makes sense because the demands of the body are low during sleep.

The setting of the whole system will determine whether, at any given blood pressure, the central control systems decide that the pressure is higher or lower than it should be. One major theory that attempts to explain programming suggests that the set point of the central mechanism that controls blood pressure is programmed by prenatal events such as suboptimal nutrition. This idea is not at all far-fetched. We have already seen how hormones can permanently reset the controls of the stress system by altering the level of receptors in the brain. Research is now ongoing to determine whether exposure to excess amounts of steroid before birth results in setting of the system to work at higher blood pressures.

Maternal Health, Small Livers, High Cholesterol and Abnormal Blood Clotting

Heart attacks are caused by the development of plaques in the smaller coronary arteries as a result of damage to the lining of the vessels. This damage is often due to increased amounts of cholesterol in the artery wall. A major factor in the progression of the disease is the deposition of fibrin on these plaques to form a blood clot. The clot narrows the coronary arteries even further and the amount of blood supplying the heart muscle becomes inadequate. At best, this deficiency gives rise to pain in the chest on exercise. This pain is called angina. At worst, there may be a sudden fall in blood flow so marked that the oxygen-deprived heart muscle beats irregularly, making it impossible for the heart to pump blood effectively and smoothly around the body. If this happens, death follows rapidly unless the poorly coordinated muscle function can be reorganized by shocking the heart with a defibrillator.

Fibrinogen is one of the major clotting factors that circulate in the blood, ready to plug up any leaks in blood vessels. Levels of fibrinogen in the blood directly determine the size of the blood clot that forms once the clotting process starts anywhere in the body. Fibrinogen is formed in the liver. The liver also plays a major role in controlling the amount of cholesterol in the blood. Fibrinogen levels in the blood are as closely associated with coronary artery disease as blood cholesterol, yet it is cholesterol that has received all the attention. Old ideas have a great tendency to dominate thinking.

Smoking increases blood fibrinogen levels. High fibrinogen in the blood is likely one of the ways smoking causes heart disease.

However, the harmful effect of smoking can be separated from adverse effects of other lifestyles on the levels of fibrinogen in the blood. The epidemiologists in Southampton showed that the level of fibrinogen in the blood of men between the ages of fifty-nine and seventy was very closely related to their weight at one year of age. Men who weighed 18 pounds or less at one year of age were compared with men who weighed more than 27 pounds at the same age. Men who had grown slowly up to one year of age had a significantly higher blood fibrinogen level in their seventh decade of life. The increase in fibrinogen levels in the men who had been lighter babies was equivalent to a 40 percent higher risk of death from heart disease.

It is also possible to relate blood fibrinogen levels in adult life to birthweight, but only when the weight of the placenta is taken into account. Baby boys who have relatively large placentas for their birthweight have high fibrinogen levels at age fifty. As we have seen repeatedly, a large placenta relative to birthweight is a sign that the baby has developed in a suboptimal world in the womb and tried to compensate by growing a larger placenta. Much further research needs to be done in both humans and animals before we understand just how the suboptimal world in the womb alters fibrinogen and cholesterol production by the liver throughout later life.

However, it is already very clear that fetal and early infant life both program production of these two important factors that determine susceptibility to heart disease. Protein deprivation during pregnancy in the rat results in marked changes in the structure of the fetal liver. The liver is divided into hundreds of little lobules fed by blood vessels that enter at the outside of the lobule and pass to the center. In fetal life, the blood from the placenta also drains to the outside of the liver lobule. The blood washes along columns of cells as it flows to the center of the lobule where the blood drains away in a large vein. Under an ordinary microscope all the cells look very much alike, but they are very different functionally. Lobule cells perform very different functions according to their precise location in the lobule. At the edge of the lobule where the blood enters, the enzymes in the cells are geared to producing glucose and secreting it into the blood. In the center, the main function of the cells is to store glucose. Compared with adult rats whose mothers received a normal protein diet, livers of adult rats whose mothers had been fed a protein-deficient but adequate-calorie diet during development are programmed to release more glucose than they store. Even the gross structure of the liver is different in the two groups. In adult rats who have been protein deprived as fetuses, the total weight of the liver is the same as in normal adults, but there are only half as many liver lobules. The whole structure of the lobules and their relationship to each other is permanently programmed by exposure to a low-protein diet as fetuses. Observations such as these show how maternal nutrition can alter the function of the liver in ways that lead to deficiencies in how the body handles glucose. Poor preparation leads to diabetes and abnormal function of the heart and blood vessels in later life.

It has often been said that you are what you eat. Perhaps this truism should be changed, at least in part, to you are what your mother ate. Rats whose mothers are fed a high-fat diet during pregnancy and the period in which the pups suckle show a decreased ability to deal with the cholesterol in a high-fat diet when they themselves reach puberty. This occurs even when the rats are fed a normal diet from the time they are weaned until challenged with a fat diet later in life. We can conclude that the activity of genes that regulate how the body deals with cholesterol can be permanently modified by the fat in the mother's diets.

Proper function of the mother's heart and circulation is indispensable for the correct development of the fetal cardiovascular system. This is a very important heart-to-heart relationship. Yet again we see the specter of transgenerational issues. When the mother did not grow a good heart and blood vessels in her own life before birth, then she will have a more difficult job supplying her own babies adequately in their life before birth.

However hard your heart pumps, the ability to deliver oxygen to all the cells in your body depends on the amount of hemoglobin in the blood. To make good red blood cells with adequate hemoglobin, we need iron, protein, glucose for energy and a slew of vitamins. Good maternal nutrition is vital in pregnancy. One study using records from five countries clearly connected maternal anemia with an enlarged placenta. Placental volume is increased as early as the eighteenth week of pregnancy when the mother is anemic. The increased placental size is a clear indication that the fetus is trying to compensate for suboptimal conditions that occur when the mother is anemic. In a study published in 1991, it has been shown that the effects of maternal anemia have pronounced effects on the blood pressure of children as early as four years after birth. This is an arresting observation. If further studies confirm this observation, it lends weighty support to the view that our cardiovascular function is programmed to a marked extent before birth.

Each one of us is unique in the way we respond to poor nutrition, stress and the lack of exercise, the triad of predisposing factors to heart disease. For a fourth, add smoking. The basis of these individual differences is being strenuously sought by geneticists. While in no way suggesting that genetic factors should be ignored, we need also to detail how the developmental program through which each of us passed in the womb has critically modified the way our heart muscle performs and our clotting factors are regulated throughout life. We cannot change the set of genes with which we are endowed, but we can change the environment in which the fetus develops and the baby grows up.

The immediate view that genes will always give us the answer is certainly the currently conceived wisdom. A recent article in the *New York Times* reports the views of Dr. Ralph Hegle from the University of Toronto in relation to the ability to detect those at risk for cardiac disease. "Dr. Hegle envisions a day, not too far in the future, when people are tested for a battery of genes when they are 18, a time when their cholesterol, blood pressure and weight may be normal, but when their genetic blueprint might point to particular risk from unexpected directions, like blood clotting, proteins or weight gain." Dr. Steve Humphries, the British Heart Foundation Professor of Vascular Genetics at University College in London, takes this view even further. He is directly quoted as saying, "A battery of eight or nine of these [genetic] tests would probably be able to give you something useful."

The whole rationale of high-tech, gene-based medicine is that a few tests in the laboratory can detect susceptibility to cardiovascular disease and hence catch it at an early, treatable stage. Early diagnosis of heart disease (or better still, a likelihood of suffering from it) would not only decrease the cost of treatment over the years but also allow the patient to lead a more normal life for longer and avoid a premature death. But the ultimate in prevention lies in the avoidance of the whole problem. To avoid the problem, we must first understand it. The view that there are major antenatal causes of heart disease is completely compatible with ideas of genetic regulation of bodily function. The overwhelming weight of epidemiological evidence, animal-based research and clinical knowledge points to the central role of developmental programming in determining whether we enjoy good—or suffer from bad—cardiovascular health throughout life. We should never forget the old saying, "A good start is half the battle."

DIABETES: THE THRIFTY GENOTYPE AND THE THRIFTY PHENOTYPE

Diabetes occurs when there is not enough insulin in the blood. Insulin deficiency may occur because the pancreas has failed and is not producing enough insulin or in situations such as obesity, when the activity of insulin is blocked by other compounds in the blood such as fats. In these situations, not enough glucose enters the muscle's and other cells to maintain their normal activity. Insulin also plays a central role in the uptake of amino acids into cells, thereby providing cells with the key building blocks needed to make proteins and grow. Not surprisingly, as we saw in chapter 5, insulin is also a major growth hormone in the fetus.

There are two very different forms of diabetes. About 10 percent of diabetics have insulin-dependent diabetes mellitus (IDDM, pronounced id-em). This is the dramatic onset form of the disease that occurs in young people, generally before thirty years of age. Untreated IDDM can result in death within a matter of weeks. IDDM is an autoimmune disease, which means a disease in which the body produces antibodies that recklessly destroy cells in the individual's own body. In this case, the antibodies damage the cells in the pancreas that produce insulin. The tendency to produce antibodies that destroy the pancreas runs in families and is very likely under genetic control. The only treatment for IDDM is to administer insulin directly to the patient by injection. Insulin- dependent diabetics must take insulin, usually by injection, every day of their lives.

In contrast to IDDM, the inheritance of the second form of diabetes, noninsulin-dependent diabetes (NIDDM, pronounced nid-em) has been hotly debated. NIDDM is by far the commoner form of diabetes, accounting for roughly 90 percent of diabetics. To date, no firm genetic markers have been detected for NIDDM, and the jury is still out as to whether this type of diabetes is a genetic or an environmentally induced condition. Probably both genes and the environment are involved. If we are to have a better understanding of these conditions, we must look for the relative contributions of genes and environment, nature and nurture.

NIDDM occurs in some human populations at a much higher incidence than others. The Pima Indians of Arizona and northern Mexico have one of the highest incidences of NIDDM of any ethnic group. About 30 to 40 percent of the adult Pima population is affected in some areas. A similar high incidence of NIDDM occurs among inhabitants of the Pacific islands of Nauru. As always, this ethnic or family distribution raises the immediate response from some observers that the cause of NIDDM must be genetic. However, we must never forget that family and ethnic groups living closely together are also an environmental group in which nurture can have similar impacts on many, even all, individuals within the group.

Those who favor the genetic origin of NIDDM have proposed a very fascinating theory that NIDDM is caused by selection of a particular set of genes in ethnic groups of people exposed to repeated periods of food shortage. This is *the thrifty genotype* theory. According to the thrifty genotype theory, at times in human evolutionary history when nutrition was poor, selective advantage was conferred on the inheritance of genes that regulated mechanisms that decrease energy usage and nutrient need. The thrifty genotype theory fits modern post-Darwinian concepts, which consider that evolutionary survival is due to transgenerational passage of genes that are better adapted to the existing environment. Those who favor a genetic origin point to studies that show that when one twin of a pair of identical twins develops NIDDM, there is a very high likelihood that the other twin will do so, too. When both twins have a condition they are said to be concordant for the condition. If only one twin is affected, the pair is said to be discordant. When one identical twin suffers from NIDDM, normal incidence of the disease would suggest that the other twin would have the disease in less than 10 percent of cases. In one study, the concordance rate for diabetes in identical twins was found to be 58 percent, or nearly six times as high as would be expected if there were no genetic tendency. This connection between twins has lead some authorities to conclude that since identical twins have an identical genetic makeup, therefore NIDDM must be genetically determined. This simple mistake in thinking is made time and time again by the media and by many researchers. We must never forget that identical twins also share a very similar intrauterine environment, often even sharing the same placenta. It is not only their genes they hold in common. Identical twins also have lower birthweights than babies who have the womb all to themselves. This observation suggests that their environment in the womb is not as good when the womb is shared as when one baby has sole occupancy. It may be a little premature to put everything down to genes.

Another recent Danish study provided strong evidence to suggest that NIDDM, even in identical twins, is more related to impaired growth before birth than it is to the genes. When twins were discordant for diabetes, only one having the disease, the twin with the diabetes was much more likely to have had the lower birthweights—by 270 grams (0.61 pounds). This significant but remarkably small difference brings to mind the similar small decrease in weight in the babies born to mothers pregnant during the Dutch Hunger Winter—approximately 250 grams (0.55 pounds). Both the Dutch babies and the smaller identical twins have a higher incidence of diabetes in adult life than occurs in the general population. So identical twin studies can actually be used to separate genetic factors from environmental factors in the womb.

One further argument can be used against a purely genetic cause of NIDDM. In some areas of the world where a rapid change has taken place from a rural to a urban environment, often from a relatively subsistence level of nutrition to times of greater affluence, there is a marked increase in the incidence of NIDDM. One classic example is the great increase in NIDDM after the arrival in industrialized Israel of Ethiopian Jews born in a low-nutrition-level peasant economy in Ethiopia. These changes have taken place far to quickly to be accounted for by a change in genetic distribution of the populations involved. In addition, NIDDM is more frequently associated with diabetes in the mother than in the father. This does suggest that maternal environmental factors operating during pregnancy are likely to play a role.

A solely genetic origin of NIDDM does not seem to fit the bill, so some researchers have suggested that adverse and suboptimal conditions in the womb result in the development of a *thrifty phenotype*. The thrifty phenotype theory proposes that in times of inadequate nutrition, fetuses develop a more economical way of regulating their energy needs. In times of food shortage, being thrifty in the womb has one immediate and one delayed advantage. First, the fetuses can use the precious resources at their disposal to protect the organs that are vital to survival in a suboptimal environment during life before birth. Secondly, after birth, this preparation will be useful for an environment in which nutritional resources will be limited. According to the thrifty phenotype theory, the deficient nutritional state of the mother and possibly the hormonal changes that accompany reduced nutrition during pregnancy program the fetus to be ready for a suboptimal nutritional environment after birth. Individuals who develop a thrifty metabolism in the womb will be better conditioned to survive harsh environments. They are likely to have developed a hyperactive adrenal gland. Steroids from the adrenal gland play a large role in reacting to times of food shortage. The development of insulin resistance will also mean that there is some degree of protection from use of glucose by the muscle thereby saving existing glucose stores for the brain. At every opportunity during times of plenty, people who developed the thrifty phenotype store fat in their middle regions around the waist. These central stores of fat are the first we put on because they are the easiest to take off. As mentioned above, the problem comes when the fetus grows in a suboptimal environment in the womb, develops a metabolism adjusted to be appropriate for periods of low nutritional intake and then as an adult is presented with abundant food throughout life. This mismatch of preparation imposed by suboptimal conditions in the uterus and postnatal plenty can result in obesity and an increase in NIDDM.

The Pima Indians and the inhabitants of Nauru Ocean can give us some clues to both the thrifty phenotype and the cause of these areas in the world with a high incidence of NIDDM. The island of Nauru is not very well endowed with natural resources, and food supply has often been at a premium. This was particularly so during the Japanese occupation in the Second World War. After the war, Australian and American companies moved in to mine the vast quantities of fertilizer on the island. Suddenly Nauru was affluent. Islanders who had been used to low nutritional levels were suddenly able to buy and eat whatever and however much they wanted. But prosperity appears to have come at a price. As many a 30 percent of the population became diabetic. Why? The answer may lie with the work of Nicholas Hales and David Barker who showed that men who develop NIDDM tended to have been of low birthweight.

According to the theory proposed by Hales and Barker, babies who were born before the boom in prosperity that resulted from mining the fertilizer had developed a thrifty phenotype to cope with the suboptimal nutrition to which they were exposed in the womb. But then, after birth, came food in plenty, and not always food of the best sort. Feasting instead of fasting, the islanders became obese and the obesity led, as it generally does, to the inability of the pancreas to cope. As a result, the incidence of diabetes among the islanders rose steeply. A similar pattern of obesity is seen among the Pima Indians.

The incidence of NIDDM is now dropping in Nauru. This fascinating switchback rise and fall in the occurrence of NIDDM cannot be due to genetic mechanisms. The increase and decrease occurred too fast. The more likely explanation is that better nutrition of young women results in a better home in the womb for their children so that they do not need to develop a thrifty phenotype with the attendant increased risks of diabetes. Only time and more research will show whether this explanation is correct, but it does hold out hope that better nutrition in young women before and during pregnancy will help to reverse the unwanted trends of diabetes, as well as obesity and heart disease in modern times.

Several factors will affect the rate at which better maternal nutrition will reverse the epidemic of diabetes throughout the world and in places like Nauru, where it is highest of all. Perhaps the most interesting issue is the extent to which the studies of transgenerational passage of diabetes produced experimentally in pregnant rats will be reflected in transgenerational persistence of the condition in humans. Offsetting any gains from nutrition will be the tendency of high blood sugar in diabetic mothers to cross the placenta and cause damage in the developing pancreas of her baby. Fortunately, this tendency can be minimized by good management of the diabetes during pregnancy.

Much of the experimental work on the effects of maternal nutrition on the development of insulin sensitivity has been carried out in rats by Nicholas Hales at Cambridge University. In one study he showed that, compared with normally nourished rats, undernutrition of fetal rats before birth decreased their life span whereas undernutrition in the period of suckling increased the life span of the pups by the equivalent of twenty years for a human being aged sixty. When undernutrition occurred at both times, the effects canceled out. What was startling was that overfeeding of rat pups that had been deprived in the uterus was not only unable to recuperate the longevity, overfeeding further shortened their life span. These effects were only seen in males. These studies have major lessons for how we arrive at a better understanding of the causes and consequences of human growth retardation and define treatment procedures that enable the baby to catch up safely.

This thrifty approach to adverse prenatal conditions enables the baby to protect the developing brain. But as with all compensations, there is a price to pay. A take-home message from this book is pay now . . . or pay later. A thrifty approach to adverse conditions in the womb does enable the baby to survive suboptimal conditions in the womb and prepare for an environment in which food is not plentiful. These biological responses may have had enormous evolutionary value over many millennia. They may have been one of the major reasons for the success of our species. However, we have developed food production methods that allow for conspicuous consumption, rendering unnecessary the protective adaptations evolution achieved. Indeed, without intending to, we often fool the system. A baby that was disadvantaged prenatally but who subsequently grows up in an environment of plenty, particularly with an overabundance of the wrong sort of food, is ill prepared for the change. The cellular processes of such a baby will be confused. Being programmed in the uterus for a world of scarcity, she or he may not be able to cope with the confusion of a world of excess. In a sense, the world has duped the baby. The baby made extensive and appropriate adjustments before birth for poor nutrition and then was given good nutrition after birth. When one considers the personal, social, and economic consequences of diabetes and obesity, surely society must wake up to the importance of an increased understanding of our biological needs, from the cradle to the grave, the womb to the tomb. Anything else is shortsighted in the extreme. We cannot afford to bury our heads, ostrichlike, in the sands.

The epidemiological data on the lifelong effects of the prenatal nutritional environment on health and disease throughout life are overwhelming. But we do not need to rely on epidemiological data only. Again, let us remember the classic example given in chapter 1 of programming the sexual function of the brain to be cyclic (female) or not to be cyclic (male) by hormones at a critical period of brain development. There are many powerful studies in animals that show the importance of these systems and with further study will enable us to unravel the abnormal mechanisms that are operating. Once we understand the abnormal mechanisms, we will be able to develop strategies to avoid the conditions in future pregnancies. For those of us who have completed our own prenatal development, a deeper understanding of the mechanisms is also literally vital. We need to know how our own body functions were affected during our own prenatal development in order to live the sort of lives that will minimize and, if possible, reverse the adverse effects of the habits our bodies have adopted.

Obesity

We live in expansive times. Opportunities for all sorts of activities increase as a tribute to the inventiveness of our species. There seems to be no end to growth: financial, personal, intellectual. Our bodies seem to want to be in on the act, too. According to the precise definition of obesity, 50 percent or more of individuals in Western society are overweight. This is the modern battle of the bulge. Here again, the epidemiological data confirm the concept that prenatal life plays a key role in the ultimate shape of our bodies. The paradox is that it is the baby of low birthweight who is at risk of becoming obese. In the Dutch Hunger Winter, the lifetime effects of undernutrition of the mother differed according to the time at which the undernutrition occurred. We have seen that if the fetus is exposed to suboptimal conditions in the early part of pregnancy only, there is an increased tendency to obesity in later life. If the exposure to undernutrition was in the last third of pregnancy or the first few months of postnatal life, the tendency to obesity was decreased. This fascinating difference in outcome fits with our first rule of programming that there are critical periods at which different systems are adversely impacted. It seems as if undernutrition early in fetal life resets the centers in the brain that control appetite so that the affected individual has a greater tendency to overeat. This is in keeping with the thrifty phenotype concept. Why then should the babies who were undernourished late in fetal life have a decreased tendency to obesity? It is suggested that they have developed fewer fat cells because the insult came at a time when their fat cells were dividing rapidly. If you have fewer fat cells in your body, it is more difficult to become fat. However, there is something about this idea that smacks of wanting it two ways, and we must await further studies currently being carried out to determine the exact mechanisms. One thing is certain: obesity is not good for your health. Being overweight is associated with an increased risk of heart disease. The nurses health study in Boston, Massachusetts, concluded that the risk of death from cardiovascular disease was four times as high in the women who were at the extreme of the obesity scale. Cancer risk was increased twofold by obesity.

Fatalism or Activism?

Does the concept of intrauterine programming of health and disease of the cardiovascular system mean we must inevitably be fatalistic, accepting whatever cardiovascular deck of cards we were dealt before birth? On the contrary, there is much that can be done. We may not be completely in charge of our own personal destinies, but we do have an enormous potential to influence how we live and how we die. We are both the products of our lifestyles as well as the producers of those lifestyles. Although the history of our own intrauterine life is critical to the function of our vital organs, brain, liver, and pancreas, there is much that happens after birth that either improves our situation or makes it much worse. Nowhere is this message clearer than in how lifestyle affects our heart and blood vessels.

We began this chapter with the conventional wisdom that heart disease is caused by three major postnatal factors: poor diet, lack of exercise and environmental factors such as stressful situations and pollution (including smoking). It is not my intention to discredit the importance of these factors—far from it. All I wish to do is to show that these lifestyle factors play out against the consequences of the prenatal conditions to which the fetus was exposed during fetal development. Even a healthy cardiovascular system at birth needs to be treated with respect throughout life. Misguided and erroneous understanding of the cause of disease conditions can lead to improper, unnecessary therapies. No better example can be found in recent times than the dramatic change in understanding of the origins of stomach ulcers. When I was a medical student in the 1960s, surgeons firmly believed that stomach ulcers were caused by excessive secretion of acid in the stomach. Reaching for their scalpels, they removed large portions of the stomach, thereby decreasing the secretion of stomach acids. Almost everyone with a stomach ulcer experienced the surgeon's knife. It is now known that the major cause of stomach ulcers is a bacterium, *Helicobacter,* for which the best treatment is a course of antibiotics. Quite a change as a result of a better understanding of the condition. Certainly easier on the patient.

EIGHT

ENVIRONMENTAL INFLUENCES IN THE WOMB

*The fault, dear Brutus, is not in
our stars, but in ourselves.*

William Shakespeare, *Julius Caesar*

We are who we are not solely because of the genes we inherited but also because of the environment we inherited. Few would dispute that, after birth, our surroundings influence the course of our lives. Epidemiologic, clinical and animal research data on how our home in the womb affects our brain, heart and body shape shows that our earliest surroundings have a lifelong effect on who we become.

In the womb, all fetuses inevitably experience their mother's lifestyle: sounds that penetrate the abdomen, alcohol from binge drinking, nicotine and carbon monoxide from smoking, drugs of abuse, over-the-counter drugs, and exotic nutrients that pass across the placenta. Some lifestyles expose the fetus to multiple whammies. As the world becomes more concerned about the quality of the environment in which we live our lives after birth, we should also become attentive to the environment in which we as a species develop before birth.

Astrologers assert that the constellations in conjunction at our birth will control our lives. Strange as it may seem to the scientific mind, the season of the year during which we develop in the womb may indeed affect our growth and development before birth in ways that are critical to our lifetime health. The astrologer believes that the stars and planets and time of year of your birth guide your destiny. Whether the stars exert an influence or not, biological forces such as the amount of oxygen available during our fetal life and other environmental influences in the womb are powerful determinants of our destiny and the health we enjoy throughout life.

Even Clones Are Not the Same Because Their Prenatal Development Will Differ

Dolly, the cloned sheep, and now mice in Hawaii, have focused attention on the mechanisms that make each one of us unique. According to conventional dogma, all clones can be considered to be the same individual. Again we see the blinkered, determinist view of the gene dominant, which leaves little room for the equally critical effects of nurture. The intrinsic shortsightedness of gene myopia is to assume that clones will be identical in all aspects. Everyone appears to be asking the question, "What would you feel like to have one or more people identical to yourself walking around?"

Mammalian clones will not be identical in all respects when they grow up. Although their genes will be the same, the environment in the womb in which they develop will differ for each cloned individual. Aldous Huxley knew this intuitively. In *Brave New World* he describes a futuristic society in which sixty-four identical individuals are produced from a single egg by the process of Boskovskization. In Huxley's *Brave New World* there is no exposure of the fetus to the element of chance in intrauterine development, no possibility of effects of maternal hormones, no gentle squeezes from uterine contractures, no coffee, no nicotine or alcohol from mother's predilections. Huxley's futuristic clones are grown from fertilization to birth in carefully defined and controlled conditions of nutrients, light and temperature. If a less intelligent, more tractable group of individuals is required, a little alcohol is added to the medium.

Dr. Simon Walker in Adelaide, Australia, has shown that the effects of the environment on the fetus may begin very early. Treatment of pregnant ewes with progesterone on the first three days of pregnancy results in larger fetuses halfway through pregnancy. This increase in fetal weight occurs even if the embryos are transferred after the progesterone treatment to another ewe who was not treated with progesterone. To date, there is no adequate explanation for the cause of this memory effect of having been exposed to higher-than-normal levels of progesterone for just three days at the very beginning of embryonic life. The progesterone may well affect the mix of proteins and growth factors secreted by the lining of the uterus that then act on the embryo to increase its growth rate. Dr. Walker and his colleagues have put forward the idea that manipulations of the early embryo will alter the distribution of the early embryo's cells between cells that develop into the placenta and the cells that will become the fetus. As a result, following this type of manipulation, the size of the baby can be significantly modified. Whatever the mechanism, the effects on the embryo are marked.

Astrology: Do the Seasons Influence Us Even in the Womb?

"The fault . . . is in ourselves." This viewpoint is the ultimate credo of the Puritan ethic. But to what extent is it true? The eagerness and belief with which many people read the astrological notes relating to their birth sign suggests that they think their lives are not under their own control but rather controlled by their stars, the constellations that were in conjunction when they were born. Those who believe in astrology feel that much, if not all, of the happenings of their lives are predetermined and beyond their own control. According to the astrologer, the seasons of the year determine the mix of characteristics such as happiness, melancholy and stoicism that make up the personality of each individual. The astrologer charts your destiny in the stars that determine your enjoyment of good health throughout life. The scientist tends to consider the whole star-struck process as superstition and snorts, "Bah, humbug."

Scientists are trained to be skeptical of ideas that cannot be put to experimental test. One of the major requirements of scientific acceptance of any new and significant observation is that the observation is, at least in theory, open to methods that can reproduce it if true, or falsify it if indeed it is false. For many reasons, I tend to the "Bah humbug" view of the influence of the zodiac on life events and I do not read the astrology columns. However, many noted figures, not just Nancy Reagan, have been said to plan their lives according to the advice of a favorite astrologer. My skepticism arises from the following question: If you are inclined to believe in the predictions of astrologers, which astrologer should you choose? The comments of individual astrologers are often so different that I cannot but surmise that they work on the hope that, quite by chance, they will occasionally be dramatically correct about events such as a sudden superlative job offer or the arrival of a new lover. Astrologers hope that their faithful followers will remember only those predictions that bore some general relationship to what eventually occurred and will forget the countless times when none of their predictions came to pass. Astrologers play it safe. The generalities in which they deal give the perception of correct predictions. Let's take an example: "You will have an important development in your personal life." On reading this, the avid horoscope reader eagerly waits for something to happen in their world. But just what constitutes important? Just what is or isn't personal? And if we believe all of this, should parents plan the time of conception of their children so that the significant extraterrestrial forces of the sun, moon and planets will be in the right locations at birth, ready to provide the children with the best start in life?

Carl Sagan in *The Demon Haunted World* puts forward some valid criticisms of astrology. "Many valid criticisms of astrology can be formulated in a few sentences: for example, its acceptance of precession of the equinoxes in announcing an 'Age of Aquarius' and its rejection of precession of the equinoxes in casting horoscopes; its neglect of atmospheric refraction; its list of supposedly significant celestial objects that is mainly limited to naked eye objects known to Ptolemy in the second century, and that ignores an enormous variety of new astronomical objects discovered since (where is the astrology of near-Earth asteroids?); inconsistent requirements for detailed information on the time as compared to the latitude and longitude of birth; the failure of astrology to pass the identical-twin test; the major differences in horoscopes cast from the same birth information by different astrologers; and the absence of demonstrated correlation between horoscopes and such psychological tests as the Minnesota Multiphasic Personality Inventory."

Note again the reference by Sagan to the problem of identical twins. Should they have similar personalities and enjoy similar health because they have the same genes and lived in the same home in the womb? Or should they show differences because they invariably had different amounts of maternal blood available to their portion of the co-owned placenta? In a few instances, identical twin fetuses may actually share a few blood vessels between themselves. When they do share blood vessels, there may be a transfusion of blood from one fetus to the other. This transfer of blood from one twin to the other is called a twin-to-twin transfusion. If twin-to-twin transfusion occurs, the environment for each twin is very different. One twin will draw blood from the other. One twin is the donor, the other the recipient. Many of these abnormalities can be seen on the screen of the ultrasound machine. The ultrasound machine is far more accurate than astrological predictions in telling us about the complex interaction between twin babies and their mother.

My own disbelief in the power of the sun and moon to shape our lives was severely put to the test by some observations that we and others made on the production of the hormone prolactin by fetal sheep. Prolactin's best-known function is to promote lactation. However, prolactin also stimulates growth, particularly wool and hair growth. Since both males and females need to grow hair, it is not surprising that prolactin is present in the blood of both male and female fetuses.

In my laboratory at Cambridge University in the early 1970s, we examined blood samples from fetal sheep to determine if there was a change in the amount of prolactin present as the time of birth approached. We had a very sensitive measurement system that allowed us to measure the amount of prolactin down to one-billionth of a gram of prolactin in each liter of blood. To our surprise, we found that the concentration of prolactin in the blood of fetal sheep was

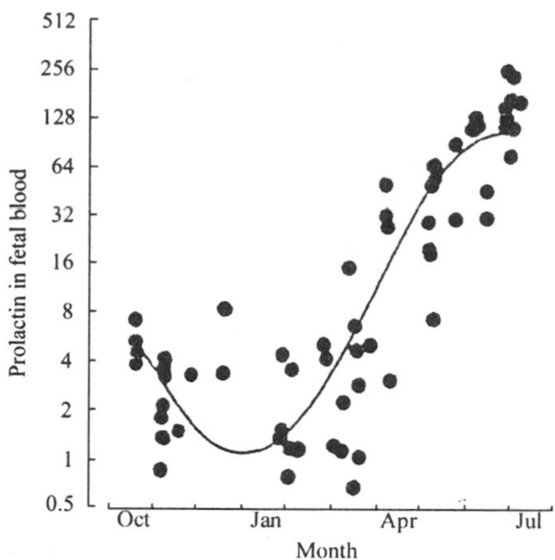

FIGURE 8.1

The changes in the concentration of prolactin in the blood of fetal sheep of few weeks before delivery at different times of the year.

extremely variable; the values were just scattered randomly over a very wide range from very low to very high. What astonished us was the finding that some fetuses had 200 units in each milliliter of blood while other fetuses at the same stage of development had as little as 1 unit. We were lost for an explanation of these enormous differences. We could find no obvious difference in the amount of prolactin in the blood of male and female fetuses. So the difference was not sex-related.

While we were puzzling over the reason for these wide differences between fetuses, two other research groups independently provided the answer. The amount of prolactin in the blood was high in fetal lambs that would be born at the beginning of the winter and low in fetal lambs that would be born in the spring. While this fascinating difference according to season does not change my views about the power of astrology, it does make me think of the differences in the signals received by the fetus destined to be born in the winter compared with the signals received by the fetus born in the spring. Clearly, it will benefit the winter lamb to be better prepared with a good growth of wool. The spring lamb does not need such a thick coat. But how on earth do fetal lambs in the womb know, before they are born, that they are going to be spring or winter lambs?

Melatonin was the wonder drug of the mid-1990s. The best- seller lists contained titles of books by respected physicians touting melatonin's ability to prevent jet lag, improve sex life, and make you live longer. According to these authors, you name it, melatonin does it. The drug stores had trouble keeping up with demand; shelves were cleaned out as soon as they were stocked. Only now are researchers sounding a note of caution regarding the variety of actions that melatonin may have on the body. But is anyone out there listening?

We are very ignorant about the function of melatonin in both the fetus and the adult. Melatonin is produced by the brain during the hours of darkness. In the winter, melatonin rises to higher concentrations in the blood each night than in the summer. The level also remains high for more hours in winter than in summer. Since melatonin crosses the placenta, the amount and the duration of time over which melatonin passes from mother to fetus give the fetus some clues as to the current length of the days and nights, and hence the season. Melatonin is one of several clocks the mother provides the fetus. The fetus can then make preparation for spring or winter according to whether the days are lengthening or shortening. This may be seen as an astrological signal, but I prefer to view it as yet another example of how closely mother and baby are linked together.

Melatonin is one of the factors that regulate the secretion of prolactin. In this way, the amount of prolactin in both mother's and baby's blood reflects the season of the year. Now we can see a little more clearly how the seasons will affect the woolly coat on the newborn lamb.

Consider these differences in the coat of the spring and winter lambs to be the result of the influence of the zodiac if you wish, but these observations leave unanswered the question: Does the season of our birth play a role in who we are and who we become? Given the present extent of our knowledge of developmental processes, all we can say at present is that we just do not know. In the words of Hamlet, Prince of Denmark, "There are more things in heaven and earth than are dreamt of in your philosophy, Horatio." But we can dream, and the knowledge we need is accumulating rapidly.

Tobacco: Our Children's Future Going up in Smoke

Big tobacco corporations and we, their customers and stockholders, continue to conduct a major assault on the bodies of the unborn. The tobacco industry is a corporate Houdini. Every new revelation on the powerful effects of tobacco products on the delicate machinery of the cells that make up our bodies seems to tie the giant tobacco industry up in webs of irrefutable information that clearly show the damage smokers do to themselves and those around them. But each time the great escape artists are able to turn the argument. They wiggle and wriggle out. Clever attorneys exploit the scientist's reluctance to be as dogmatic as the defenders of tobacco. Focusing on small difficulties researchers have in providing complete proof of the addictive properties of nicotine in cigarettes and the carcinogenic nature of tobacco smoke, the industry ignores the overwhelming power of the cumulative evidence. Like Houdini, the great escape artist, the tobacco industry repeatedly bursts free. The parallel is imperfect in one important regard. Houdini did no harm to others. He entertained and enthralled. Each time he escaped, he lived to enthral again. Each time the tobacco barons escape, they survive to continue killing and destroying the health of millions. The conscience of the tobacco barons, if it exists, does not care about the harm they do, even to children as yet unborn. If they did, they would immediately cease and desist from making and marketing tobacco.

Numerous research studies in pregnant animals show that tobacco products, especially nicotine, have unwanted effects on how the mother's body works. It has been repeatedly shown that nicotine decreases the amount of the mother's blood going to the placenta to feed the fetus. This is a major whammy for the baby. Smoking during pregnancy delivers several other whammies to the fetus: tobacco smoke contains high concentrations of carbon monoxide, a gas that is actually lethal in relatively low concentrations. Carbon monoxide combines with hemoglobin in the mother's blood and her baby's blood, decreasing the ability of red blood cells to transport oxygen to developing tissues in the fetus, including the brain. The tobacco barons and the advertizing industry just cannot deny these adverse effects of nicotine on fetal development.

In addition to the hard scientific data on the harmful effects of nicotine on both mother and fetus, numerous epidemiologic studies consistently show that smoking during pregnancy results in an average reduction in birthweight that is generally placed at around 150 to 320 grams (0.33 to 0.70 pounds). The effects of this apparently small degree of growth retardation should be evaluated in relation to the average birthweight reduction of 150 grams of the babies of mothers who were pregnant during the Dutch Hunger Winter. Few experts would say that pregnancy during the Dutch Hunger Winter provided the best possible home in the womb for the developing child. We saw in chapter 2 that there were multigenerational effects in the adverse health outcomes of babies who were the children, especially the daughters, of the Dutch Hunger Winter. Among all the bad news, the good news about smoking is that it is always advantageous to stop. Since most fetal growth occurs during the final third of pregnancy, quitting smoking even late in pregnancy does help to lessen the adverse effects on growth. This is true even as late as the seventh or eighth month of pregnancy. It's best not to smoke at all, but if you are a smoker, your baby will begin to benefit the very moment you stop.

In response to this well established demographic and scientific evidence that tobacco smoke is an environmental pollutant responsible in a major way for intrauterine growth retardation, the tobacco industry swings into its Houdini act. The defenders of tobacco claim that there is a multitude of factors responsible for low birthweight babies. They are, of course, correct in that comment, but they are erecting a smoke screen to deflect the argument. There is one critical question we should ask: What are the major and preventable causes of prenatal growth retardation? Cigarette smoking is one of the most preventable causes of growth retardation. The industry's defenders follow up the many-factors defense by answering that a 250-gram (0.55 pounds) decrease in birthweight is so small that it is irrelevant to future health. Let us never forget two things: the small decrease in weight reflects how hard the baby had to work to keep growing at nearly the normal rate. There is certainly a price to pay later in life for that effort, that attempt to compensate for a suboptimal home in the womb. We have seen that this degree of growth retardation at birth can have consequences that are permanent. In addition, not only is any catch up growth incomplete, but we have seen that attempting to catch up may present its own long-term problems.

It is clearly detrimental to smoke at any time during pregnancy, and we should remember that women are pregnant before a missed period tells them so. The evidence is overwhelming: Smoking during pregnancy is harmful to the baby. Women who smoke are twice as likely to have a low birthweight baby. In 1990, the United States Surgeon General reported that smoking was the major cause in 26 percent of all low birthweight children born in the United States, about 14 percent of premature deliveries and 10 percent of fetal and infant deaths. The decrease in birthweight that can be attributed to smoking increases with the number of cigarettes smoked. Passive smoking has also been associated with low birthweight. Fathers who smoke may affect the growth of their as-yet-unborn child independently of a smoking mother. When this information is integrated with the knowledge of the biochemical effects of nicotine on blood flow and the developing nervous system, we have powerful evidence from each of the three routes of information—epidemiology, basic research and clinical findings—upon which biomedical knowledge moves forward.

Epidemiology is the demographics of medicine. The tobacco barons should be able to comprehend epidemiological and demographic information. They are businesspeople. Big business understands demographics. Wall Street is built on demographics. Hollywood focuses its productions on demographics. Politicians pore over demographics. Demographics also tell us that the nation is getting older and that elderly Americans have been moving to the Southern sun states where the physical act of living is easier. The commercial and political response to this demographic information is seen in the efforts of Wall Street and the political parties to pay attention to the needs of the elderly. No such luck for the unborn. They have no checkbooks or votes.

Despite the unborn baby's lack of economic clout, politicians and business leaders would be wise to pay attention to the demographics of the unborn. The unborn will greatly alter our lives. On the creativity of the most recent newborn as well as those as yet unborn will rest the comforts of our own old age. The intelligence of the young will determine the success of the business community, on the calmness of their minds will depend the safety of the streets and on their willingness to see their own debt to posterity will depend the future of their own children.

The Family Circle of Smoking

Quitting smoking is not easy. Only one fourth of smoking women are able to stop when they find out they are pregnant. Of those who stop smoking, a third will begin smoking again before their baby is born. Here we have the remarkable situation where the women who have quit apparently know full well that smoking will harm their precious babies, and yet they cannot stay away from cigarettes. In comparing the addictiveness of smoking and alcohol, it is of great interest that women who were both smokers and drinkers before pregnancy found it more difficult to stop smoking than to stop drinking alcohol. So much for the claims by the tobacco industry that smoking is not addictive.

A recent review article in the *British Medical Bulletin* developed the concept of the "family circle" to describe how the damage of smoking impacts development at multiple stages. The harmful effects on the fetus, including low birthweight and increased risk of respiratory diseases, are carried forward into childhood. The higher incidence of frequent minor ailments in the children of mothers who smoked during pregnancy can cause absence from school and falling behind with schoolwork, which can lead to underachievement. Children of mothers who smoked during pregnancy are likely to have smaller stature. Being smaller than one's peers can also affect a child's self-esteem. Passive smoking in the home exacerbates these effects and adds others. The child may become disenchanted with school and reject the values and goals of learning and trying to be healthy. She or he is then at increased risk of becoming a smoker. These young smokers are most likely to leave school early, to start families early and to smoke during pregnancy, thus continuing the "family circle" or "cycle of deprivation." If we left out the last three words, this summary might pass as an internal memo within one of the giant tobacco companies depicting a successful scenario for encouraging the habit in the next generation (maintaining the transgenerational effects of smoking) and keeping up sales. Not addicting indeed!

Preconceptual effects of smoking, or any other maternal or societal behavior, are very difficult to tie down in the complicated picture of social class, varied maternal diet, paternal and maternal smoking. However, it would be prudent to remember that the very same damage smoking causes in the arteries of the heart that lead to the well-established increase in heart disease in smokers is likely progressing slowly, insidiously, blocking and slowing the flow of blood in the arteries all over the body. The uterine arteries may already be damaged in smokers, even before they become pregnant. The uterine arteries are the baby's vital supply line to the placenta.

The health hazards of passive smoking have become a major concern not just of environmentalists but of all those who inhabit smoky social settings where they wish to be with their friends but not other people's vices. It was not so long ago that it was considered offensive to complain that your meal was being spoiled by tobacco smoke wafting across one's dinner table, even in the most expensive restaurants. Fortunately, times have changed, and California is even about to prohibit smoking in bars. The issue is complex. It pits the rights of the individual to do something against the rights of another individual not to have to endure that activity and suffer from it. One report of the Environmental Protection Agency concluded that secondhand tobacco smoke is responsible for 3,000 lung cancer deaths each year.

Nicotine, a drug in every sense of the word, acts on the same receptor as one of the most important molecules in the body, acetylcholine. Acetylcholine is a major neurotransmitter used by nerve cells to tell other nerve cells or gland cells what to do. The nerves to the heart secrete acetylcholine in situations in which it is necessary to slow down the rate at which the heart beats. As so often happens, different cells have slightly different receptors for important signaling molecules. One of the major forms of the acetylcholine receptor was named the nicotinic receptor as long ago as 1904. Regardless of a century of information to the contrary, the tobacco industry continues to state that nicotine is not a drug. I suppose, like Humpty Dumpty, they want to use a word to mean what they want it to mean. Nicotine's actions in the body are in large measure due to the fact that one of the most important receptors on cells, especially brain cells, cannot distinguish nicotine from acetylcholine.

One of the popular current diagnoses for failure to progress in the early years at school is attention deficit hyperactivity disorder (ADHD). Some reports suggest that ADHD may affect as many as one in twenty-five children. As with so many other developmental problems, the condition affects boys more often than girls. This sex difference could, of course, be genetic. However, we have constantly seen that adverse programming effects occur in tissues and organs that are growing fast. Boys do seem to be at higher risk than girls for many developmental deficits, an observation that may be due to the fact that boys grow faster than girls during fetal life.

A recent study found that while 22 percent of mothers of ADHD children smoked a pack of cigarettes a day in the final third of pregnancy, only 8 percent of mothers of children without ADHD smoked at all. As with all epidemiological studies, there may be other differences between the mothers in these two groups, but the study did everything possible to ensure that both groups were balanced for other factors such as parental IQ and parental ADHD. Perhaps we should add a third N word when we are considering prenatal programming in today's society: nature, nurture and nicotine.

Smoking has been associated with sudden infant death syndrome (SIDS). SIDS kills 8,000 babies a year in the United States alone. Although the fundamental cause of SIDS is unknown, it is clearly a sleep-related disorder. Babies who die of SIDS do so during sleep. For unknown reasons, these unfortunate babies fail to arouse during some challenge that occurs to their nervous system in the early months of life. Prenatal nicotine exposure has a very high correlation with SIDS when compared to other drugs of abuse such as cocaine.

Good sleep is fundamental to good health throughout our lives. When asked how we slept last night, we may well respond, "I slept like a baby." Sleep research is a fascinating area that is moving forward fast. In any one night of sleep, we go through several different levels of sleep. The two most marked phases are rapid eye movement sleep (REM) and non-REM sleep. Both these phases are important to our well-being.

Using the power of the ultrasound machine to look into the human uterus during pregnancy, it is possible to see that the human fetus is passing through phases during which the baby's eye movements are very similar to adult eye movements that occur during REM sleep. Studies in fetal sheep permit the investigator to placc electrodes near the fetal eyes and record the patterns of eye movements to register the different types of fetal sleep throughout the last third of pregnancy. Many external and internal factors affect the amount of REM sleep the baby is taking. Contractures, the gentle squeezes or womb hugs which the uterus performs repeatedly every thirty minutes or so, will switch the baby out of REM sleep. Thus it is possible that an active uterus throughout pregnancy will alter fetal sleeping patterns in the womb.

Sleep, particularly REM sleep, is important for brain function. Interrogators who wish to break down prisoners to obtain information have known for years that REM sleep deprivation greatly confuses an individual. When denied the opportunity to indulge in bursts of REM sleep, the brain becomes overloaded. Sleep is even more important for a developing baby than a grown adult. Nearly twenty years ago, Dr. Majid Mirmiran from the Netherlands Institute for Brain Research showed that REM sleep deprivation of newborn rats just from the age of seven to twenty-one days of life led to abnormal behavior patterns, particularly altered exploration and sexual mating behavior when the rats reached adulthood.

It will be no surprise that Dr. Mirmiran and others have shown that the richness of the environment in which young rats grow up can program their behavior in adult life. Further studies show that environmental enrichment during the early weeks of a young rat's life enhances brain development. REM sleep deprivation of young rats prevents these beneficial effects of environmental enrichment. This important observation shows how interactive are the effects of the environment in determining our well-being in later life.

In adults, acetylcholine can wipe out REM sleep. Nicotine at doses that are absorbed into a smoker's blood will markedly alter the sleep-wakefulness patterns of newborn rats at day twelve of life. The frequency of bouts of REM sleep is halved. What is the consequence of a lack of REM sleep during fetal development? We just don't know.

We need to know how the fetus develops because fetuses perform many critical, vital functions very differently from adults. That was number eight of our ten principles of programming. A recent study of fetal rats has highlighted how little we know about the effects of nicotine on the developing baby. Like all drugs, nicotine exerts its effect by combining with receptors on the surfaces of cells that are affected. Researchers at Stanford University have recently shown that the fetal rat has a receptor for nicotine that is unique to fetal life. The fetal nicotine receptor has a different chemical structure from the adult receptor. The consequences of this structural difference in the receptor may be profound. Nicotine may have completely unanticipated effects on the fetus. In the fetal rat, nicotine has a marked effect on one of the major genes that regulates the function of the circadian clock in the developing brain. This nicotine effect is present three days before birth but is lost two days after birth. Nicotine has no effect on this gene in the clock in the adult pregnant rat. So we must be very careful when we say that drugs like nicotine have no effect on the baby in the womb. The effects may be restricted to very small critical time windows during development. Even if there is no effect of the drug on systems researchers are used to studying in the adult, before we can dismiss the possibility of any effects before birth, we need to study the effects of the drug in the fetus because the fetus has some unique jobs to do in the womb. The fetus performs many activities that the adult no longer needs to do, so fetal systems may be vulnerable in a way that we cannot study and understand by looking at the phases of our lives that occur outside the womb. Where is the old conservative philosophy, "In ignorance, abstain?"

Alcohol: "Another Little Drink" Will Do Us (and Our Baby) Quite a Lot of Harm

As the soldiers marched along the battlefields in the First World War, they sang "Another little drink, another little drink, another little drink won't do us any harm. . . ." Perhaps not if the likelihood is a bullet in the head in the near future. But for the fetus, whose whole future life lies ahead and has much growing and developing to do, alcohol is a dangerous chemical, a very potent drug that gives rise to fetal alcohol syndrome (FAS). FAS is the end result of repeated prenatal exposure to alcohol, particularly during early development. FAS was first described in France in 1968 by Lemoine and colleagues. Landmark papers from the United States followed in 1973. The U.S. Surgeon General first issued warnings against the dangers of alcohol in pregnancy in 1981. FAS has been called the only known 100 percent preventable birth defect.

There is very little information on what are safe levels of fetal alcohol exposure. Some studies suggest that as little as two drinks a week may result in increased agitation and stressful behavior in newborn babies. We just don't know, so, "In ignorance, abstain," is probably the optimal course.

The effects of alcohol on body systems are extensive, so it is no surprise that alcohol is bad news for the fetus. Investigators have labeled alcohol problems *ethanol teratogenesis.* Studies in pregnant sheep show that alcohol decreases the amount of blood flowing to the fetal brain. This fall in brain blood flow is very dangerous. If the mother who drinks alcohol also smokes, the amount of oxygen in her blood and the blood of the fetus will be even further decreased. So a cigarette-smoking lifestyle can expose the baby to multiple whammies. There is both less blood going to the baby's brain and less oxygen in that blood. No wonder the effects of alcohol on the developing brain are so severe. The totality of effects on the fetus over nine months will be modified by a wide range of factors in the environment: maternal nutrition, frequency and intensity of episodes of exposure (binge drinking), the critical periods of development at which the fetus is exposed, genetic susceptibility and many other factors that have already affected fetal well-being for better or worse (smoking being an additional problem). However, the lack of current understanding is clearly stated by the Institute of Medicine in the United States: "At present, there is uncertainty whether minimal alcohol intake during pregnancy could be associated with any degree of injury to the baby." The Institute of Medicine also strongly recommends that every effort is made to reduce any exposure to alcohol in mother's milk immediately after birth.

FAS is diagnosed by the physician from a set of physical characteristics that are usually easily discernible at birth. If not immediately obvious, FAS fetuses are easily recognized within a few months after birth. The cluster of features are slow growth during fetal and postnatal life with a lack of ability of the baby to catch up after birth, even when provided with excellent nutrition. Failure to catch up is probably due to a decrease in the number of cells in the baby's body as a direct consequence of alcohol inhibiting the division of cells in early development. FAS babies are characteristically small and thin. Brain damage is clearly shown by a small head and brain accompanied by mental retardation, behavioral irritability, hyperactivity, bad coordination and learning problems. There are characteristic malformations of the face. These include small, widely spaced eyes, a small, upturned nose with a wide, flat bridge and flat cheeks and small chin caused by impaired growth of the major skull bones that go to make up the face and jaw. The growth abnormalities are not limited to the head. Heart defects are very common in FAS. The kidneys and genitals may be small. All this adds up to the poor outcome that results from exposing dividing, migrating cells to alcohol.

To date, it has not proved possible to demonstrate a specific receptor for alcohol on the membrane of cells. How then does alcohol alter the function of cells? Alcohol is very soluble in the fats that make up a large portion of the cell membrane. When it gets into the cell membrane, alcohol may well alter its strength as well as other functions. Changes in this vital outer envelope of cells are likely to have very profound consequences on the movements of cells as they travel to their rightful place in important organs such as the brain during the various stages of development. Some of these effects may be very subtle. A mother's alcohol binge at a critical time of development of the brain cortex could possibly alter exactly where one neuron decides to settle down. As a result, the wrong communications between cells will have been established locally with potential permanent consequences. It is the subtle effects of alcohol that need attention. The extreme effects of alcohol on the fetus are well documented. We need more information on the moderate effects rather than the extreme effects. Because these moderate effects are more subtle, they will be more difficult to determine. Even if they are subtle, they may yet be important in the complex, twenty-first-century world.

While the majority of children with FAS are only mildly mentally retarded, with IQs around 65, there is much variability. Binge drinking, defined as five or more drinks at one time, has been linked with low IQ and learning difficulties at the age of seven years. IQs even as high as 85 can be a great impediment to social integration and acceptable performance in our complex society. The FAS child may show the following unwanted characteristics: failure to grow at the normal rate and associated feeding difficulties and delays in motor development. Preschool FAS children often show hyperactivity, and behavioral disturbances such as ADHD, language difficulties and communication problems. In school, these unfortunate children have severe problems dealing simultaneously with the many things going on around them. They have specific problems with hearing-related functions. FAS children generally fail to make friends, are aggressive and are unable to learn from their mistakes. Importantly, they have difficulty connecting punishment with the wrong deed.

Overall incidence of FAS in the United States ranges from 1 to 3 per 1,000. However, the incidence can rise as high as 10.7 per 1,000 in some groups of Southwestern Plains Indians. There is clearly a complex mix of cultural, nutritional and other factors that influence the incidence of FAS and its milder relation, a syndrome called fetal alcohol effects (FAE). The very existence of FAE reminds us of the need to look for harmful marginal effects that occur at the low end of exposure to alcohol.

Cost estimates for FAS babies in the United States are difficult to make because of problems in diagnosis and the existence of all ranges of level of effect. The lifetime cost of treatment and care of a typical FAS baby has been calculated as nearly $600,000. The total estimated cost has been placed as high $9.7 billion a year. Regardless of whether this is a gross overestimate, the costs in terms of lowered quality of life and increased risks to society from deviant behavior are high.

In *Brave New World,* Aldous Huxley tells of a future in which different types of humans are mass-produced in varying numbers required for different positions in society. Embryos are grown in hatcheries tended by scientists dressed in "white, their hands gloved with pale corpse-colored gloves." Eggs produced in the fertilization room are grown in special broths and budded until ninety-six buds are produced from each embryo. The buds are then placed in incubators. In the book, the director of the Central London Hatchery and Conditioning Center describes the process as, "Two, four, eight, the buds in their turn budded; and having budded were dosed almost to death with alcohol . . . thereafter—further arrest being generally fatal—they are left to develop in peace."

The director is proud of this ability to produce batches of multiple clones to order. "For the first time in history . . . millions of identical twins. The principle of mass production at last applied to biology." Various embryos received treatments to produce individuals completely suited to their future function in life. Embryos destined to become tropical workers receive immunizations against typhoid and sleeping sickness at optimal stages of prenatal development. Chemical workers are trained before birth to tolerate lead, caustic soda tar and chlorine; embryos of future rocket-plane engineers are submitted to constant rotation. The director explains that the goal of the constant rotation is "to improve their sense of balance . . . doing repairs on the outside of a rocket in mid-air is a ticklish job. We slacken off the circulation when they're right way up, so that they are half starved, and double the flow of surrogate when they are upside down. They learn to associate topsy-turvydom with well-being; in fact they're only truly happy when they are standing on their heads." Aldous Huxley clearly did not need to be convinced about prenatal programming. His words here fit the concept, now based on a firm experimental basis, that those structures receiving good nutrition while they are active develop in one way, restricting nutrition to other structures can literally lead to imbalance.

Huxley was also well aware that the developing fetus needs an adequate supply of oxygen. "The lower the caste, . . . the shorter the oxygen. The first organ affected is the brain. After that the skeleton. At seventy per cent of normal oxygen you get dwarfs." As we have seen, the first organ affected is probably not the brain. We can excuse Huxley for not knowing about the clever way the fetus can shunt more blood to the head to spare the brain as much as possible. However, the overall idea is correct: The quality of life, the prenatal origins of health and disease, depend on the environment to which the baby is exposed during development. In the brave new world described, the preparation of individuals is divided into high-class, achieving alphas, through betas, down to the lowest form, the gammas. Gammas are smaller than alphas and are "conditioned to associate corporeal mass with social superiority." Certainly, there is a relationship in our own society between being tall and success in life. Gammas were conditioned by adding alcohol to their incubation medium during fetal life. Aldous Huxley had great prescience when it comes to FAS and FAE.

Relatively few years—in terms of human history—have elapsed since the writing of *Brave New World*. There have been enormous advances in assisted reproductive techniques that have brought us face-to-face with the issues Huxley addresses. The concept of mass-production of identical individuals by repeated splitting of the embryos has now been taken a stage further. In the cloning of Dolly, researchers took a mammary gland cell from a donor adult sheep, removed the nucleus and put it in an egg whose own nucleus had been removed. The egg was then incubated in a recipient mother to produce a clone of the sheep that provided the mammary gland cell—not the one in whose womb Dolly developed. In reporting the achievement, it was often stated in the media that such clones would be identical with the donor when they grew up, the only qualifier being that the "mother," the adult who had furnished the nucleus, would have been born at an early date and grown up in a different environment. True. But Dolly's mother and Dolly also developed in different wombs. Thus, they would not be identical, even at birth.

Drugs of Abuse

One study reported in 1991 that 15 percent of women delivering in teaching hospitals and 3 percent of women delivering in private hospitals admitted to cocaine use during pregnancy. Cocaine users were more likely to use other illicit drugs, to smoke and to drink alcohol during pregnancy. Twenty percent of black mothers, 24 percent of single mothers and 21 percent who did not graduate from high school had taken cocaine during pregnancy. The figures for alcohol binge drinking were 9, 19 and 15 percent, and for smoking cigarettes, 52, 63 and 58 percent. For cocaine abuse, these figures represented as much as a fifteenfold increase over a twelve-year period.

Pay now or pay later. This is the inevitable rule of pregnancy. If society does not pay adequate attention to prenatal care, society will be called upon to pay the bill during the whole life of the individual. On Sunday, November 20, 1994, *Sixty Minutes* aired a program on the effects of crack cocaine on the developing fetus. The early images in the program were of several premature babies delivered to women who had used cocaine during pregnancy. The small babies were shown surrounded by the blinking and beeping instruments of the modern, high-tech neonatal intensive care unit. Not only are these crack-exposed babies small and very much at risk, but they are very irritable and prone to all sorts of crises if stimulated to even the slightest degree. Therefore, nursing staff leave them alone for fear of stimulating a bout of irregular movement. These poor, unfortunate children are deprived of the touching and bonding that we saw in chapter 8 is so important to good brain development.

These babies are not like other premature babies. They have been assaulted in the uterus. They have been prisoners of their mothers.

They have been beaten and battered just as surely as if their parents had taken a stick to them after birth. The *Sixty Minutes* program focused on the attempts of the Medical University of South Carolina to stop mothers from taking crack cocaine during pregnancy by threatening the mothers with arrest if they continued the cocaine habit.

Sixty Minutes reported that the American Civil Liberties Union (ACLU) had become involved in the case and that the ACLU was taking the university to court on behalf of the mothers. Many legal, ethical and moral issues were raised. Most of the mothers taking cocaine were black and the accusation was made that the Medical University of South Carolina was being racist. We should leave the legal issues to attorneys trained to deal with them, but we may well ask, "Would it be acceptable for the mothers, white or black, to give their babies cocaine after birth?" The police chief, an African American, disagreed with the ACLU and did not see the hospital's action as a racial issue but an attempt to protect the unborn children.

Society must wake up to the needs of children before they are born just as it takes care of their needs after birth. Cocaine is a major assault on the children in the uterus. An assault far worse than hitting a small child with the palm of your hand in a fit of anger. Yet parents can be charged for smacking their children once the children have exited the uterus. Should they not be equally responsible for drug-induced physical assault before the child is born? Society has reached a stage in its evolution at which it is considered acceptable to step in if parents fail to educate children. We do not appear to be ready to intervene when parents damage babies prenatally to a state at which they are essentially uneducable. If possession of cocaine is an offense, then surely its possession within one's bloodstream is the ultimate possession. Why can a person be charged if the cocaine is in their pocket but not transported to their baby's bloodstream?

The ACLU always tries to stand up for the underdog, the minority view. I also believe that defense of individual rights of the minority is fundamental to our free society. But with freedom comes responsibility. The individual is responsible for her or his actions, especially when others are damaged by these actions. Cocaine in the blood of the mother produces major damage in the fetus.

The saddest thing for me about the *Sixty Minutes* program was the utter ignorance of the lawyer who had traveled from New York to take the case of the women who had been made to give up the cocaine habit. The attorney was asked whether she had been in the neonatal intensive care unit to see the small, irritable, inconsolable babies. She had not. She might have been asked whether she had seen one-year-old, badly affected babies whose mothers had taken crack cocaine. These are children with short attention spans, disorganized abilities to relate to others, a disposition to cardiovascular crises, prone to die young.

The young lawyer displayed a complete ignorance of biology. She passed off the poor health and poor prognosis of the crack cocaine babies as being no different from the other unfortunate babies in the neonatal intensive care unit. She claimed that such units are always places with sick babies, implying that there is nothing unusual about crack babies. The evidence, she said, "does not support the notion that cocaine constitutes any special danger. It is like getting out of breath when pregnant or too much or too little exercise. It is similar to the risks of changing cat litter. What we see here is a police state." It may be that trying to bring some sense to the situation—to stop mothers from abusing their babies in the uterus—reminds her of the police state. But intelligent people like this lawyer should stop twisting the facts to their own purposes. Cocaine is a very potent chemical. It decreases blood flow on both sides of the placenta, in the mother and in the fetus. Cocaine causes unwanted uterine contractions that leads to premature labor. It stimulates the baby to move and breathe in the uterus even at times when the baby is short of oxygen. When short of oxygen in the womb, normal babies stop breathing and moving to conserve oxygen for their brain. By increasing the energy needs that result from movement, crack babies expose their brains to further oxygen lack.

The developing brain, like your or my brain, is full of nerve cells that secrete catecholamines. Catecholamines are a group of compounds called neurotransmitters because they pass messages from brain cell to brain cell. The actions of these neurotransmitters are fundamental to normal brain development. Cocaine, by virtue of its chemical similarity to the catecholamines, interferes with the interactions between nerve cells as they develop. The effects are obvious for anyone who has the time to look at the babies in the neonatal intensive care unit. The lawyer involved in the *Sixty Minutes* program apparently did not. She should learn some physiology before she starts equating the risk of changing cat litter while pregnant, or inappropriate exercise, with the damage caused to the fetus by cocaine.

The ACLU lawyer criticized the approach of making the mother (and one hopes the father) responsible for endangering the welfare of the child as a "way station on the way to jail." She is correct to some degree. In one sense, we can consider the home in the womb as a jail since the baby did not go there as an act of personal will. The maternal uterine jail can be a pleasant, comfortable, hospitable place or it can be made into the most life-threatening of environments from which the baby has no immediate hope of escape and will suffer the consequences for a lifetime. I repeat, the ACLU lawyer would do well to learn some fetal physiology.

Over-the-Counter Drugs

About ten years ago, Dr. Dick Swaab, the director of the Netherlands Institute for Brain Research, was invited to the United States to address a very active scientific society interested in fetal and newborn development. He was asked to speak on his special area of interest, the harmful effects of drugs, both approved and illicit, on the developing brain. The meeting took place in the fall at the idyllic location of Chatham Bars on Cape Cod. At the end of his talk, as we were walking along the New England shoreline, talking about the mechanisms whereby these strong chemicals may alter brain function, Dr. Swaab was approached by a very senior obstetrician. "All you do is provide evidence for lawyers to make trouble. You shouldn't be researching the effects of these drugs on the fetus. I hope I never see you in court, Dr. Swaab," the obstetrician said with some malice.

The medical profession feels beleaguered by attorneys who wish to blame them for all the things that go wrong with pregnancy. This obstetrician we met on the beach clearly felt that unscrupulous attorneys would seize on Dr. Swaab's research to make yet more claims of medical negligence. The obstetrician feared that Dick Swaab's findings would be used to attack the pharmaceutical industry for making profits from dangerous drugs or the obstetrician for prescribing them. The physician's concerns that he might be sued sometime during his career were probably very well-founded. When will society wake up to the fact that we are all in this together? We all share responsibility. Drug treatments are used in obstetric care, as well as other branches of medicine, when there is already an abnormality. It would, of course, be best if none of us were ever sick, especially in pregnancy. The use of antiepileptic drugs may be life saving for some pregnant women. Drugs that lower blood pressure may be urgently needed by pregnant women with increased blood pressure in late pregnancy. However, we cannot administer these powerful medications, these very active chemical compounds, without a careful cost-benefit analysis. At the same time, society, requesting treatment as it does, must share the burden of responsibility. It is morally indefensible for a society to ask for treatments and then blame those who tried their best to ameliorate the condition for which the treatment was prescribed.

Effective drugs that bring relief to specific abnormal conditions in both the pregnant and nonpregnant state are very active chemicals. These compounds often last longer in the blood than the similar chemicals that the body normally produces. Their very potency probably means that they will have side effects by acting on other biological processes similar to the one the physician wishes to alter. The problem of side effects from drugs used to combat all medical conditions must be addressed at several levels: the avoidance of the conditions that bring about the need for the drugs; adequate animal testing before the drugs are used for treatment of human conditions; carefully controlled clinical trials to demonstrate the effectiveness of the drug, the correct dosages and the possible side effects so that meaningful cost-benefit analysis can be undertaken; education of the patient to permit her or him to evaluate the benefits and costs of taking the drug. It is of interest to consider each of these issues separately.

Drug development has become a dangerous, complex and expensive task for the pharmaceutical industry. The drug industry, like any industry, should not be criticized for wishing to make a profit. Pharmaceutical companies certainly cannot operate at a loss and survive. Developing a new drug is an extremely expensive activity, more so today when there are, rightly, so many considerations of documentation of safety, so many studies demanded before the drug is even released for human trials.

One of the major steps in the discovery and evaluation of new drugs is the testing of potentially useful agents in animals. Studies on drugs that have potential as treatments for human disease must be tested in animals first. Nowhere is this more true than in the identification of drugs that have a use in pregnancy. The pregnant state involves a complex interaction of mother, placenta and baby. Studies in cell systems can indicate effectiveness and suggest that side effects are rare. But it is only by finally testing the drug in pregnant animals that we discover such features as whether the drug crosses the placenta, whether the fetus destroys the drug faster or slower than the mother, whether the drug or some of its by-products accumulate in the amniotic cavity. With respect to this last highly critical issue, it is clearly impossible to evaluate drug accumulation in amniotic fluid in studies conducted solely with cell suspensions in a test tube. In the womb, the distribution and effects of the drug are affected by the fetal kidneys that produce the bulk of the amniotic fluid. The fetal membranes that surround the amniotic cavity also play a role in production of the body fluids of the fetus. Fetuses swallow amniotic fluid, reabsorbing it through their gut. Each of these pathways may greatly modify the effects of any drug when compared with the effects in a nonpregnant woman or even in the mother herself during pregnancy.

The search for safe treatments leads many to health food stores. While it is admirable that we are concerned about good health, the very existence of special health food stores does suggest that other stores are unhealthy. However, we are often completely ignorant of the composition and activities of the active ingredients of health foods. Herbal remedies contain powerful ingredients. Digoxin, one of the most useful compounds for treating the failing heart, was first extracted from the foxglove plant. Drugs are powerful compounds that work on cells by attaching to receptors on the cell surface and instructing the cell to work harder or to stop working so hard. Many drugs either stimulate or inhibit the activities of cells that have receptors on their surface that recognize the drugs. Other drugs can act on enzymes, increasing or decreasing the rate at which they function. There is nothing unique in the mode of action about any one drug. All drugs are simply compounds that interact with our bodily functions in some way. They have potential benefits as well as potential to do harm. It is the way they are used and when they are used that can cause health problems. It is important to understand their actions on our bodies.

The worrying aspects of health foods and herbal remedies is the relative lack of regulation. In America, the Federal Drug Administration carefully monitors the sale of drugs produced by the pharmaceutical industry. We all insist on this oversight. In contrast, health food stores can sell virtually anything. The composition of the products offered is often totally unknown. I am intrigued why the very people who are so often skeptical (correctly so, since skepticism is not a bad attitude when taken in moderation) about the claims of the pharmaceutical industry, are so blindly trusting of health foods.

In both America and Britain you can buy health food pills marketed as containing "healthy" bacteria that the makers claim will populate the gut of those taking the pills and thereby improve their health. Studies have shown that these pills may contain antibiotic-resistant bacteria. Some of the bacteria are even resistant to the super antibiotics that are kept in reserve as a last line of defense to treat very sick individuals when all other antibiotics have failed. While these bacteria may not do harm to healthy people, they are potentially lethal to the very people who might be wanting a tonic to pick them up.

There is still much to learn about the normal functional changes in a woman's body during pregnancy. Recent research shows that adaptations occur in her heart and blood system as early as the fifth week of pregnancy. It appears that the early changes are critical if the pregnancy is to proceed normally. The implications of this statement are very profound. All women considering pregnancy (and their partners) should be aware that they can be several weeks pregnant before they actually realize that they are pregnant. It is preferable to start any required lifestyle changes before pregnancy than to wait until one is six weeks pregnant. The environment in the womb is critical from the very first day—and before.

NINE

YOU ARE YOUR BRAIN

You are your brain.

Dick Swaab, Director,
The Netherlands Institute for Brain Research

The significant observation that certain functions of our brain and our behavior are programmed to a considerable extent by prenatal events was clearly demonstrated over forty years ago. Studies in rats showed that a brief period of exposure of the female brain to male hormones conditions the brain's reproductive activities to be the male continuous, acyclic form for life. In chapter 6, we saw how prenatal and immediate postnatal events alter the level at which the interrelationship of brain activity and production of stress hormones is set. In a similar way, suboptimal nutrition and unfavorable environmental factors acting at critical periods of brain development during fetal and newborn life can program other brain functions and behavior.

Brain development is activity-dependent, and the environment in which the fetus develops in the womb plays a major role in the birth, connection and activity—the siring, wiring and firing—of newly formed neurons. The interaction of many different types of cells is vital to good brain development. It is crucial to grow a good blood supply to the brain during fetal development. Even the brains of identical twins will not have exactly the same structure in part because they will not develop exactly the same blood supply. The conditions under which the brain develops will modify how the genes function.

In the uterus, the fetus cycles through periods of different behavioral activity. One phase resembles adult rapid eye movement sleep (REM sleep). The duration of bouts of REM as well as non-REM sleep is altered by changes in the baby's intrauterine environment, the home in the womb. Suboptimal environments in the womb lead to problems in later life. Development of cerebral palsy and other neurological problems are more likely to be caused by slowly progressing, insidious shortages of oxygen during fetal life than by sudden, short-term oxygen deprivation at birth. Intelligence is as greatly affected by environmental influences during fetal development as it is by genetic endowment. The development of sexual orientation and personality involve an interplay of genes and environmental factors in the womb that program brain function during critical periods of development. We, and our brains, are products of nurture in the womb just as much as our genetic heritage.

The Siring, Wiring and Firing of Fetal Nerve Cells

"Billions and billions" was a catch phrase that Carl Sagan used frequently to indicate that the heavenly star count was, in practice, uncountable: vast, awe-inspiring and overwhelming. We do not need to travel to galactic space to consider the prospect of billions and billions of interrelated entities. Within your brain you have one hundred billion nerve cells, each one closely related to hundreds of other nerve cells. In an act of creation rivaling the origin of the universe, every single cell in the mature nervous system arises from the division of a small cluster of primitive nerve cells. Every nerve cell has a specific time to be born. In the early phase of development of the brain, nerve cells are moving restlessly around the brain searching for their unique home. Their movement towards their individual, personalized, final resting place in the mature brain bears a close resemblance to the explosive dispersion of the stars at the original big bang that saw the start of our own universe.

Three critical events occur as the brain gradually forms its multitude of complex structures and establishes connections between them. Brain cells are born, they connect together and begin to fire.

These developmental processes are often referred to as siring (birth), wiring (connection) and firing (activity).

In addition to the nerve cells, the brain contains one hundred billion support cells called *glial cells*. Each glial cell also has to be sired from specialized precursor cells. For normal brain development to occur, all the support cells must station themselves in the correct location with respect to the highly mobile neurons. Glial cells surround, protect and nourish the conducting cables, or axons, that carry impulses to and from the neurons. Glial cells wrap themselves around the nerve fibers to produce a many layered insulating tube. These tubes form the pathways that direct the wiring diagram of the brain. By insulating the nerve fiber from its surroundings, the tubes also help to speed the transmission of messages between the neurons.

Growing good neurons during fetal life is only one part—albeit an important part—of growing a good brain. Recent research shows that proper development of nonnervous structures in the brain is also critical to good brain function. It is impossible to develop a healthy brain without good interaction between glial cells and neurons. It is also extremely important that the right number of good blood vessels form throughout the whole brain. We have seen in chapter 4 how poor development of blood vessels in the fetal pancreas can set an animal up for diabetes in later life. So, neurons alone do not make a brain. It is important that the glial cells are carefully nurtured during their development. The membranes around the glial cells contain special fat molecules that the fetus cannot synthesize. It is, therefore, critical that these essential fats are present in the mother's diet in adequate amounts. The baby is totally dependent on adequate transfer of essential fats across the placenta from the mother to grow good insulation around nerve cells and enable them to function well. The siring and wiring of neurons is critically dependent on maternal diet.

Just as mariners have to use instruments to chart their way through the oceans, developing neurons must chart their way through the complex, ever-changing jungle of cells and fibers that

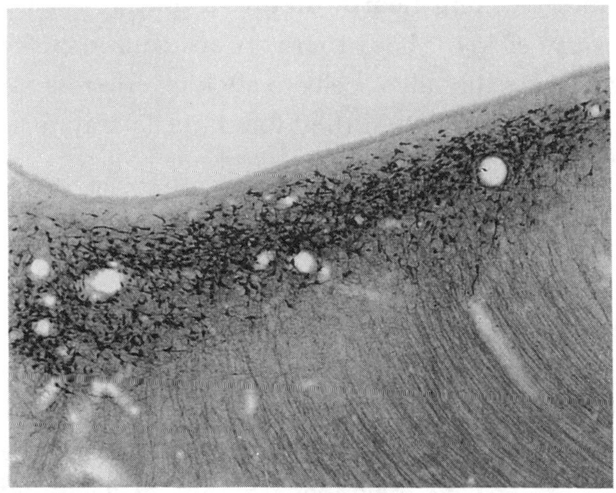

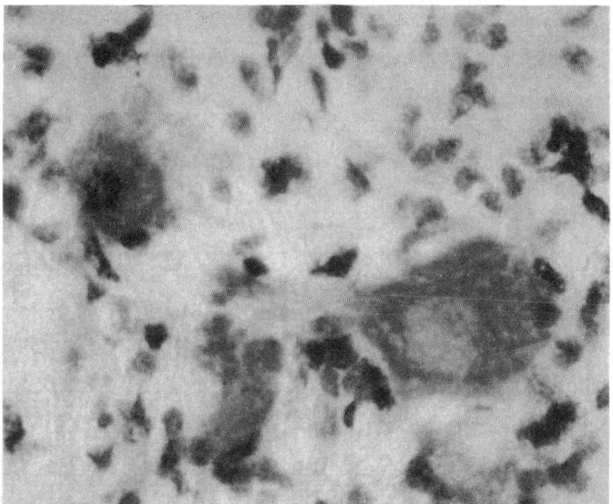

FIGURE 9.1

Top: Large neurons and their smaller glial support cells. Bottom: Neurons with their fibers sweeping away to another part of the brain.

make up the rapidly growing fetal brain. Cells migrating to new areas of the brain need signposts in the same way mariners use islands and coastlines to steer by. These youthful traveling nerve cells look for specific signpost molecules on the surface of nearby cells in the thicket of intermeshing nearby neurons and glial cells. On the surface of every cell in the body there are specialized molecules called *adhesion molecules* that allow cells to stick together as they crawl by each other. Sometimes, when they touch, cells stay together in the same place permanently. Other cells indulge in brief encounters, as if they are airline passengers waiting at the same airport for connecting flights to different cities before they move on to their final destinations. If a cell makes a mistake in timing or doesn't have the right ticket, it may never reach its correct final home. It is imperative that nerve and glial cells secrete the correct adhesion molecules at the correct times and in the correct amounts. It is also important that the cells that want to interact with the surface adhesion molecules on a specific neighboring cell, however briefly, have receptors to the adhesion molecules. If the required adhesion molecules are not present in the correct places as one nerve cell passes the nerve cell or glial cell that should rightfully be its lifetime neighbor, the migrating cell may wander on by and end up in the wrong location. As in our adult life, being in the right place at the right time is everything. Your neighborhood friends as well as your distant contacts have a lot to do with who you are and what you accomplish in life. It is the same in the brain. The single feature of the brain that distinguishes humans from all other mammals is the complexity and size of the cerebral cortex, the outer layer of the most recently evolved part of the brain. The cerebral cortex is full of very highly connected nerve cells. The diversity of different types of cells, their staggering number and the intricacy of the interconnections are all critical to the complex higher functions of thought and creativity. As the brain evolved, the size and complexity of these higher areas increased faster than the size of the skull. The only way to house the number of cells that develop in the human cerebral cortex was to fold the nerve cell layer to produce the highly convoluted appearance of the two cerebral hemispheres. During this folding process, grooves (sulci) form to separate the elevated folds (gyri). The major sulci on any human brain are easily identifiable with the unaided human eye

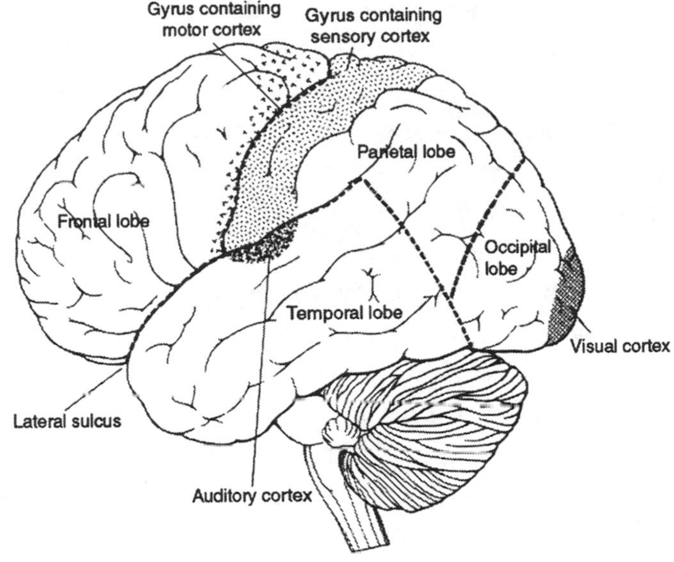

FIGURE 9.2

Brain convolutions with location of the areas of the brain that processes auditory, visual and sensory information marked.

No two brains are exactly the same. Even the brains of identical twins are not identical. This is further evidence that the processes that control the development of the brain are not solely genetic. Nutritional and other factors such as prenatal stress at key stages of development may permanently alter the number and fine interconnections of neurons and glial cells in the cerebral cortex and other parts of the brain.

Heavily folded in on itself, the outer layer of nerve cells in the cerebral cortex is extraordinarily complex. The different regions of the cortex are given names according to their function: the motor cortex (the area responsible for controlling the body's movements), the auditory cortex (the area that receives and analyzes sounds), the visual cortex (responsible for visual analysis of the world about us) and the primary sensory cortex (the area that receives messages from the skin all over the body). There is a fundamental pattern of six layers of neurons in all of these areas of the cortex, but the mix and detailed interrelationship of cell types differ from region to region. When we look down a microscope, we can easily distinguish the visual cortex from other areas such as the hippocampus, the part of the cortex that plays a major role in memory functions and our body's response to stress. Part of the hippocampus has a collection of nerve cells arranged in a crescent very much like a sharp tooth. For this reason, this particular area of the hippocampus is called the *dentate gyrus.* The various cell types and their relationship to each other in the visual cortex and the dentate gyrus are just as recognizably different and easy to distinguish for a trained neurologist as a desert landscape is from the Rocky Mountains. The hippocampus is directly connected to the hypothalamus, the brain's major computer center for controlling the body's hormone responses. It is the intricate connectivity and interaction of these various different groupings of cells that permit humans to undertake the myriad sophisticated, specific brain functions that underlie our behavior. Development of mental ability and competent behaviors depends on good brain development during fetal life.

These layers of the cerebral cortex develop from the inside out. As the embryo develops, the first nerve cells to arrive in the cortex take up their stations in the innermost layer. The next group of cells that move in use these pioneering first arrivals as signposts to direct them as they climb out to their own permanent locations farther out toward the surface. If one set of cells is slow to take up its location—or worse, gets into the wrong place—the whole structure of the brain can be compromised. Each cell must be in the right place at the right time. Permanent changes in location and connections may occur in neurons and glial cells exposed to a variety of insults during development. Lack of glucose and other nutrients, too much cortisol in the blood of the developing fetus as a result of maternal stress, poor oxygenation and excessive exposure of the developing brain to alcohol are all unfavorable conditions that may result in permanent alterations. Because normal completion of each phase of development depends on successful completion of the previous phase, suboptimal conditions, even for a very short time during development, can result in permanent alteration of brain function.

ACTIVITY DEPENDENT MATURATION

Like other important structures in the fetal body, development of brain structure and function is *activity-dependent*. For example, the growth of the fetal lungs has been shown to depend on the periodic breathing movements the fetus makes in the womb. Studies in animal fetuses have shown that fetuses that do not spend a good proportion of their time undertaking breathing movements are born with smaller lungs. Likewise, in order to form properly, developing nerve cells require a constant stream of stimulating messages from other nerve cells. This activity dependence has been well demonstrated when nerve cells are grown in culture in a dish in the laboratory. Nerve cells stimulated electrically while being grown in culture develop more connections with their neighbors than nerve cells that do not receive electrical stimulation. As a consequence of activity dependence, the correct completion of one stage of brain development helps to stimulate the next process in the progression. The conditions in the womb must be right for development to unfold in precisely the correct sequence. Correct and timely interaction of genes and the environment is fundamental to normal brain development. If the conditions are inappropriate, even for a limited period of time at a critical stage of development, nature and nurture may interact inappropriately and the correct unfolding of the whole genetic blueprint for the brain may be impeded. As a result, a critical stage may be missed.

Developmental neurologists who study the siring, wiring and firing of the brain seek answers to the following critical questions: What factors regulate the precise timing when nerve cells are born or sired? How do nerve cells find their way through the mass of developing structures to hook up correctly with their correct partners? What signposts do the traveling nerve cells use to ensure that the brain is correctly wired? Since it is clear that different parts of the brain have very different firing patterns, what types of molecules regulate the firing of the neurons?

The siring, wiring and firing of nerve cell activity are activity-dependent processes, each interacting with the other. As they fire, developing neurons release growth factors from their terminals that influence the growth and division of other nerve cells nearby. These newly formed cells then contribute to the wiring. Thus siring affects wiring, which is necessary for firing. At the cellular level, normal development of the brain is clearly activity-dependent.

The environment that exists within the womb modifies the level of activity of the organs of the developing fetus, including the brain. The activity of the fetus in turn alters the environment in the womb. Thus fetal development is a highly interactive developmental situation, not one that is just determined by the genes. This is our principle number three of the ten principles of programming described in chapter 1. There may be some purely genetically driven events very early on in development that are not at all activity-dependent. Special sets of genes called *homeobox* genes—or *hoxgenes,* for short—control the development of bilateral symmetry of the embryo. Hoxgenes also provide instructions for the formation of the primitive body segments that give the embryo its early earthwormlike appearance. These early events lay down the framework for future brain development. However, I have a hunch that it is wrong to conclude that even these early events are controlled solely by the genes. We have seen how growth in the first three days of life in sheep embryos can be affected by the amount of progesterone in the fluids in the uterus. The functional capabilities of the genes will interact with nutritional factors, environmental pollutants and drugs of abuse such as hard drugs and alcohol.

Why am I so skeptical about the idea that genes alone are responsible for shaping our health throughout life? There is abundant evidence that a whole mix of chemicals in the environment can cause irreversible alteration to even the very earliest stages of development of the brain and spinal cord. We have seen the asymmetry of the faces of babies affected by fetal alcohol syndrome. Another example is the association of vitamin deficiency with spina bifida. In spina bifida, the tube that forms the spinal cord fails to close during very early stages of development. As a result, the spinal cord, one of the most critical early developmental midline structures, remains exposed to the outside world. It is one of a group of malformations collectively called *neural tube defects.* Folic acid is one of many factors needed for correct closure of the neural tube. This unfortunate nerve tube abnormality shows that early genetic programming can be influenced in major ways by the environment.

Chemicals in the environment that disorganize early development of the embryo are called *teratogens.* The effects of teratogens on the developing brain generally occur at very early stages in the formation of the brain, but the eventual outward signs of the damage may be delayed for weeks, months, or even years. In my book, *Life Before Birth,* I described the effects on the fetal brain of a toxin from the corn lily plant. If a pregnant sheep eats the corn lily on the fourteenth day of her pregnancy, a toxin in the corn lily deforms the developing fetus's brain. As a result, five months later, the brain of the fetal lamb is unable to send the hormone signal to the placenta that starts the birth process. Normally, this signal is sent about thirty days before birth. The deformed brain of the fetus that was exposed to the toxin from the corn lily five months earlier cannot send the required signal. As a result, the birth process does not start. Some of these affected fetal lambs are still in the uterus after two hundred and fifty days. This is equivalent to a women carrying her pregnancy for fifteen months and showing not the slightest sign of going into labor. These delayed effects of early exposures to toxins are a dramatic example of the impact that abnormal brain development can have on how the baby lamb's life turns out.

The corn lily deformity holds another important lesson. If the pregnant ewe eats the plant on a different day of early pregnancy—say day twelve—a different deformity will occur. This story is very reminiscent of the tragic thalidomide story. In the 1950s, pregnant women experiencing the nausea of early pregnancy were given the antinausea drug thalidomide. We now know that thalidomide is also a teratogen. Exposure to thalidomide predominantly results in fetal limb deformities. The actual deformity that develops depends on the precise embryonic stage at which exposure occurs. In some children, thalidomide caused abnormalities of forearm development. In others, their legs, and in some cases, all four limbs were malformed.

Nerves Program the Speed at Which Muscles Contract

Nerve cells use electrical signals to stimulate or inhibit other nerve cells, gland cells and the muscles that we use to move our bodies. If during development the nerve fiber that normally connects with a muscle cell is prevented from arriving at the muscle cell in time, the impatient muscle cells send out guidance molecules that act as signals to nearby nerves—often the wrong ones—to sprout and try to make connections to join the muscle. The lonely muscle cells are desperately trying to ensure that they are connected with the brain and spinal cord so as not to be left without connections to provide them with the information they need. Without any instructions from nerves, limb muscles are unable to contract at all, let alone perform precise, delicate, controlled tasks. However, hooking up with just any nerve fiber will not do. It is important that the correct connections are made. Different nerve fibers come from different parts of the brain and carry very different messages. If muscle cells hook up with the wrong nerves, they will get the wrong messages, and the whole character of their function can change for life.

The muscles that move our limbs are called *voluntary* muscles because we are able to control their function. Voluntary muscles are completely dependent on nerves for their activity. If the nerve is severed, the muscle is paralyzed. There are two major types of voluntary muscle fibers that we use to control movement: white muscle and red muscle. The major difference between these fibers is the speed at which they contract. White muscle contracts fast but fatigues easily. Red muscle contracts more slowly but can keep working for a long time because it contains more of the pigment myoglobin that helps to store some oxygen. It is myoglobin that makes this type of muscle red. If during fetal or early newborn life a nerve that would normally have connected with a developing white muscle is dissected out and sewn onto a muscle that was going to develop as a red muscle, the impressionable muscle fiber gets a different set of messages from the brain and develops as a white fiber rather than the red type of fiber, which would have been its normal fate. This is an excellent example of how the development of cells in all parts of the body can be controlled by the pattern of input from the nervous system.

Early Events Alter the Rate at Which the Brain Ages

The scientific evidence for the notion that prenatal and immediately postnatal conditions have effects on the lifelong function of the heart and blood vessels was discussed in detail earlier. What about the brain? There are very interesting studies conducted in rats that indicate that programming alters the rate at which the brain ages. We have seen how dietary restriction during prenatal development shortens the life span of rats while restriction immediately after birth results in increased longevity. The mechanism may be connected with that ability of prenatal stress to program lifelong increased activity of the adrenal stress system. When the level of adrenal steroid activity is increased, the brain ages faster. Stress in the immediate postnatal period appears to have the opposite effect, resulting in a decrease in the level of activity of the hypothalamus, pituitary gland and adrenal gland in later life. As a result, the brain ages at a slower rate. So much for the "slings and arrows of outrageous fortune." They even determine what's going on in our heads.

The hippocampus is very important in our memory processes. When we are young, memory is crucial to learning tasks and progressing in our developing relationship to the outside world. The hippocampus forms slowly over a lengthy period of time. In rats, the dentate gyrus develops relatively late and some of its neurons are even born postnatally. The hippocampus is particularly involved in spatial learning and memory; it plays a role in matching what is expected with what actually happens. The hippocampus is important in putting events in one's life in the context of previous events remembered. Thus, anything that disrupts normal hippocampal development will likely have marked effects on brain function that will determine our emotional responses, memory and intelligence.

Fetal Attempts to Spare The Brain in Times Of Adverse Challenges: Brain-Sparing Is Not Total

We have seen how competently the fetus responds to many challenges posed by suboptimal conditions in the uterus. However, we should not assume that these clever responses come without a price. As in so many other activities in our lives, we pay now or we pay later. Fetuses exposed to suboptimal conditions in the womb attempt to spare their brains at the expense of the rest of their bodies. It is important to realize two things. Because there is an overall shortage, some tissues in other parts of the body pay the price for these attempts to spare the developing brain. Also, brain sparing in times of adversity is not complete. The sparing of the brain should only be considered as relative to other organs like the liver that suffer much more. The extent to which fetuses can protect their brains depends on the nature and extent of the challenge, as well as past events during development. In experimental studies it is possible to reduce the amount of oxygen available to a fetal sheep in the uterus in several different ways. First, if the mother breathes less oxygen, there will be less oxygen circulating in her blood going to the placenta. Also, there are experimental ways to lower the amount of maternal blood going to the placenta; this also results in less oxygen being available to the fetus. Finally, we can decrease the amount of blood flowing in the umbilical cord to the placenta with the result that the less fetal blood reaches the placenta to carry oxygen back from the placenta to the fetus. In each of these situations, fetuses respond by increasing their blood flow to the brain at the expense of other organs in the body like the skin, muscle and liver. However, when the concentration of oxygen in the fetal blood falls significantly, the total amount of oxygen available to the brain will be decreased, regardless of how hard the fetus tries to compensate. When oxygen and nutrient deficiency is marked, the developing brain begins to suffer, and nerve cells may not develop properly.

Studies on the fetus in a large number of species show that the brain does pay a price for nutritional deprivation. In one study in sheep, when one group of pregnant ewes was undernourished both before conception and until the end of the first month after conception, as might be expected, their fetal lambs were growth-retarded, but their brain weights were protected. In a second group of ewes undernourished for ten days in late pregnancy, fetuses were also of low body weight but again, their brain weights were protected. However, brain weight was reduced in fetuses whose mothers were exposed to both the early and the late under-nutrition. Neither period of maternal undernutrition by itself was enough of an insult to alter brain weight. However, early maternal nutritional compromise rendered the fetal brain susceptible to damage by the second insult. This study clearly shows that fetal development is a continuum, and nutritional and other events at one stage interact with challenges at other stages of development.

Nutritional Challenges and Brain Development

Undernutrition is a stress to the mother. As a result, the amount of adrenal steroids circulating in her blood will rise. Feeding a diet in which the amount of protein was cut in half during pregnancy in the rat results in the growth of a small placenta. This small placenta is not able to protect the fetus from passage of adrenal steroids from mother to fetus. We have seen on several occasions how increased passage of steroids across the placenta from mother to fetus is able to program the developing fetal cardiovascular and hormone systems. Dr. Simon Langley Evans from Southampton in England also noticed that the brains of the fetal rats whose mothers were protein-deprived showed multiple enzyme abnormalities in the hippocampus and hypothalamus. When studied at four weeks of age, the rats who had been exposed to protein deficiency as fetuses had abnormal twenty-four-hour rhythms in their secretion of ACTH, the hormone that drives the adrenal gland to secrete its steroid hormones. In humans, abnormal rhythms and levels of activity of the brain adrenal axis are related to depression and other long-term neurological problems.

Impaired brain development as a result of suboptimal maternal nutrition can be passed down across the generations. Female rats exposed to undernutrition when they themselves were fetuses give birth to pups whose brain weight and cell number is reduced. One study conducted twenty years ago examined the short-term and long-term effects of maintaining pregnant rats on either adequate dietary protein or a marginally deficient protein diet for thirteen generations. Pups born in the malnourished colony were ten times more likely to be growth retarded and their brains were about 5 percent smaller. Some parts, such as the cerebellum which controls fine movement and balance, was as much as 10 percent smaller. The words the authors use to summarize their findings are alarming in the extreme to those who study aberrant behavior and learning difficulties in young children. "The young malnourished rats showed increased exploratory behavior, transient head tremors and an increased sensitivity to noise, the latter being long-lasting if not permanent. When adult, they showed marked differences in behavior and learning patterns and it was difficult to attract and hold their attention. In situations demanding a choice the animals were very excited, emitted loud squeals and tried to escape from what was clearly a stressful situation. However, a casual examination of the malnourished adults revealed a rather small, badly groomed, excitable rat without gross abnormalities."

The study cannot separate the effects of low protein in the mother's diet during pregnancy from the effects later in life because at weaning, the rat pups were put on the same low-protein diet given to their mothers. It is likely that the quality of their mother's milk was also poorer than control animals given a normal diet. However, the study does highlight the effects of chronic malnutrition on the group receiving the poor-protein diet. Also, since the unwanted effects on the nervous system showed early in life, it is quite clear that the adverse and suboptimal conditions in the womb played at least a part in the abnormal brain and behavioral function.

After thirteen generations of a poor-protein diet, the investigators carried out a study to see how quickly they could rehabilitate the growth-retarded rats. Here, their experimental design was able to evaluate the role of poor conditions in the womb. Female rats from a colony that had been exposed to ten to twelve generations of low-protein diet were fed a normal diet during pregnancy, and there were pups compared with a second group of pups whose mothers were fed the normal diet from after delivery. A third group of pups were

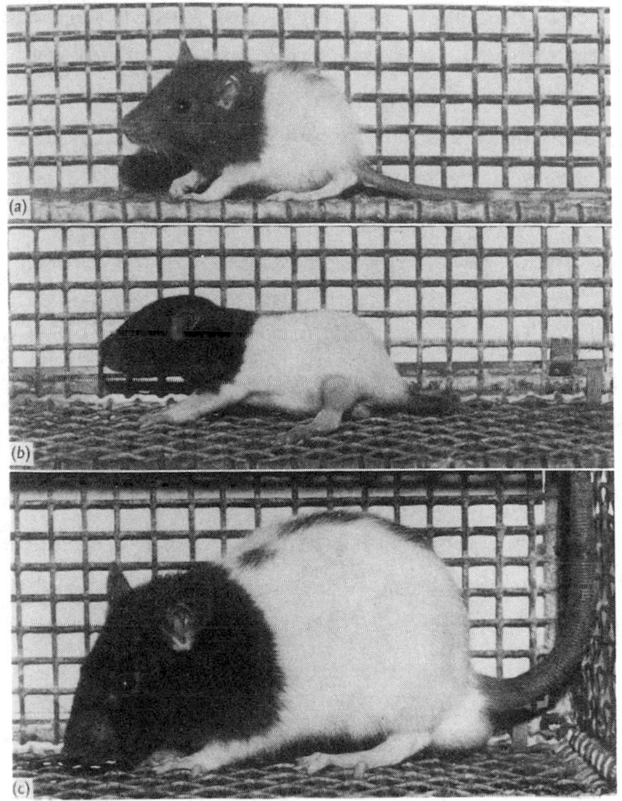

FIGURE 9.3

The upper panel shows a forty-two-day-old rat from the colony exposed to a low protein diet; middle panel: a twelve-day-old rat from the normal colony—it is the same size as the forty-two-day-old rat from the poorly nourished colony; lower panel: a forty-two-day-old rat from the normal colony.

rehabilitated from four weeks of age. The pups who were already four weeks old before they were given the normal diet showed no improvement in their growth, behavior or learning ability. In contrast, the pups whose mothers were well fed throughout pregnancy not only improved but eventually overgrew the normal pups by nearly 20 percent in weight. This finding is not surprising. Here again we see the effect of a sudden return to normal diet in a situation in which mother and fetus had been programmed over several generations to adapt and compensate for a suboptimal pregnancy situation. The colony of rats was so well adapted to times of deficiency that in times of excess, the fetus was able to grow faster than normal.

However, tests of learning ability showed that the pups who had been rehabilitated in the womb, while performing better than those rehabilitated at four weeks of age, still learned more slowly than the pups of mothers from the group that had received an adequate protein diet over the previous twelve generations. Rehabilitation of fetuses prenatally for a total of three generations completely corrected growth and behavior, but the offspring still had a residual learning deficit.

It is not surprising that malnutrition before birth carries a major price. But there is a second, even more critical message for society in this study. It reminds us that we should not expect all of the consequences of previous deprivation to be put right at once within one generation.

Intrauterine Hugs: I Love You, Baby

Studies have shown that in species as different as sheep, rats, guinea pigs, monkeys, baboons and cows the uterus contracts periodically throughout pregnancy. These bursts of uterine muscle activity are called *contractures* to distinguish them from labor and delivery *contractions*. Contractures are much weaker than the contractions of labor. In addition, contractions last less than a minute while contractures last several minutes. Throughout pregnancy in sheep, a contracture occurs about every half hour and lasts three to fifteen minutes. Contractures are likely to be the same events that many women feel throughout late pregnancy. In pregnant women they are often called Braxton Hicks contractions after the British physician, John Braxton Hicks, who first described them in 1872.

This type of spontaneous activity is very common in muscle of the nonvoluntary type that makes up the uterus. Unlike voluntary muscles, which need a constant stream of instructions from nerves, the involuntary muscles of the gut, the heart and the uterus will continue to contract without any outside influences from nerves. The nerves to the heart can slow down or speed the rate at which our hearts beat, but the heart is totally able to beat at its own appointed steady rhythm without the need of any help from the nerves. If this were not so, transplanted hearts would not function in the recipient. When a heart is transplanted, the nerves to the heart cannot be removed from the donor and transplanted with the heart, and the recipient's nerves are not able to regenerate and connect up with the heart muscle fibers.

In late pregnancy, as the amount of amniotic fluid decreases, the fetus comes more and more into contact with the wall of the uterus. She is no longer swimming in a private pool of fluid. Her situation is more like someone in a narrow bath, shoulders and hips touching the sides. As a result, contractures squeeze the fetus at the points of contact. Measurements made during a contracture in late pregnancy show that the dimensions of the fetal lamb's chest can decrease by as much as a third. A contracture is quite an experience for the fetus. My friend Tom Kirschbaum calls contractures "intrauterine hugs."

The Importance of Sensory Stimulation and Good Prenatal Sleep

Sleep states and behavioral changes can be studied in the human fetus using the ultrasound machine and, in a wide variety of animal fetuses, using much more sophisticated techniques. The study of fetal behavior in the uterus provides very important information that can be evaluated in relation to the work of pioneers of study of behavior in the newborn period such as T. Berry Brazelton. The baby is born with well-developed behavior patterns that have been maturing over the last ten weeks of fetal life and are more and more like the newborn baby's behavior as birth approaches. These periods of changing behavior are likely to be critical to the activity-dependent maturation of the brain. It appears that sleep states gradually change in the uterus in late pregnancy as the fetus prepares for the world outside. Every mother hopes that her baby will develop a good,

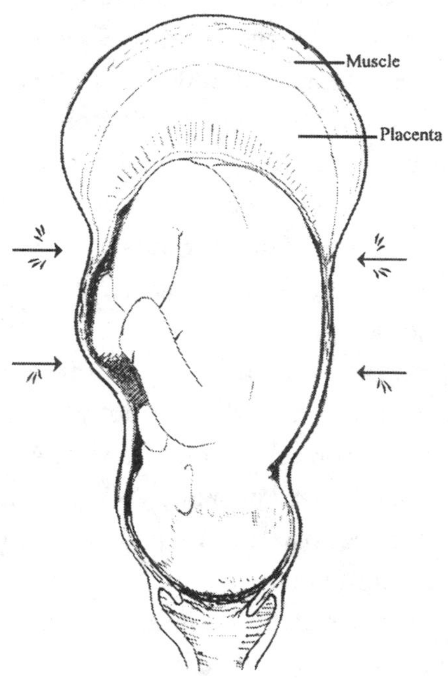

FIGURE 9.4

Contractures of the womb give the baby a hug and a squeeze.

regular sleeping pattern. When a newborn baby has regular sleeping patterns, it certainly makes mother's life easier. Correct alternation of sleep and wakefulness is of critical importance to normal brain function after birth. It is certainly of great importance during development.

Throughout life in the womb, the fetus is subjected to many influences. Sound penetrates the uterus easily, especially low-frequency sound in the frequency range of the father's voice. Although there are elegant studies that demonstrate the various sound patterns that reach the ears of fetal sheep in the womb, there is no evidence that the fetus can learn while still in the womb. This has not stopped several unscrupulous companies from selling tapes to strap to the belly of the pregnant woman so that the environment of her fetus can be enriched. Studies by Dr. Peter Hepper in Belfast, Ireland, have shown that newborn babies will change their heart rates when they hear tunes that their mothers listened to frequently throughout pregnancy. However, the newborn baby very quickly forgets these tunes and the heart rate change is lost very quickly. I have been approached for an endorsement of the learning value of prenatal sound stimulation by more than one company that sells tapes to strap to the pregnant mother's abdomen to stimulate the baby and speed up mental development before birth. I know of no evidence that this type of external stimulation will have a lasting effect on the fetal brain. There might even be a possibility of brain damage if the sound is too loud or prolonged. Fetuses need sleep, so waking them up with sound at inappropriate times may be a harmful event. We just do not know enough to make any firm statements about prenatal learning.

Contractures stimulate the fetus by squeezing him. Very often, when a contracture starts, the fetus alters several forms of activity. In one study in late pregnancy in sheep, altering the contracture pattern of the uterus altered the development of fetal brain waves and increased the rate at which the levels of cortisol rose in fetal blood. Cortisol is normally rising at this phase of pregnancy in fetal sheep and we do not yet know the consequences—good, bad or indifferent—of a faster rate of rise of the level of cortisol in the blood of the fetal sheep at this stage of development. We do know that cortisol plays a key role in the preparation of the lung for air breathing, in preparing the fetal kidney to take care of the baby's urine production and readying the baby's gut to allow her to digest the foods she never received when she was in the womb. We have seen in chapter 6 that changes in adrenal activity before birth produce long-term effects that are very different from the programming that occurs when the rat experiences stress after birth. Even the effects after birth are different according to the nature of the stimulus; stress of infection compared with handling, for instance. Handling even has different effects if it is short-term or long-term, frequent or infrequent. But the effects are there and need to be characterized and understood so we can help children and adults with mood disorders. The help needed is both preventive and restorative.

Contractures also decrease the amount of blood flowing through the wall of the uterus to reach the placenta. As the uterus contracts, it squeezes the uterine arteries and slows the flow of blood through them. As the blood flow to the placenta falls, the delivery of oxygen to the baby decreases a little. In normal pregnancy, this fall is no threat to the baby. In fact, just as you and I like a change in our surroundings every now and then, a little variety, the changing oxygen climate in the baby's blood probably plays a good role in toning up the baby. In any event, we do know that the baby experiences that a contracture has occurred. How can we be so sure of that? Recording directly from the fetal sheep shows that if the fetal sheep is in a period of REM sleep when a contracture occurs, the fetus switches out of REM sleep. This change in fetal behavior tells us that the baby's brain registered what was going on and changed the level of its brain activity.

SCHIZOPHRENIA

Some researchers claimed to have discovered the gene responsible for schizophrenia in 1988. That claim is now discounted. The controversy has been rekindled by recent reports of links of schizophrenia with genes on chromosomes 6, 9 and 20. Only time will tell whether these more recent linkages of genes to schizophrenia are any more secure than the 1988 report. One of the major problems with genetic linkage studies is that researchers focus very sharply on close family members of affected individuals. As a result, linkage of genes between the individuals studied is inevitably going to be high. Given the complexity of the condition, the causes of schizophrenia will require much more study before the full story is understood. If there is a genetic component in schizophrenia, it is important to evaluate the strength of that component in relation to prenatal and postnatal environmental factors that bring out the susceptibility to the disease. One of the recent studies only claims that the genetic linkage they have demonstrated underlies 15 to 30 percent of the schizophrenia cases in the families studied.

There is a difference in the age at which schizophrenia manifests itself in the two sexes. Male onset is earlier than female. Thus, sex hormone changes at critical times during development may bring out a tendency to schizophrenia later in life.

The use of magnetic resonance imaging shows that the area of the brain known as Broca's area is activated when a schizophrenic hears voices. We use Broca's area in our brains when we are producing inner speech such as when we rehearse a public presentation silently to ourselves. The problem for schizophrenics is that they do not understand that their own brain is initiating the activity. Instead, schizophrenics think that the voice they hear belongs to someone else. It appears that schizophrenics have lost the normal connections between the different language areas of their brains. The siring, wiring and now the firing of nerve cells in the brain have gone wrong.

Much evidence clearly indicates that schizophrenia is a developmental disease that is markedly affected by conditions experienced by the fetus before birth. In schizophrenics, brain size is about 2 percent lower than normal. At birth, head circumference is significantly smaller in babies who will eventually develop schizophrenia. To compensate for this decreased size, there is an increase in the amount of the fluid around the brain. The corpus callosum, the major collection of fibers that connects one side of the cerebral cortex to the other, is thinner in schizophrenics, and the hippocampus can be smaller by as much as 15 percent.

One of the most interesting theories about the cause of schizophrenia relates the incidence of the condition to viral infections such as influenza during pregnancy. According to epidemiologic studies, more babies born in late spring and early summer will suffer from schizophrenia than babies born at other times of the year. Mothers who spent the early months of their pregnancy in the winter months are more exposed to winter viral infections. Schizophrenia is also more common in children born in late spring and early summer in years following winters of high incidence of influenza than in years following winters in which influenza incidence was lower. One of the leading world authorities on schizophrenia told me that he originally laughed at this suggestion of a connection between schizophrenia and viral infection. He thought it was rubbish. But studies in England and Wales of data collected over a period of eighty-eight years convinced him of a very high correlation. Once again, though, we must not confuse correlation with causation.

Thus schizophrenia has been thought by some to be a good example of the worst form of programming, doom from the womb. According to others, adverse conditions later in life bring out a predisposition. As we have seen time and time again, there is no real dichotomy here. Both early and late influences may be active. The brain changes caused by prenatal events, both genetic and environmental, may set the stage for schizophrenia to occur if the conditions in the environment precipitate the condition. If infection is involved, we might conjecture—and supposition is all it would be—that the high incidence of schizophrenia that supposedly occurred in the Middle Ages might have been due a rampant viral infection caused by lack of hygiene. The picture of the village idiot or madman that has come down from preindustrial times has many of the hallmarks of schizophrenia. There is certainly an enormous mythology relating to schizophrenia. At least we now have methods like magnetic resonance imaging to look into the brain at times when a schizophrenic experiences the symptoms of the disease and so begin to learn about its physical basis.

The concept that the seeds of schizophrenia and other forms of mental disease are in our genes is strongly imprinted in our minds. In literature and common folklore there is an abundance of anecdotes that mental illness tends to run in families. If, for a moment, we accept this notion, we must again recall that the family is an environmental unit just as it is a genetic unit. We must remind ourselves that a congenital condition, something that we are born with, does not necessarily mean it is solely genetically inherited. So, it is no surprise that researchers continue to haggle over the degree to which inheritance is responsible for complex conditions such as schizophrenia. Mental illnesses are notoriously problematic to classify precisely, and hence the diagnosis of each case is difficult. In fact, the very variability of many mental illnesses argues against a single cause. It is easy enough for a medical textbook to define a condition precisely. It is less easy to place a particular individual affected by the condition into a box narrowly defined by a book.

The Bell Curve Revisited: The Interplay of Nature and Nurture in Determining IQ

In the preface to *The Bell Curve: Intelligence and Class Structure in American Life*, Herrnstein and Murray describe the division of our society into economic haves and have-nots. To any student of history, this division is not a new social phenomenon. Such divisions have been present in every past human society. Feudal lords hunted with their hawks and addressed themselves to "the lascivious pleasing of the lute," while their poverty-ridden peasants provided them with the best food available. Mayan priests enjoyed the good things of life while the peasants toiled in the fields to deliver the bounty for sustenance of the priesthood. Social stratification and economic exploitation was the bedrock of slavery in America and remains so in the sweat shops of modern-day Asia.

Herrnstein and Murray lay the explanation for this stratification at the door of genetic differences in intelligence. Their claim that the most intelligent and the best connected get accepted at better schools and colleges, go on to better-paying jobs and end up with more control over their lives cannot be refuted. However, the claim that the intelligence to be successful is the restricted attribute of an intellectual elite with a definable genetic endowment merits very close inspection of the biological origin and basis of intelligence. The concept that the recipe for success lies almost completely in genetic inheritance of IQ ignores the interplay of nature and nurture. Genes clearly are a major determinant of the function of the brain, and functional capacity of the brain has a lot to do with intelligence. However, very little is known about the connection between brain function and intelligence other than the certain knowledge that myriad factors are involved. I would contend that one major dimension is missing from the extensive discussion that has dogged this controversial book since publication in 1994. Neither the book nor any of the review articles about the book that I have read have evaluated the role of the quality of development during prenatal life on intelligence. In all the discussions about nutrition, heritability and other influences on intelligence in *The Bell Curve,* there is virtually nothing said or written on the role played by the conditions to which each of us is exposed during prenatal life.

Congress has designated the 1990s the decade of the brain. Enormous advances are being made almost daily in our knowledge of how the brain works, but the fundamental factors that determine the many features of intelligence still elude analysis. Intelligence is not a single characteristic. There are many forms of intelligence; different brain components are used in the performance of quantitative, visual and verbal tasks. The factors that regulate development of these functions and how they interact are poorly understood. The existence of idiot savants who can listen to a lengthy piece of music for the first time and then replay it without error, note for note, but who cannot perform the simplest of day-to-day tasks, leaves everyone searching for a working definition of intelligence.

Herrnstein and Murray's argument has been exposed time and time again as being unsupported by facts. Indeed Herrnstein and Murray acknowledged that correlation between two characteristics is just that: a correlation. We must continually remind ourselves not to confuse correlation and causation; the very best epidemiologists such as David Barker constantly warn us of this danger. Cause and effect can only be definitively proven by controlled scientific studies in which the putative cause is changed (preferably in a graded fashion) while all other factors in the environment remain unchanged. If a causal link truly exists, these studies will show a graded change in response as we change the suspected causative factor in a graded fashion. Given the complexity and continuously changing nature of human society, such a controlled study of the proportional regulation of intelligence by nature (the genes) and nurture (the environment) is immensely difficult and may even be impossible in any given human population. The data in *The Bell Curve* do nothing to get at the fundamental issue: the relative contributions of nature and nurture.

To arrive at that synthesis, we must bolster epidemiologic data with carefully controlled animal studies.

Let us look at some of the comments that Herrnstein and Murray make.

"To try to come to grips with the nation's problems without understanding the role of intelligence (in succeeding in life) is to see through a glass darkly indeed, to grope with symptoms instead of causes, to stumble into supposed remedies that have no chance of working." Agreed. To attempt to treat the disease without knowing the cause is not the best way to proceed. But what are the critical causative factors that mold intelligence? The statement that intelligence is needed to succeed in life is like saying that we cannot survive for very long without water to drink and an even shorter time without oxygen. This all-embracing truism advances our knowledge of the underlying biological basis of intelligence very little. To then turn around and very subtly tell us that everyone who has not succeeded in life is *by definition* unintelligent is like saying that the poor benighted English must always live with cricket and can never enjoy baseball. It ignores the fact that the British have never really had the opportunity to play baseball or even to see it played well. Earlier this century, the British might have scoffed at the soccer capabilities of the Dutch, Germans, Italians, French and Brazilians. Any fan knows that British soccer teams now lose more frequently to these latecomers than they defeat them.

The insidious suggestion of Herrnstein and Murray's core argument is that we should all accept the overwhelming—if not even complete—role of genes in determining the potential intelligence of an individual. This conclusion is not supported by the biological evidence currently available. We must not discount the enormous effect of the environment, before and after birth, in modifying the genetic protomap. Consideration of prenatal environmental factors is almost totally ignored in *The Bell Curve*. In the thirty-page chapter on parenting, the section "Maternal IQ and Well-Being of Infants" totals just four and a half pages: prenatal care is given just half a page, low birthweight merits two pages and infant mortality only a page.

The central theme of *The Bell Curve* is an important half- truth. This is the book's terrible danger: half-truths are often more difficult to combat than clear, outright lies. The half of their thesis that is true is that intelligence is important in determining success in life. The half that is not true is that how an individual is likely to perform in society is completely—or even mostly—determined by their genes.

In the chapter entitled "Steeper Ladders, Narrower Gates," Herrnstein and Murray do discuss the portion of intelligence that is inherited. Intelligence as a whole (whatever that may mean) is given a value of 1.0. Thus, if heritability is 0.5, then 50 percent of intelligence is inherited, due to the genes, and 50 percent is the result of the environment. I want to look first at how these fractions are calculated and then at what exactly they mean in relation to the importance of prenatal life.

The classical method of determining the heritability of any characteristic in contrast to the effect of the environment has been to compare the intelligence of related individuals. The closeness of the relationship determines the proportion of their genes that the individuals share. Thus, identical twins have exactly the same genes. As a consequence, investigators attribute differences in their eventual size, abilities and intelligence to factors in the environment. It is here that we see the first gaping hole in the authors' calculations of heritability. I quote Herrnstein and Murray: "Except for the effects on their IQs of the shared uterine environment, their IQ correlation directly estimates heritability." What a small word is *except*. We have already considered the weakness of the identical twin approach. Although identical twins coexist in the same uterus, it is very unlikely that they obtain exactly the same amounts of nutrients and oxygen. As we have seen already, the relative amounts of the single placenta shared by the two fetuses may be very different. Identical twins rarely have the same dimensions at birth.

Herrnstein and Murray continue: "The most modern study of identical twins reared in separate homes suggests a heritability for general intelligence between 0.75 and 0.8, a value near the top of the range found in the contemporary technical literature." Now comes the information that should have been discussed in depth because it shows that the *environment*, not *heredity*, plays the major role in determining intelligence. "Other direct estimates use data on ordinary siblings who were raised apart or on parents and their adopted-away children. Usually, the heritability estimates from such data are lower but rarely below 0.4." So it seems that some of the studies suggest that just 40 percent of intelligence is determined by heritability and the larger portion, 60 percent, by the environment, including the prenatal environment when all the nerve cells vital to intelligence are getting their act together.

There are so many logical flaws in the arguments put forward by Herrnstein and Murray that arise because the arguments are circular and self-serving. They would have us believe that we cannot improve the divisive distribution of intelligence in society by improving the environment. "This . . . point is especially important in the modern societies, with their intense efforts to equalize opportunity. As a general rule, as environments become more uniform, heritability rises. When heritability rises, children resemble their parents more . . ." They are saying that if you eliminate every effect of the environment, the only factors that will affect intelligence will be genetic, heritable factors. That banal, obvious conclusion does nothing to tell us how much of the currently existing difference is inherited. Unless we undertake human genetic engineering, the only way we can improve intelligence, or any other human characteristic, is by improving the environment, the nurture of our children. In order for any improvement to occur, we must understand the prenatal factors that affect the full expression of intelligence.

The authors of *The Bell Curve* fully believe that the majority of the factors that regulate intelligence are heritable. They prefer the estimates of 0.8 but concede that the data available to date would only permit an estimate somewhere between 0.4 and of 0.6. Let us leave aside the flaws in the calculations and accept for the moment the 0.6 factor. This means that 40 percent is due to environment. Moving the intelligence curve for the whole population up 40 percent certainly will not remove the disparity, but it can only help the disadvantaged. But what happens if the figures are wrong? The authors' failure to separate prenatal environmental effects from genetic effects is one good reason why the heritability figures may well be wrong.

Finally, what if the real figure is 40 percent of intelligence due to heritability, the figure that Herrnstein and Murray say is the lower one found in their nontwin studies? Then improving the environment will have a bigger effect on those of low intelligence. The authors do not note this consequence anywhere in their book. The authors prefer to state the consequences of dealing with the environment in the negative fashion. They say, "As environments become more uniform, heritability rises." So, if they are right and 60 percent of the difference in intelligence is due to the environment, equalizing the environment, although it does not remove the difference, leaves the difference as a smaller part of the whole. Herrnstein and Murray do no justice to their own intelligence by omitting to state this fact.

In conclusion, the current data put forward by Herrnstein and Murray stating that 0.4 to 0.8 (yes, the figures vary throughout the book) of intelligence is inherited is too wide a spread to close the discussion on whether modification of the environment will have any effect on human intelligence. For the developmental biologist the epidemiological, animal and clinical studies on the programming of organ function, heart, liver and the brain point strongly to a need to learn more about the long-term consequences for health and disease of prenatal life.

Sexual Differentiation: Brain and Behavior

Is there a relationship between the structure of the brain and sexual orientation? Few issues can be calculated to raise the temperature of debate more than this sex-related part of the nature-against-nurture debate. I have referred to the studies in newborn rats in which a very brief exposure of the female brain to male hormones can permanently condition the brain to function in a male fashion. The male hormone programs or imprints critical brain structures to function in the male fashion although the genetic makeup of the rat is female.

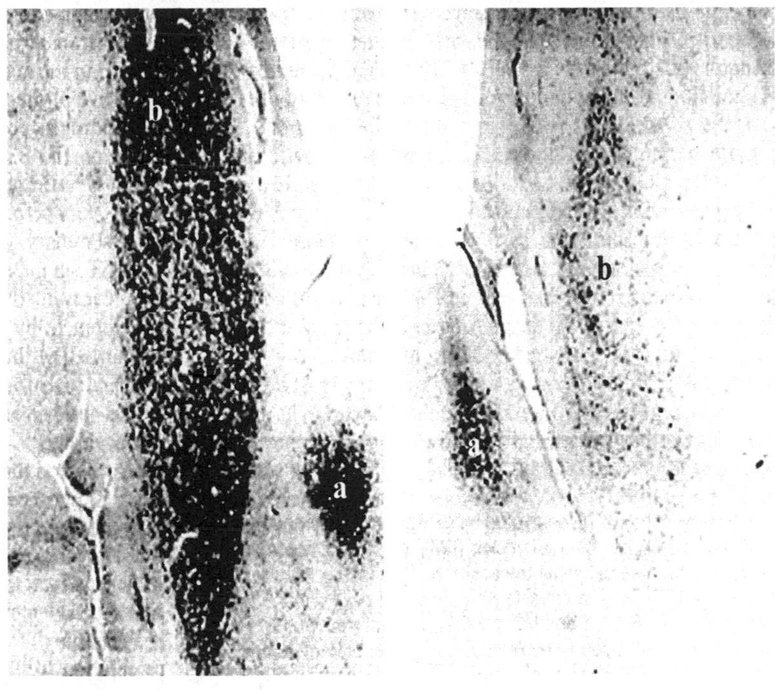

FIGURE 9.5

The structure of many brain areas differ between men and women. On the left is one of the groups of nerve cells in the hypothalamus in a male brain; on the right, the same group in a female brain. The nerve cells have been stained for their hormone vasoactive polypeptide. There are two subdivisions to this group of cells—a and b.

In humans, there are peaks of sex hormone production at three stages of development. The first occurs during the first half of fetal life, the second around the time of birth and the third at puberty. The major change in some of the collections of nerve cells in the hypothalamus that differ between males and females is not complete until four years of life and may be related to either of the first two peaks. The programming by the hormonal changes appears to take a long time to complete. We should not be surprised that the biology of sexual differentiation in humans is regulated by more protracted and complex mechanisms than observed in the rat. This difference follows from the fact that our brains are much more complex from the structural and functional viewpoint than the brains of rats.

Significant sex-related differences in the structure and function of the brain are described by some researchers and not by others. When a region is different in the two sexes, the region is said to be sexually dimorphic. This literally means that the region takes two forms, a female and a male form. One needs to be an expert to resolve the differences between various reports and the findings in various species. If we look at the causes of differences between research studies, what we find depends very much on the technology and approaches used in different laboratories.

First, we can differentiate nuclei in different regions of the brain by cell counts. This way we can demonstrate whether there are differences that might be present even if there is no difference in the size of the region. It is of course possible to have two collections of nerve cells that occupy the same amount of brain space but are composed of different numbers of cells. Again, we see that size is not everything. We need to know the exact number of cells in the different critical areas their interconnections to other nerve cells within the area and their functional connections to distant areas of the brain. Not all researchers who have commented on sexual differentiation of brain structures have counted the numbers of cells in the areas of interest. Counting cell numbers under a microscope is a tedious process, but it needs to be done.

The second way that we can show differences between collections of nerve cells is to use staining techniques to see if there are different signaling molecules in the nuclei in the two sexes. Dr. Dick Swaab and colleagues at the Netherlands Institute for Brain Research have shown that significant differences begin to appear between the male and female sexually dimorphic nuclei in the human brain around four years of age. There are no major changes in the sex hormones in males and females at this time. A surge in male hormones did take place at the time of birth, four years earlier. By puberty, the nuclei contain twice as many cells in males as in females. So some researchers think that that the surge in male sex hormones that took place at birth four years earlier protects the male brain from the programmed cell death that takes place in these structures at four years of age.

The critical question that many would like answered in a much more definitive fashion than currently possible is whether there are clear differences in the hypothalamus associated with homosexuality. Dr. Swaab has shown that there are marked differences in the suprachiasmatic nucleus in the brain of homosexuals with AIDS. The suprachiasmatic nucleus is the location of your internal clock. However, we do not know the significance of this difference in homosexual men. Was it caused by the AIDS virus? Was it the cause of the homosexuality, or was it a result of a homosexual lifestyle?

The central issue here is that we can see structural differences in the brains of homosexual men that differentiate them from heterosexual men. We do not know what is cause and what is effect. As in all areas of knowledge, there are factions who would interpret the findings to suit their feelings and preferences. To some, the fact that sexual preference appears from animal studies to be in large measure programmed is a reassurance. Many people consider that this view removes sexual orientation from the arena of guilt or undesirability. According to this school of thought, sexual preference is programmed, so there is nothing one could, or indeed should, do about it, and society must recognize a wide range of differences, just as society recognizes people of different heights and different physical capabilities.

The other school of thought would hold that sexual preference is just that, a preference controlled solely by our will. This is in many ways the more polarizing view in that it leads to two confrontational viewpoints. One group, who sees homosexual (gay or lesbian) behavior as abnormal, feels that if such behavior is a matter of choice, then those practicing it must bear the consequences of disapproval by those in society who believe homosexual behavior to be abnormal. Homosexuals who would believe that their behavior is totally a matter of choice may do so because to them is more pleasing to feel that they totally control their individual destiny. The truth probably lies somewhere in between. Dick Swaab has shown that collections of brain cells critical to gender identification are larger in males than in females and are smallest in transsexuals. This is the first indication that there are anatomical differences that relate to sexual preference rather than just plain sexual makeup (or the genetic complement). Only more research will give us the answers.

TEN

BORN TOO SOON, BORN TOO LATE

There are many events in the womb of time which will be delivered.

William Shakespeare, *Othello*

Events that occur as we are ushered into life are major influences in how we are ushered out of life. This connection between birth and death is particularly strong for those born prematurely. If all goes well in pregnancy, it is the fetus who decides that it is time to take on the challenges of the outside world. At the end of a normal pregnancy, the fetal adrenal gland secretes hormones that circulate in the fetal blood to the placenta and change placental function, starting off a cascade of events that leads to birth. These same fetal hormones play an equally important role in maturing many organ systems such as the lungs that the newborn baby will need to function competently in the world outside the womb. Babies born at the end of the full forty weeks of pregnancy have made all the necessary preparations in the correct sequence and at the correct time. In contrast, babies born prematurely may not yet be ready for the complex challenges posed by an independent life. If the fetus has inadequate time in the uterus before birth to prepare thoroughly for the great adventure of life, there can be long term consequences for health throughout life after birth.

Prematurity occurs in about 10 percent of all pregnancies but is the cause of 75 percent of infant deaths that occur during labor or in the first month of life. Prematurity is also a major cause of lifelong disability. Fifty percent of long-term handicap is related to prematurity. The major as yet unsolved challenges of prematurity are to anticipate, diagnose and prevent premature labor. Currently there are no well-accepted methods of anticipating which pregnant women will go into premature labor. This unfortunate weakness of modern medicine is due in large measure to a lack of understanding of the causes of both normal and premature labor. However, there is a growing body of knowledge that indicates that chronic infection in the reproductive tract is a major cause of prematurity. This close link between infection and premature birth may explain the increased incidence of prematurity in association with lower socioeconomic status in the United States and other countries.

The currently available methods for diagnosing, monitoring and treating women in premature labor are inadequate. This scenario of ignorance needs to be addressed by a concerted research effort. The economic benefits that will flow from decreasing the incidence of premature birth will be large and occur rapidly. There are two aspects of our lives that are vital to our health: the choice of our parents, especially our mothers, for the home they provide us in the womb, and the length of time we stay in the womb before we each journey out on our own personal adventure.

The Baby Normally Decides the Time to Be Born

Getting it right at the start is often the key to success in life. This is certainly true for choosing the time to be born. Studies in animal species such as sheep and monkeys in which the young are born at a mature stage of development have shown that the baby very cleverly controls the time of delivery, ensuring that she or he is adequately prepared for the great challenge that lies ahead. At the same time as babies mature the various systems needed for an independent existence, they send out hormonal signals to the placenta that play a central role in starting the birth process. In sheep, the signal is the steroid hormone cortisol, produced by the adrenal gland of the fetus.

The cortisol instructs the placenta to switch from producing progesterone to producing estrogen. As a result, the amount of progesterone in the mother's blood falls and the amount of estrogen rises. It is the baby who throws the switch for this very clever change in the placenta's function. Throughout pregnancy, progesterone has acted to quiet the muscle wall of the womb, thus helping pregnancy to continue. Estrogen, in contrast, stimulates the muscle to contract. Estrogen also powerfully recruits many other mechanisms that bring about rupture of the fetal membranes, and it causes the cervix to soften and dilate. So, very cleverly, the fetal lamb makes sure that at one and the same time, the block to labor is removed and the powerful stimulators of labor are produced in large amounts.

This self-promoting and independent activity of the fetus in determining the length of development he or she needs in the womb is cleverly linked to the maturation of the organs the newborn baby will need to survive after birth. In addition to telling the placenta to change its function, cortisol gives instructions to the fetal lungs, gut, kidneys and other organs to make detailed preparations for an independent existence after birth in the liver, lungs, gut, brain and kidneys. Therefore, under normal circumstances, when a baby is born after at least thirty-seven weeks of pregnancy, everything is ready and there is no mismatch between being delivered and being ready for life after birth. This is a very elegant and clever system.

In some ways, primates, including pregnant women, do not seem to be as clever as sheep. The levels of progesterone in the mother's blood do not fall at the end of pregnancy. There is no removal of the blocking action of progesterone at the end of pregnancy in any primate species studied. However, the fetal adrenal gland in monkeys and human babies secretes a large amount of a slightly different steroid hormone, androgen, in the last few weeks of pregnancy. This androgen circulates in the baby's blood and is converted by the placenta into estrogen. So, with respect to the rise in concentration of estrogen in the mother's blood, there is considerable similarity between the pregnant sheep, pregnant monkeys and pregnant women.

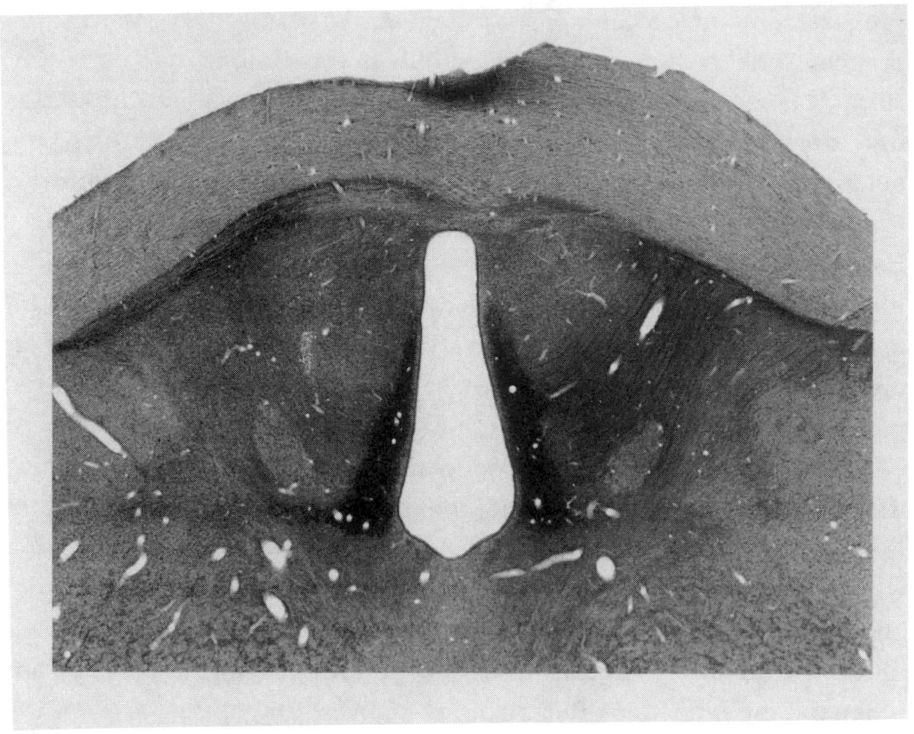

FIGURE 10.1

Nerve cells in the hypothalamus of the fetal sheep that send out the signal to begin the birth process lie on either side of the ventricle. The granules that contain the hormones involved are darkly stained with an antibody.

In order to understand the abnormal mechanisms of premature labor, we must first understand how normal labor occurs. Labor involves three main processes: biochemical changes that lead to the rupture of the membranes that surround the fetus; softening and dilatation of the cervix; and efficient, regular contraction of the uterine muscle. The same hormones and local factors within the uterus regulate these three processes. Not surprisingly, these processes are very closely linked, and for birth to be normal, they must proceed in step with each other to an orderly conclusion.

In every species studied, the uterus is not quiescent throughout pregnancy. Contractures are occurring at infrequent intervals. At the time of birth, contractures switch to contractions. In monkeys and baboons, the switch is very dramatic, occurring one night around the time darkness falls. Even more striking, on the first night that the switch from contractures-to-contractions occurs, contractions only last a few hours and then the muscle activity returns to the contractures mode throughout the following day. The contractures-to-contractions switch then repeats itself for several nights before birth. This is the normal progression that occurs at the end of a normal pregnancy. Often, a pregnant woman will not feel the nightly switch until the last night of her pregnancy when she is finally going to deliver.

There is no need to point out to women who have had children that it is most common to go into labor in the evening or the nighttime. This repeated nighttime switch has considerable value. First, it is a way of synchronizing the fetus to the outside world for a few days before birth. That way, the baby has some preliminary indication of the existence of a twenty-four hour day. The baby has been receiving other clues about the twenty-four hour day in the uterus for some time, but the effect on the baby of the powerful contractions are a last-minute reminder to get as much in synch with the mother as possible before birth. Good synchronization prepares babies for feeding and other activities they will perform with their mothers after birth.

The other significance of the repeated switch, increasing in intensity for several nights before delivery, is that it provides an opportunity for the fetus to perform more gradual preparations for the outside world than if the whole process takes place precipitously at one time. Immediately before delivery, the fetal head has to mold itself into the correct shape to go through the birth canal. The bones of the skull are still soft and can slide together to some extent. It would be advantageous to the baby to do this very gently over several days rather than rapidly and explosively in just one night. Indeed, in rapid and explosive deliveries there is always the possibility of hemorrhage into the baby's brain. To prevent damage to the baby's

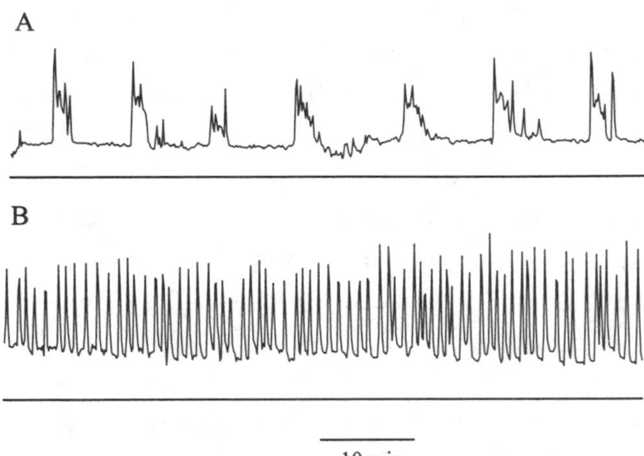

FIGURE 10.2

Electrical recording of (A) contractures and (B) contractions of the muscle layers of the womb.

head, the cervix must also be softened and dilated to allow the baby through. Correct softening and dilatation of the cervix are crucial to a normal delivery. These critical changes in the cervix are brought about by a gradual change in the hormones produced by the placenta as well as within the cervix itself.

Born Too Soon: Causes and Consequences of Premature Birth

When one or all of the three fundamental processes of labor begin early, the mother is in premature labor. Premature birth is unfortunately defined in two somewhat different ways. The most valuable method defines premature birth as birth before thirty-seven weeks of the normal forty weeks of pregnancy. Another definition is to consider the baby as premature if she or he is born weighing less than 2,500 grams (5.5 pounds). However, classifying babies as premature by size is misleading. It is possible for a baby to deliver at the right time but to be small because he or she is growth-retarded. Growth-retarded babies born after a pregnancy of normal length have

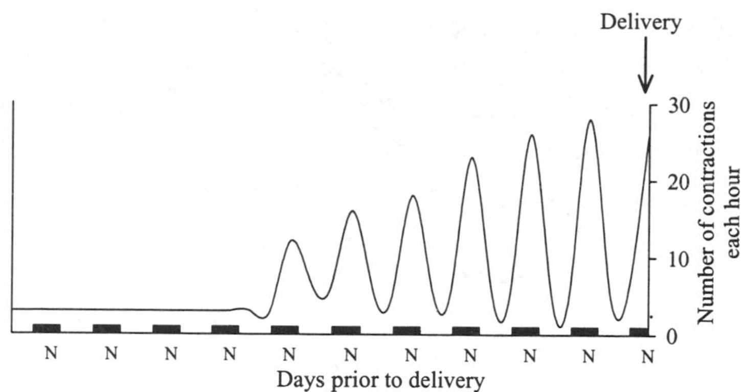

FIGURE 10.3

In pregnant monkeys, the switch from contractures to contractions is a nighttime event with more contractions occurring each night for several nights before birth occurs. This well-designed system results in a gradual preparation for birth. It is also the reason why labor most often begins in the evening.

their own mix of immediate and lifetime health problems that differ from the problems of prematurity.

In the United States and other industrialized countries, approximately 10 percent of babies are born prematurely. Since four million babies are born in the United States each year, that means about 400,000 babies are at risk. The unwanted consequences of premature birth are both short-term and long-term. This small proportion of babies born prematurely account for 75 percent of the babies who are born dead or die in the first month of life. Premature babies also account for 50 percent of all of long-term handicaps. Being born too soon adds significant problems to the early life of the baby. It is thus very important that the baby is given the best chance to make the right decision on the time to be born.

There are many causes of premature birth. It is therefore unfortunate that we use the same term for a variety of conditions. No one would consider fever to be a disease in itself. A high temperature is certainly a sign that not all is well, but it does not tell you the cause of the illness. The multiple nature of the origins of prematurity is a major reason why premature birth is so difficult to anticipate, diagnose and treat. Expectations of finding a drug that is a silver bullet able to stop all forms of premature birth are probably inappropriate because of the multiple causes. The treatment of premature labor will only be successful when the different processes that start premature labor are better understood. Obviously, prevention is better than cure. However, the multiple causes of premature labor pose as many difficulties when we try to develop strategies for prevention of prematurity.

Some causes of premature labor are better understood than others. Premature labor occurs with a greater than usual frequency in women carrying more than one fetus. The larger the number of fetuses, the greater the risk. The cause of the premature onset of contractions of the uterus when twins or triplets are present is quite easy to understand. It is stretch. Stretch unstabilizes the muscle of the wall of the uterus, tilting the balance away from the factors that maintain pregnancy toward those that tend to start labor. The more babies, the greater the stretch on the uterus and the more likely the uterus is to go into labor prematurely. This form of premature labor can be considered to be fairly normal. Rest and avoidance of stress will help pregnant women with multiple fetuses to carry their babies as long as possible. However, carrying quadruplets, quintuplets or even sextuplets is not a normal human reproductive pattern Twins only occur normally in 1 in 80 pregnancies, triplets roughly once in every 6,400 natural pregnancies. The modern explosion of multiple pregnancy and the associated increase in premature labor is almost entirely due to the assisted reproductive techniques that are being used in fertility clinics. The most famous multiple births are the McCaughey septuplets born in 1997 in Iowa, who are the first known set of sextuplets to have all survived the perils of early delivery. Their survival is a tribute to what has been learned about the changes babies undergo around the time of birth, developments in modern obstetric care and the skills of nurses and neonatologists in the neonatal intensive care unit, the NICU.

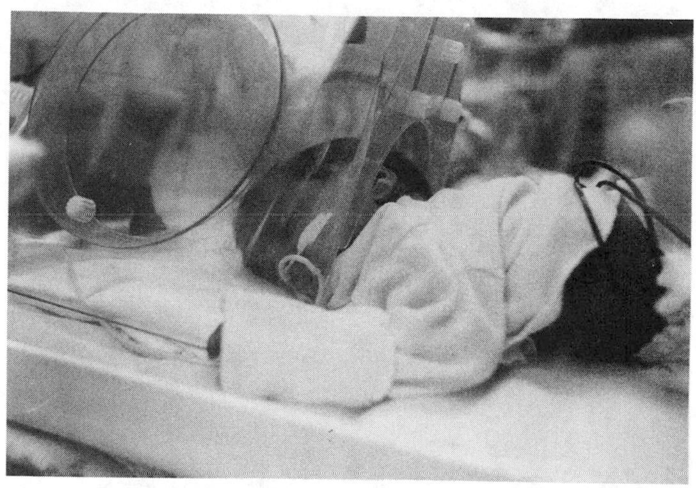

FIGURE 10.4

When a baby is born prematurely the Neonatal Intensive Care Unit must take the place of the womb.

In recent years it has become clear that there are at least two major causes of premature birth: maternal infection and stressful situations of different types. Infection in the vagina and uterine cavity can lead to premature labor in the period around twenty-four to thirty weeks of pregnancy. This view is strongly supported by evidence of infective organisms in the placenta and fetal membranes of women delivering at this stage of pregnancy. Bacterial vaginosis is the name given to the presence of abnormal numbers and varieties of bacteria in the vagina and reproductive tract. Bacteria may also be present in the amniotic fluid. Bacterial vaginosis may increase the likelihood of premature delivery by as much as 40 percent.

Some experts are of the opinion that women who eventually go into premature labor may have this type of low-grade infection even before pregnancy starts. Bacteria can produce powerful chemicals that stimulate responses in the defending white cells in the uterus and throughout the body. Some of these defense systems are very similar to the mechanisms used at the end of pregnancy to rupture

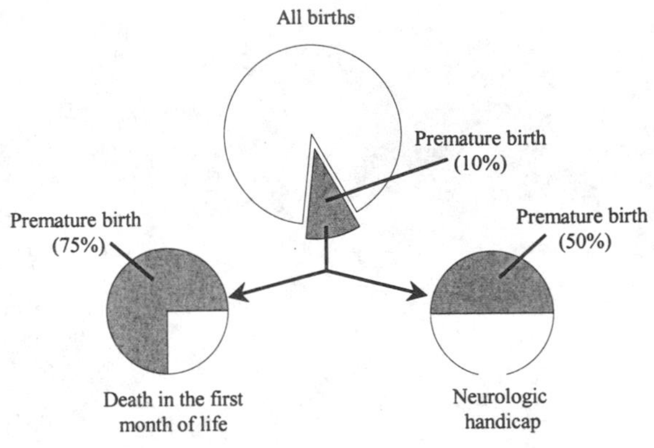

FIGURE 10.5

Only about 10 percent of births occur prematurely, but this 10 percent of all births accounts for 75 percent of early deaths and 50 percent of long-term handicaps.

the fetal membranes, convert contractures to contractions and dilate the cervix. This link of infection to premature birth is a major area of current research. Very interestingly, recent studies have even shown that pregnant women with dental infections and gum disease also have a higher incidence of premature delivery. So the bacterium does not need to be in the uterus or even nearby to cause trouble.

There are several valuable lessons to be learned from this recent research. First, maternal health and resistance to infection *before* pregnancy is a key factor in preventing premature birth. Secondly, some preliminary attempts to treat premature labor with antibiotics have shown some promise. Antibiotic treatment of premature labor due to infection also decreases the likelihood that the newborn baby will be infected during delivery. In one study, antibiotic treatment reduced premature delivery by over one-third. This encouraging approach shows just how important it is to understand a condition in order to start rational methods of prevention and treatment. The idea that many instances of prematurity may be due to infection is somewhat reminiscent of the gastric ulcer and helicobacter story described in chapter 7. Forty years ago, the surgeons who were removing large parts of the stomach to treat gastric ulcers would have scoffed at a suggestion that they should have looked for a simple bacterium.

Cigarette smoking is associated with gum disease since smoking impairs the ability of the normal defense mechanisms in the mouth to kill bacteria. In addition, smokers often have poorer nutrition that can lead to a decreased resistance to infection. So the adverse effects of poor oral hygiene is another whammy delivered by the tobacco industry to the poor fetus. It must be said that the level of association of cigarette smoking with premature birth is low. Smoking only increases the likelihood of premature birth by about 25 percent. Did I really say only 25 percent? Twenty-five percent of the babies born prematurely in the United States adds up to 100,000 premature babies. Smoking damages blood vessels, and there is a feeling among some researchers that decreased blood flow to the uterus may also play a role in setting the stage for premature birth. So again, smoking is not good news. Smoking is sadly increasing in young people, especially teenage girls, and may be one of the factors why prematurity is higher in adolescent pregnancy.

The premature birth of babies born after only thirty to thirty-five weeks of pregnancy is now thought to result from the baby's stress responses to insufficient nutrients or other key factors such as oxygen. We have seen that stressed fetuses increase the activity of their adrenal glands, the very glands that make the preparations for birth at the end of a pregnancy of normal length. These babies may be giving signals to get on with the preparations for the birth process early because things are getting a little stressful inside, and they think that it may well be better out than in. These stressed babies may be the babies Bill Cosby was considering in his comedy act I mentioned right at the beginning of chapter 1. Recently, researchers in Australia have suggested that the baby monitors food resources available in the womb. They suggest that when food supplies begin to run short, the baby sends out a "Let's get on with it," signal. The baby's start signal may play a role in both normal labor and this form of premature labor.

Maternal stress may also set in motion endocrine changes that start premature labor. Major life events such as death or loss of a partner or close family member, loss of employment, poor home conditions, economic worries of single-parent mothers and other forms of elevated psychological stress with no apparent resolution in sight can all increase the level of activity of the maternal stress systems. Although it is unclear which factors are directly responsible, we do know that even under normal circumstances, the maternal adrenal gland produces about a third of the androgen hormones the placenta uses to make estrogens. The other two thirds of the androgens come from the baby's own adrenal gland. Any stress related increase in maternal androgen production will lead to increased estrogen production. There are several studies that show that some forms of premature labor are accompanied by a rise in estrogens circulating in the mother's blood.

In premature labor, the muscle of the uterus switches from the contractures to contractions mode prematurely. However, the progression of premature labor will differ from case to case. Each instance of premature labor will require different methods of diagnosis and treatment, according to its cause. Each pregnant woman in premature labor provides the obstetrician with unique problems. The challenge of monitoring the activity of the uterine muscle is to precisely define the patterns and strength of uterine muscle contraction throughout the whole day and night. While this type of recording can be made in animal studies using sensors directly attached to the muscle wall of the uterus, equally sensitive techniques are not available for use in pregnant women. How do we identify the patient at risk for premature labor, and having identified her, how do we monitor her progress? If we cannot diagnose, we cannot treat. The current inability to accurately monitor the course of premature labor at all times of the day is a great limitation in the attempts to decrease the incidence of prematurity.

It is very difficult to treat a disease if the cause is unknown. While progress has been made in understanding the role of infection and stress in precipitating premature delivery, much more needs to be discovered before we even understand the many cellular processes that combine to produce normal delivery. Then we need to try to understand how pathological processes such as infection activate some parts of the system prematurely. Because the birth process is so important for the survival of the species, nature has developed a number of interlocking and often redundant processes that are progressively recruited to ensure that, once started, the birth process goes through to completion as rapidly as possible. If not caught very early, this formidable array of self-supporting and enhancing systems is difficult to stop. That is the way it was designed, to come to completion effectively and rapidly once started.

Deficiencies to Which the Premature Baby Is Exposed: Lungs, Gut, Kidneys

Neonatologists are pediatricians who look after very small babies, some born as early as twenty-four weeks of pregnancy. The last twenty years has greatly advanced our knowledge of the needs of the very small baby who has prematurely left the safety of the womb. As a result of studies conducted in fetal sheep by Sir Graham Liggins, we now know that treating women in premature labor with a synthetic form of the adrenal steroid hormone cortisol will accelerate the maturation of the fetal lungs. As a result, a premature baby will be more able to breathe adequately and survive. Treatment only needs to last as little as two days before birth. The steroids stimulate the production of the surface active compounds that help to keep the little balloonlike air sacs in the premature baby's lungs.

Prematurely delivered babies have not had time to complete their preparations for independence. Shakespeare has King Richard the Third attribute his bodily deformities to the fact that he was "brought before my time into this breathing world scarce half made up." Premature babies have not yet developed their lungs, gut or kidneys completely, and neonatologists and nurses in the intensive care unit must exercise their knowledge to tide these precious and precociously delivered babies over until their essential organ systems function fully.

The ability of the premature human baby to survive at 60 percent of the normal length of pregnancy, twenty-four weeks of a normal forty week pregnancy, is truly remarkable, compared with babies born at this stage of development in other species. In one way, this ability to overcome a shortening of the stay in the uterus attests to the toughness of the human race. In another, it may be a disadvantage. At very early stages of development, this overall resilience of the body may not be exactly paralleled by the ability of other specific body functions, particularly the higher activities of the brain to survive without major consequences. Certainly survival has been greatly enhanced by the technologies of the neonatal intensive care unit, but there may be a price to pay. The baby may survive but with a mix of residual challenges that will continue throughout life.

What will be the ultimate fate of these small graduates of the NICU? One of the major risks associated with prematurity is cerebral palsy. The term *cerebral palsy* covers a very wide range of brain damage that affects both voluntary movement and behavioral activity. It is much easier to observe and quantify the degree to which movement is affected in babies than to test intelligence or learning ability. Cerebral palsy is a chronic disability that involves abnormal control of movements and posture, it appears early in life and generally does not become worse as the child grows. One of the leading pediatric neurologists Richard Naeye clearly states his opinion that there is very little association of cerebral palsy with asphyxia during the birth process. Dr. Naeye's view is that cerebral palsy is a condition that precedes premature labor. That view of someone who has studied this condition for a lifetime does not stop the flood of legal action that tries to connect the brain damage to mismanagement of delivery. Mismanagement may indeed sometimes occur. However, many researchers now consider that prematurity is not usually the cause of the brain damage. Rather, the brain damage comes first and causes the prematurity. It is of considerable interest that Dr. Roberto Romero, the head of the NIH Intramural Pregnancy Research Branch, considers that infection in midpregnancy has the dual effect of causing brain damage and stimulating the fetal brain activity that starts the birth process. If this dual effect of infection is true, far from being a result of prematurity, brain damage is part of the actual cause of the prematurity.

The best time for a baby to be born is when he or she decides to make the journey. There have to be very good reasons for the obstetrician to start labor off before it starts spontaneously. One good reason for using medical methods of starting labor is knowledge that the pregnancy has definitely lasted over forty-two weeks. When a pregnancy continues past forty-two weeks, there is a real risk that the placenta may fail to provide the baby with enough oxygen and nutrients. There are many other good reasons for obstetricians to start labor at different times of pregnancy, but starting labor off must always be weighed against the possibility that the baby is not yet ready for the great adventure of being born. The timing of labor should be baby-driven, not doctor-driven.

The main danger when an obstetrician uses one of several methods available to start labor is that labor may go partway to completion but then fail to progress. If this happens, the only thing to do is to perform a cesarean section. Cesarean delivery is quite safe but it short-circuits some of the preparatory processes for life after birth that nature has evolved. It is clear that the route of delivery is a major factor in the baby's adaptation after birth. For example, cesarean section compromises the newborn baby's ability to regulate body temperature, an activity the baby did not have to undertake in the uterus. The baby also takes longer to establish regular, efficient, air breathing after a cesarean section delivery.

Premature babies are just not ready for the outside world in many ways. They are exceptionally sensitive to all types of stimuli. Dr. Maria Fitzgerald at London University has conducted studies on the development of the various types of nerve fiber immediately before and after birth. She has shown that it is very easy to overstimulate premature human babies and rat pups with sensory stimulation. Prematurely born babies are hyperexcitable by touch. It appears that at early stages of development, there is a different balance of maturity of nerve fibers. Before the normal end of the preparation for birth, the baby has a predominance of fibers that produce irritable responses. Babies need the full forty weeks in the womb to mature all their sensory functions before being exposed to the multitude of stimuli that will bombard them in the busy outside world. Chapter 6 considered how the complex pattern of inputs to the fetal and neonatal brain can permanently alter the level of function of the adrenal stress axis. It is therefore highly likely that being born prematurely alters the input to the developing brain at a time when brain development is very activity dependent. As a result, mood, behavior and intelligence may all be changed permanently.

Allergies and Being Born Too Late or Too Small

Allergies can greatly affect the quality of life in many ways. Children with allergies miss days at school, and on many days, even when they are able to attend, they cough, sneeze, and itch. All these distracting activities are hardly conducive to concentration. Skin allergies can increase self-consciousness in the young. Adults with allergies may miss days at work, decreasing their efficiency and employment potential. The collective impact of allergic disease is seen by the vast array of over-the-counter and prescription medicines that have been developed by the pharmaceutical industry to alleviate these conditions. There is also a thriving industry in sensitivity testing and treatment against suspected dusts and other factors to which an individual may be considered allergic.

What are the major causes of allergies? How much effort is being put into prevention rather than cure? Is there indeed a financial incentive to prevention when treatment is so lucrative? It is unarguable from the allergy sufferer's viewpoint that considerable financial advantages would flow to the individual and to society if we knew more about the cause of allergies, and we developed mechanisms for preventing them.

There has been a been a pronounced rise in the occurrence of allergic diseases such as asthma and hay fever during the last quarter of a century. Allergies arise when there is an imbalance of the two major cell types in the thymus gland that respond to infections, the so called T-helper cells. One of these types of cells produces antibodies that are responsible for allergic reactions. There is now considerable evidence that early life events modify the proportions of these two types of T-helper cells and the balance of their activity. As a result, there is increased production of a particular group of antibodies called IgE. Epidemiological studies have shown that in a group of men and women studied at the age of forty-seven to fifty-five, the concentrations of IgE were highest in those who had been born after 41 weeks and in those who had the largest head size at birth. The findings of this earlier study have been confirmed by researchers in Denmark.

Experimental studies in rats show that protein restriction during pregnancy also produces fetuses with heads that are disproportionately large for the size of the body. Later in life, these rat pups have abnormal proportions of the different white blood cells in their circulation. The prenatally deprived rats also have abnormal responses to bacterial products. So it appears that nutritional conditions present during prenatal life may program lifelong responses to infection and sensitivity to the many products in our environment that can give rise to allergies.

Can't We Do Something to Anticipate and Prevent Prematurity?

Treatment of premature labor will continue to be difficult until it is possible to make an early prediction that any individual woman is likely to begin labor before thirty-seven weeks of pregnancy. There are many factors in a woman's past medical history that may give a warning clue. However, what the obstetrician needs are tools similar to those used in the diagnosis of heart disease. After all, heart function depends on normal function of its muscle cells, just as contraction of the womb depends on muscle cells. As a result of years of study of the heart, cardiologists have a wide array of tools to help them, laboratory tests to measure chemicals released from the damaged heart and the ability to record the electrical activity of the heart on the electrocardiogram. By contrast, the obstetrician has few such powerful tools. In the '50s, '60s and '70s, heart disease was the daily fear of powerful male executives. There was an enormous incentive to develop methods of diagnosis and treatment. The unborn child has no such clout.

Biochemical Tests For Prematurity

There has been some progress in the discovery of biochemical tests that will predict premature delivery. Work by Dr. Gillian

Lachelin at University College Hospital has shown that during the final days of pregnancy, the amount of estrogen in the mother's saliva rises faster than normal when she has a higher than normal risk of going into premature labor. This intriguing finding has led to one of the most promising biochemical tests to monitor whether a mother has an increased risk of starting labor early. The test is very simple. The pregnant woman just thinks of her favorite food, begins to salivate and collects the saliva into a small tube. The sample is very stable and can be taken to the obstetrician later the same day. A quick laboratory test is available to measure the amount of estrogen in the mother's saliva, and the obstetrician can have the result within a few hours. The best results come when several samples are taken on successive days and a trend can be established.

Another promising test is to measure the molecule fibronectin in the secretions that can be collected from the mother's cervix during pregnancy. Fibronectin is one of the constituents of the glue that sticks the fetal membranes to the wall of the uterus. In the first weeks of pregnancy, the membranes around the fetus gradually adhere to the wall of the uterus. At normal delivery, the membranes must peel away from this attachment. When the membranes separate from the wall earlier than they should, this may be the first step toward premature labor. When the membranes become unglued in this way, fibronectin appears in the cervix and vagina. Since it is not normally present at these locations early in a normal pregnancy, measuring fibronectin taken in samples from these sites can be used to help predict premature labor.

These two simple tests have only recently become available, but they do show promise in identifying women at risk for premature delivery. However, there is no cause for complacency. Further tests are needed because of the very complex nature of premature delivery. There is also the need to know what to do once it is clear that the risk of premature delivery is increased.

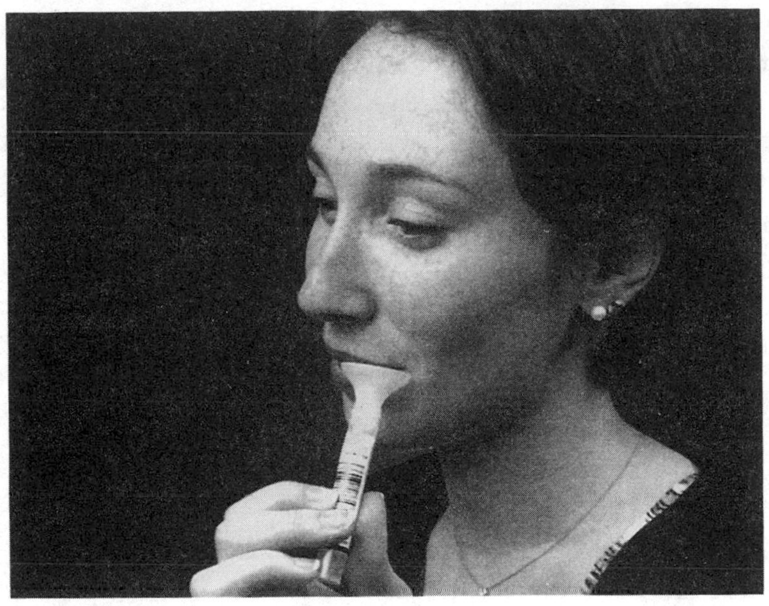

FIGURE 10.6

It is very simple for a pregnant woman to collect a saliva sample in a small tube for a test which may help to predict premature labor.

Promising New Methods Which Involve The Cervix

It is too-simple a view to think that good contraction of the womb is the sole requirement for birth to occur safely. The cervix, the outlet from the womb, is firmly closed throughout a normal pregnancy. As the time for birth approaches the hormonal changes that occur in the mother make the cervix soften. During labor the cervix will dilate and shorten. If shortening of the cervix occurs too soon, there is a likelihood that delivery may occur prematurely. Recent research indicates that measurement of the length of the cervix using the ultrasound machine can provide useful information on the risk that a pregnant woman will go into premature labor. If the cervix is longer than three centimeters (1.2 inches) the likelihood of premature delivery is extremely low. This new use for the marvelous capabilities of ultrasonography holds great promise for monitoring women at risk for premature delivery. A major advantage of the ultrasound is that the result is available immediately—no need to wait for a test result to come back from the laboratory.

The recent focus of attention on the risk of early softening and dilation of the cervix has led to increased interest in methods of preventing problems with the cervix. Several new drugs are able to alter the rate at which the cervix softens and dilates but much more research in both animals and pregnant women is needed before these approaches can be used clinically. In the meantime, obstetricians sometimes can stop the early opening of the cervix by encircling it with a stitch to hold it closed. This method is called cervical cerclage.

The Big Sell: Home Uterine Activity Monitoring

There are two major deficiencies of biochemical tests compared with continuous monitors. Unfortunately, biochemical tests usually require some hours for analysis. The result is not immediately available to the physician. Fortunately, this delay is rapidly becoming shorter and shorter as chemical assays are combined with smart computer chips. The second limitation of biochemical tests is that they only give a snapshot of the situation at one small moment of time. Electronic monitors like the electrocardiogram machine can give a continuous picture second by second of what is going on in the heart muscle. Unfortunately, there is no similar monitor available to tell the obstetrician what is happening in the muscle of the uterus during normal pregnancy and as premature labor progresses. There is a pressing need for a monitor than can register and report the muscular activity of the uterus whenever premature labor is likely.

We humans are very bad at going to the root of problems. When we have a system that is muddling along, appearing to work, we hide behind the old view, if it works don't fix it. But what do we do when the only available methods really don't work, or at least not as well as we would like? It is often difficult to gather up enough energy and resources to find a way of doing a job properly, especially when there

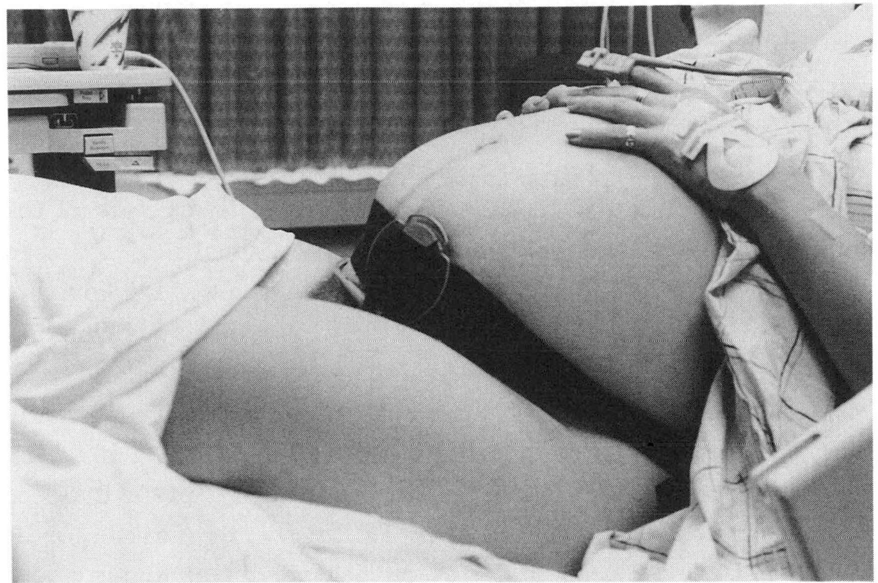

FIGURE 10.7

The belt of the tocodynamometer is strapped tightly to the pregnant mother's abdomen to record contraction of the womb.

is plenty of money to be made in the way the job is currently being done. In this search for a monitor that would help the obstetrician know exactly how strongly the uterus is contracting, I am going to describe an example of commercialization of an application with very limited ability to precisely determine what the muscle of the uterus is doing in both the low activity contractures mode, a pattern of uterine activity that is innocuous, and the ominous high activity contraction mode that threatens to lead to premature delivery. Don't expect too much thoughtful, enlightened discussion of merits, just watch this space for the dollar bottom line.

A simple instrument with the complex sounding name the Smyth guard ring tocodynamometer—the toco for short—is currently the only monitor in wide use for studying the patterns of contraction of the uterus in women who are threatening to deliver prematurely. This instrument and its widespread use, despite its major limitations, has always fascinated me. It's inventor, Dr. Norman Smyth, worked at the hospital at which I trained, University College Hospital in London, England. He was a small, white-haired boffin who would appear into his electronics laboratory in the dark recesses of the hospital and tinker away on his invention. The medical students used to call him The White Rabbit because of his rapid walk, the fact that he had white hair and his habit of repeatedly looking at his watch to catch up with time.

The full name of the device, the Smyth guard ring tocodynamometer, may sound high-tech, but the principle on which it works is simple. Take a flat disc like an ice hockey puck and core out the center. Place a small pressure-sensitive element in the cored-out center, strap the puck to the pregnant woman's abdomen above the uterus and wait. The theory is that when the uterus contracts, it pushes against the belly wall and will push the sensor into the outer ring. A small gauge in the center of the ring then registers the degree of pressure.

In order to obtain a good registration of the contraction of the uterus, it is very necessary that there is not too much fat and other belly wall tissue intervening between the wall of the uterus and the sensor. It is not surprising that it has been demonstrated that the tocodynamometer is not much use in women who are over 60 percent above ideal body weight. In experimental animals, we are able to place sensors directly on the pregnant uterus and record its activity patterns very precisely. We know that when the uterus is contracting in the contractures mode, labor is unlikely to occur. This pattern is innocuous. It is when contractures change to contractions that labor begins to threaten. In most women, the toco is able to register strong, well-established contractions but cannot measure contractures. By the time contractures have changed to well-established contractions, the many interactive, self-stimulating and reinforcing processes of premature labor may be very advanced. So we have a detection problem. Unless the pregnant woman is very thin, there is very little chance that the toco is able to reliably distinguish between contractures and contractions. More sensitive techniques are required.

In an article entitled "Pregnancy Monitors: Life Savers or Costly Gadgets?" Elisabeth Rosenthal of the *New York Times* described her own use of the tocodynamometer in a home uterine-monitoring program. What she wrote is very honest and very enlightening. She first describes her situation. "Because this reporter was at high risk of having a premature baby, my obstetrician started me on a home uterine-monitoring program in the 24th week of my pregnancy, in the hope of detecting and forestalling early labor." Already several issues have been raised. Right from the start she highlights the twin need of *detecting* premature labor and being able to do anything about it.

Elisabeth Rosenthal again: "For two hours each day for the next 12 weeks, I lay down and fastened a belt containing a pressure sensor around my abdomen to pick up contractions in the uterus underneath. . . . Once a day, I hooked the monitor into the phone and sent the signals representing the two hours of tracing to a nurse, who scanned them and reported the results. I got a few minutes of praise and encouragement if the tracings were good or advice and an order to repeat the process if there were too many contractions."

The praise and encouragement are important. Several studies have been conducted on the role played by the reassurance of the nurse contact. In one of these studies, one group was composed of pregnant women at high risk of premature delivery who were monitored and also had the contact with the nurse. A second group of similar women only had contact with the nurse. The results show that it is the contact with the nurse that seems to be beneficial. During the time the pregnant woman is being monitored daily, she feels that a trained professional is watching over her and helping her deal with the problems.

Here I should digress to the comments of Dr. Michael Katz, a professor of obstetrics at the University of California at San Francisco. I should say that I know Michael Katz well and respect his integrity. Indeed, once, many years ago, I sat on a panel that interviewed him for a fellowship at UCLA. Although, as I recall we offered him a fellowship, he decided to go elsewhere. I don't hold that against him. Here is what Dr. Katz is reported as telling Elisabeth Rosenthal. "In every study . . . randomized, non-randomized, big, small . . . the combination of home uterine-activity monitoring and daily contact with a nurse produced better outcomes. If you want to study which component helps, be my guest. But that doesn't matter to my patients. . . ."

It doesn't matter? Dr. Katz seems to be saying that since the whole package works, the whole expensive package, we should pay for the ineffective, unnecessary parts as well. We do not need to worry about any costly, ineffective parts, he seems to be saying. According to this view, it does not appear to be the healthcare provider's place to determine whether the patient is being sold ineffective remedies at a high price. This is important, even if the ineffective remedy is packaged with an effective one. Surely we should strive to get rid of the ineffective part, especially when it is the expensive component.

Elisabeth Rosenthal again: "The cost was over $11,000, almost three times the doctor's fee for the whole pregnancy. But thanks to the program . . . or was it in spite of it? . . . I delivered on my due date, at noon." With costs in the range of thousands of dollars, we definitely need to ask what parts of the procedure are necessary and what parts are simply revenue generators for the companies involved. Indeed, I believe it is incumbent on the companies themselves to demonstrate efficacy before they sell the service. Such a controlled study of efficacy has never been scientifically conducted.

Surely the vast amounts of money spent on utilizing an unproven system day after day, week after week, in a multimillion-dollar industry would be better spent producing better methods and more stringently evaluating current treatments. I do not know what Dr. Katz means by "be my guest," but if it means that he and the other companies involved in marketing these devices are prepared to put more of their profits into finding better methodology, I would be delighted.

Dr. Katz again: "I wish the various task forces-instead of beating on home uterine-activity monitoring-would study it and tell me at what daily cost it is cost-effective. I need them to say: For these types of women, it is worth it at $35 a day, or $100 a day, and for these types, it is not." Who does Dr. Katz want to provide the answers on whether the instrument works and is cost-efficient? Surely that is the responsibility of the companies themselves.

Elisabeth Rosenthal writes, "Doctors have very little information about the normal number of unfelt uterine contractions in the second half of pregnancy. Many doctors who use monitoring consider more than four detected contractions in an hour to be abnormal, but it is possible that many women with normal pregnancies have contractions that are just as frequent. Recent research has suggested that it is the pattern of contractions, not their frequency, that signals the onset of early labor."

Our closest relatives, monkeys and baboons, have very clear patterns of uterine contractility. We have learned a lot from them, but there is much more we need to know. Monkeys and baboons virtually all start the labor-type contractions at night. Since labor lasts a varying length of time, the actual delivery may take place during the day, but the switch from contractures to contractions generally occurs at night. We need to learn more about these patterns of uterine contraction and their causes. We need to develop monitors that record more precisely what the uterus is actually doing. Instead, what is happening? Millions of dollars are spent on unproven systems that have been rushed into the marketplace in an attempt to fulfill a very real need. It is sad that while the money is available to make more money commercially, the money is not available from the companies involved to obtain the information to evaluate whether the whole procedure has any real merit. Dr. Donald McNellis said, "We would like to separate the components and we have designed a trial, but we have not been able to get co-funding from these companies, and we can't afford to do it ourselves."

I hope this story, the abuse of inadequate technology for profit, is of interest at several levels. Many people have made a lot of money from this activity. There is nothing wrong with making money, but the companies making money from an unproven system have a duty to society to determine the value of their methods and if there is no value, to retire the systems. They should not take the position that they are entitled to continue doing what they do until someone else tells them whether home uterine-activity monitoring is effective. That attitude certainly seems to me to be reflected in the comments of Dr. Katz quoted above from the *New York Times*.

CAN'T WE DO SOMETHING TO PREVENT PREMATURITY?

For many years I have worked to evaluate drugs that have the potential to inhibit the uterine activity that gives rise to premature birth. One drug on the market that shows great promise is a molecule that inhibits the action of oxytocin. Our own and other research groups have shown that this drug is very active in pregnant sheep, monkeys and baboons against some forms of premature uterine contraction that occur several weeks before the normal end of pregnancy. However, there are other forms of premature labor where this agent may not be very effective. There is a constant need for more research, for better drugs and for a better understanding of their potential usefulness in the different forms of premature labor. We also need to know more about any unwanted side effects on the developing fetus.

A few years ago, I wanted to undertake some collaboration with a good friend of mine, an excellent pharmacologist who was, at that time, a rising star in one of the world's largest pharmaceutical companies located in Europe. He had a particular interest in drugs that alter the function of another major group of compounds that affect the contraction of the uterus—the prostaglandins. So I asked if we could collaborate on some research to find out why some forms of the hormones, the prostaglandins, stimulate uterine muscle to contract while other prostaglandins inhibit contraction. If we could understand the what and why and when and where and how and who of the inhibitory ones, they might be very valuable in the treatment of premature labor. Would his company support an effort to conduct animal studies to get information on how to design drugs that would block premature labor? He was very interested and wrote to his immediate supervisor. He was given a very negative reply after which he wrote me this letter, names have, of course been changed to preserve confidentiality.

Dear Peter, The problem with asking straight questions is that you often get straight answers, and they may not be the answers that you wanted. I put the case for pursuing research into potential treatments for premature labor to our new number two, Dr. William James, a distinguished medico in the field of cardiovascular disease. Then I waited. One thing is certain, and that is that I shook the tree. Dr. James contacted our Research Director, Dr. Susan Grimes, and asked her to find out whether our company should be actively involved in this area of research. Incidentally, you met Dr. Grimes last year when you visited our research unit and gave your talk on the need for better diagnosis and treatment of premature labor. She was very impressed with the progress you have made on the mechanisms that control how the pregnant monkey uterus contracts throughout pregnancy and at birth. She was as convinced, as I know you are, that you have an excellent model for studying drugs that may be of use in preventing premature birth in pregnant women. The Research Director went to our Medical Director and sought his views. The Medical Director went straight to the guts of the issue, as he saw it, probably correctly from the purely business viewpoint. The Medical Director asked the question, "If we had a compound now that prevented premature labor, would we develop it?" Unfortunately, he answered his own question with an emphatic "No!" Coming from a Medical Director, his reasons are predictable. The pharmaceutical world sees a concern for two individuals rather than one. One of the individuals, the baby, is often in a highly vulnerable state, and the possibility of complications which may have nothing to do with the drug, but which may result in potentially damaging litigation. I was told, politely but firmly that our company currently has many therapeutic irons in the fire, and does not need to take on projects that are as potentially hazardous as this one.

> *I was told in as nice a way as possible that this is not an area of collaboration that I am to follow. I expressed my extreme disappointment but was told to face facts and accept that if the company would not support the end product (and there is no arguing with the medical director), there is no point in directing resources toward it.*

I have read and reread this letter often. I do not wish to attack the pharmaceutical industry. Quite the opposite. Society must recognize the fundamental dilemma that confronts the pharmaceutical industry in their important work to provide safe, active drugs to combat disease. When it comes to each individual case of threatened premature birth, the very baby at risk, possibly already damaged, is the very baby who needs the help of the drug. We have seen that infection may be present, the baby may be short of oxygen. There are almost certainly several things that are already wrong with the baby. If the physician now uses the drug, and there is an adverse outcome, it will prove all to easy to lay the blame on the drug.

Economic Costs of Premature Birth

A report produced by the National Commission to Prevent Infant Mortality in 1988 came to the following conclusions. "Infant mortality—babies who are born alive but die before their first birthday—is one of the best indicators of the overall health of society." This statement is central to the major message of this book: the most important factors that affect both health and disease impact our lives before we are born. In fact, the statement that the death of newborn babies is an indicator of the general health of society is very prophetic, unknowingly so, when one considers that the epidemiologic findings of David Barker and his colleagues on the lifelong health consequences of poor prenatal development had not yet really come to the fore.

In 1985, in the United States, 40,030 babies died before they reached the end of their first year of life. Another 11,000 were of low birthweight and suffered long-term disability. The report continues, "If these 40,030 babies had not died in 1985, the current value of their future earnings would have been $10.2 to $18.9 billion. . . . If the United States could nearly halve its rate and achieve Japan's low rate of 5.5 deaths per 1,000 live births . . . there would have been 20,660 infant deaths in 1985 with foregone earnings of [only] $5.3 to $8.9 billion . . . . [With Japan's low rate] an additional $6.4 to $12 billion in total wages could have been earned over the children's lifetimes. Of these foregone earnings, an estimated $1.4 to $2.6 billion would have been paid in federal taxes over the children's lifetimes."

The majority of the costs incurred by low birthweight and premature babies comes in the first year of life. Estimates of first-year medical costs suggest that initial hospitalization amounts to around $55,000 for babies under 1,500 grams (3.3 pounds) and the costs for the first year are approximately $60,000. The same figures for all babies are $2,500 for medical costs in the first year and $1,100 for the initial hospitalization. From the economic viewpoint, if effective diagnosis and preventive treatments can be developed, the savings from successful prevention of premature birth will be returned to society very rapidly. Dr. Jeanette Rogowski has calculated that finding ways to improve birthweight of babies over 750 grams (1.65 pounds) by just 250 grams (0.55 pounds) produces first-year savings of as much as $16,000 per baby. If premature baby weights could be improved by 500 grams, the saving on the care for each child would be as much as $28,000. The fact that the major expenses on premature babies come in the first year suggests that top priority should be given to this area of lifetime health rather than picking up the pieces at the other end of life. The savings can then be plowed back into other areas of lifetime health care.

Although it seems logical to prevent problems at their source rather than to pay for their consequences, the question inevitably arises: Who pays for this extra initial cost before the savings start to flow? Much prematurity occurs in the lower socioeconomic strata of society. Thus funding has to come from the government through medicaid and other state and federal sources. One study in California concluded that Medicaid paid the costs for 40 percent of all very low birthweight babies in the state. We should all be prepared to contribute to the up front costs of prevention of premature birth. After all, our insurance premiums will reflect the costs of the special care required by very premature babies throughout life. There is also the family burden carried by those families in which premature babies grow up.

New advances in treatment of premature babies have the potential for both increasing and decreasing the costs of prematurity. With advancing technology, increasingly small, premature babies are rescued at a developmental stage that leaves them unprepared for life outside the womb. These diminutive children must be resuscitated and maintained in high-tech neonatal intensive care units. Costs will continue to mount.

In summary, prematurity is a story of both success and failure. The success story is our understanding of how to deal with premature babies in the NICU, especially how to keep them alive until their lungs can function better. The failure is our inability to prevent the occurrence of prematurity and its inevitable sequelae. Failure to achieve a significant reduction in the incidence of prematurity is due to many causes. The willingness to even consider drive-by deliveries, with rapid discharge of mother and baby, as being acceptable shows our impoverished mind-set concerning the need to invest in the future. We are just shifting the cost from the period of pregnancy to later life. We need a much better understanding of the prenatal origins of health and disease. Without a better understanding, we will have to pay a high price in more lifetime illness and long-term handicap for those who are born too soon and too small. Society always eventually pays the price for inattention to major problems. The issue is not whether we can afford the effort to reduce prematurity. It is whether we can afford not to.

ELEVEN

BACK TO THE FUTURE

Perhaps the roses really want to grow,
The vision seriously intends to stay;
If I could tell you I would let you know.

Suppose the lions all get up and go,
And all the brooks and soldiers run away;
Will Time say nothing but I told you so?
If I could tell you I would let you know.

W. H. Auden

The concept of prenatal programming is firmly based on information obtained from epidemiology, clinical research and animal studies. Like all new areas of knowledge, programming has been appropriately challenged by intellectual and scientific scepticism. This is as it should be. When all the evidence is taken together, the overall principles of programming can be shown to be sound. Although, as always, epidemiologic data has many criticisms, the data from animal studies are compelling. However, more information is needed about detailed mechanisms to permit prevention and treatment.

Molecular biology has transformed every aspect of late-twentieth-century modern life, not just medicine but law and commerce as well.

However, the concept that our genes are the sole determinant of who we are has led to a disabling gene myopia. The nature-nurture debate needs to be rethought and reworked in the light of new knowledge from all areas of developmental biology so that this sterile dichotomy no longer stifles thought.

Programming is a fundamental feature of our biology. Its presence highlights the need for more biological education and more research. Everyone in our society needs to be aware of how their body works. Your body is more important than your automobile or computer. We need to raise the level of education regarding pregnancy so that we understand the challenges of normal fetal development and the consequences of inadequate preparation for a lifetime of health.

An ounce of prevention is worth a pound of treatment. Americans spend more than $600 billion a year on health care. Yet we ignore the economics of failure to ensure a good start in life: Pay now, or pay later. Disease fights forward; the consequences come later.

Finally, there is a political dimension to programming. Society now has laws that attempt to prevent child abuse. We need the political will to prevent prenatal abuse and establish social conditions during pregnancy to provide each child with the best possible start in life. Knowledge of programming should lead to activism, not fatalism.

Programming: True or False?

"A hundred years ago when tuberculosis and rheumatic heart disease were common, the proposition that the childhood environment affects adult health would have been self evident. This proposition may still hold, even though infective disease has given way to degenerative disease." So writes David Barker in a *British Medical Journal* editorial entitled "The Womb May Be More Important Than the Home." After considering the extensive evidence put forward to support programming, Dr. Barker pushes the argument back into fetal life and concludes, "The old model of adult degenerative disease was based on the interaction between genes and an adverse environment in adult life. The new model that is developing will include programming by the environment in fetal and infant life."

The overwhelming weight of clinical epidemiologic data from all four corners of the world, both developed and developing nations, supports the view that the quality of our home in the womb programs our health throughout life. This burgeoning area of biological research tells us some critical truths about how our bodies work. It will also be one of great benefit to mankind in the years to come. It is of vital importance for our social and economic future that we learn the lessons of this fascinating story.

How firmly do the experimental data support the concepts put forward in this book? Are these ideas just the madcap notions of biased researchers with tunnel vision who are trying to justify funding for their own work? Or is programming a fundamental law by which our bodies work, a law as basic as the law of gravity? To answer these questions for yourselves, I ask you to suspend judgment until you have evaluated the facts that I have presented. This is a powerful and overarching story and you now have the information you need to decide for yourself. You have the numbers, so to speak. Making an emotional judgment is not good enough. Consider the triangle of knowledge: epidemiology, clinical research and animal research. As in so many things, the devil is in the details.

The story began with reflections on a small episode in a war to defeat Nazi tyranny. We traced it further in the epidemiological detective work of David Barker and his colleagues. Their sifting of detailed records in England, Holland, India and China is a fascinating chapter in both social and medical history. Ethel Burnside, the staff at the hospital in Mysore, India, and at the London Missionary Society and the Rockefeller Hospital at Beijing in China collected and archived their detailed records on mothers and their babies long before the advent of computer databases to store, sort and tabulate. They could not have conceived of the use that has been made of their meticulous records.

The full impact of the knowledge gained from lifetime health records and the demographic human history is supported and enhanced by the fact that the conclusions drawn can be shown to be consistent worldwide. We have seen, for example, the establishment of similar relationships of restricted fetal growth and an increased tendency to diabetes in later life in the Pacific Islands, Mexico, Europe and the subcontinent of India. This universality provides compelling evidence for programming.

As befits the scientific method, there are those who have urged caution in accepting the idea of programming. Thus, in a recent review, Dr. Michael Kramer writes: "Recent studies have reported associations between fetal and/or infant growth and nutrition and adult chronic disease. Based on the results of these studies, it has been hypothesized that programming in early life substantially determines the occurrence of various pathologic phenomena in later life. This hypothesis, if true, carries serious implications for clinical practice and public health policy. The large number of recently published programming studies notwithstanding, causal inference in this domain remains a serious challenge. Programming studies are unique in that potential causes are temporally separated from effects by a span of some five decades or more. Various direct and indirect pieces of evidence suggest that the reported associations may be biased rather than causal. Selection bias, failure to define, measure and adequately control for the confounding health consequences of social deprivation, and inconsistencies in the hypotheses tested and in the methods of data analysis and reporting are among the factors that weigh against a causal explanation for the associations observed."

In the same review, Dr. Kramer writes, "Clearly, more work on this phenomenon is required before the biological basis for such findings can be accepted, even in the animal domain." It is the animal studies that have been discussed here that clinch the issue. Their power is enhanced because they were obtained from a number of laboratories, in a variety of species and on several continents. The same general principles of programming apply to studies conducted in sheep, rats, guinea pigs, llamas, and rhesus monkeys. There, are of course, likely to be both similarities and differences between groups of animals. For this reason, it is always worth searching for common themes. So often when studying biological systems, we learn more from the differences between species than we learn from the similarities.

In the various chapters in this book, we have seen fundamental underlying principles emerge from animal research. I summarized them as ten principles of programming in chapter 1. The placenta acts as a barrier protecting the fetus from many environmental assaults. However, the placental barrier is incomplete. There are several situations in which the mother produces adrenal steroid hormones in quantities that exceed the placenta's ability to restrict their transfer to the fetus. In these situations maternal hormones cross the placenta in higher than normal amounts. When developing fetal tissues are exposed to these high levels of stress steroids, they may respond by permanently changing the level at which their own activity is set for the rest of life. Exposure of the unborn baby to abnormally high levels of steroids is one of the mechanisms whereby protein deficiency in the mother's diet programs the developing heart and blood vessels to function in a way that leads to high blood pressure in later life. High levels of steroids in fetal blood also alter fetal brain function permanently by changing the receptors in critical areas of the developing brain.

Fetuses who experience suboptimal conditions in the womb attempt to compensate for poor oxygen and nutrient delivery by diverting blood to the brain at the expense of other organs. The compensation does not come without a price. Several organs, including the liver and kidneys, may not develop to their full capacities. The liver and kidneys are two key organs that perform many critical functions after birth. Their failure to perform normally can result in a wide variety of lifetime cardiovascular problems and other diseases. These are two of our ten principles of programming.

In the early days of activity in a new area in science that involves a major change in fundamental ideas, there is a primary need for hard data to establish the new area, provide credibility and delineate boundaries. Then, as a solid body of evidence accumulates from several unrelated and often competing laboratories and research groups, the new field becomes increasingly firmly based in hard fact. Speculation to introduce new concepts in the area can now be built on firm, established and growing experimental data. I predict that in ten years' time or even less, there will be general acceptance by biologists of developmental programming. There will also be a much clearer knowledge of how programming for a lifetime of health or disease occurs at the cellular level.

DARWIN AND LAMARCK: ONE LAST LOOK AT NATURE AND NURTURE

The science of cellular biology has exploded over the past twenty years. One of cellular biology's major achievements has been to demonstrate the central role of genes in regulating our bodies through the blueprint encoded in DNA. Sadly, however, gene myopia has afflicted some sections of the biomedical community. The second half of the twentieth century has surely and deservedly been the era of the gene. In the mid 1950s, few could have anticipated the revolution in biological understanding that was about to cascade across all branches of biology, medicine and law as a result of this momentous finding. Even commerce and culinary art have been affected. The uniqueness of the DNA of each individual within a species is now used as powerful legal evidence. DNA has become the scientific method of choice in establishing identity. Detailed knowledge of the differences in DNA between closely related species recently enabled the use of DNA typing to show that much of what is sold as Beluga caviar is often just ordinary fish roe.

In the future, molecular biology and its application to genetics will have an ever-increasing effect on our lives at all levels: our health and even our personal lives. In some inbred Orthodox Jewish groups, testing for the gene for Tay-Sachs disease allows potential partners who possess one copy of the gene to discover whether the other partner also has a copy. The prospective couple can then make considered judgments about the impact on their lives of marriage and the risks to their children. The exciting findings of the human genome project will soon allow biochemists to track each gene in everybody's private blueprint, carefully describing the chains of bases that sit along the string of pearls that is their genetic inheritance. A change of base here or an extra base there will indicate a variable tendency to specific disease conditions. Sometimes those minor but functionally important changes can lead to crippling, even fatal illness. Fortunately, however, our bodies often have a variety of built-in safety and repair mechanisms as well as redundancies when there is trouble with a particular gene.

Gene myopia and excessive reduction of our biology to the simple unchangeable enactment of a predetermined genetic program is a narrow and misleading way of attempting to understand our normal function in health and our susceptibility to disease. For some scientists and nonscientists alike, molecular biology has actually impeded our understanding of who we are and how we got here. Genes are nothing without an environment in which to function. Genes must replicate, express themselves and function within the context of the whole organism. And, of course, the whole organism must function in the context of its environment. The reductionist approach to biology, while of critical importance in research, plays into the hands of those who want a quick fix to abnormalities and disease. Time after time, approaches to specific illnesses have blindly followed the path of "Find the gene . . . that's all we need to do to solve the problem." I can think of numerous instances in which brilliant investigator-clinicians I know have made comments such as, "I want to find the gene that produces pregnancy hypertension, the gene that causes schizophrenia, the gene responsible for alcoholism . . . " and on and on. We should never forget that the gene for schizophrenia was found in 1988, and then the claim was retracted. The root cause of schizophrenia is much more complex, much more challenging. We are who we are in all our bodily functions because of an interplay of the environment on our genetic inheritance. If we are honest, avoidance of gene myopia means that we must replace genetic determinism with a conceptual framework of environmentally modified, activity-dependent developmental programming. Fortunately, developmental programming is a brighter, more optimistic concept than genetic reductionism.

In chapter 4, I questioned the all-embracing validity of one of the fundamental ideas of modern biology: namely, that permanent changes in genes are the vehicle through which all modifications of

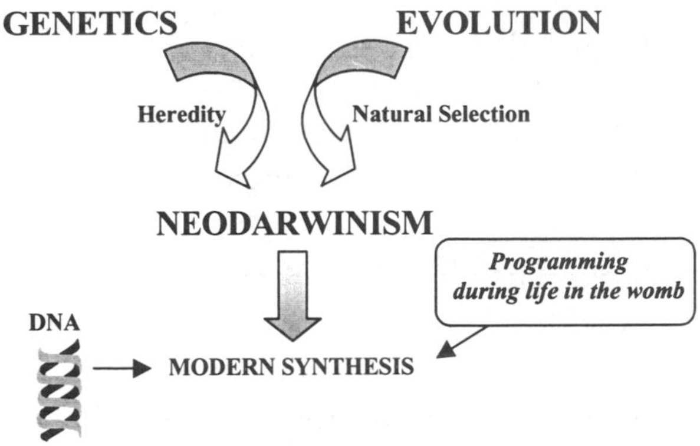

FIGURE 11.1

The modern synthesis of who we are must include the influence of our life in the womb in programming our health and disease for a lifetime.

normal function are passed from one generation to the next. Lamarck put forward the notion that some characteristics acquired during one's lifetime can be passed to subsequent generations. This idea of transgenerational passage of acquired—that means nongenetic—characteristics has been given short shrift in scientific circles. The geneticist, C. D. Darlington, called Lamarckian views, "the evergreen superstition." Lamarck's views have been considered incompatible with knowledge of the molecular biology of the gene. Acknowledgment that there might be anything in the idea that environmental effects could pass transgenerationally was also hindered by some high-profile frauds attempts to manipulate

Despite initial rejection of any novel concept, there is an inevitability that a new idea's time will come. Firm evidence is now abundantly available for the transgenerational inheritance of acquired biological processes by nongenetic factors that impact the fetus during life in the womb. The mechanisms by which transgenerational passage of characteristics occurs are dependent on the environment, though they must of course exert their actions on cells through gene-dependent mechanisms. We have seen multiple examples. Andre Van Assche and William Oh's rats that have been made diabetic by drug treatment during pregnancy pass on the tendency to diabetes through their daughters. The growth-retarded women who were themselves fetuses during the Dutch Hunger Winter of 1944–1945 gave birth to smaller babies. It took at least three generations for the rats chronically malnourished for thirteen generations to return to normal weight. Even then, behavioral function had not returned to the level of the controls.

Darwin, Mendel, Crick and Watson and the modern view of the central role of genes won the day over the ideas of Lamarck and his colleagues. However, I wonder almost daily what Lamarck would have given for knowledge of the animal studies and human epidemiology data presented here on the origins of health and disease. In science, it never pays to have ideas for which there is no experimental evidence, even if you are on the right track. It is essential that others can reproduce your results in their own laboratories. Reproducibility of any set of data is the indispensable test of knowledge that claims to be scientific. The observations must be reproducible by anyone if true, and amenable to methods that can falsify them if they are indeed false. According to Berthold Brecht, "The aim of science is not to produce everlasting wisdom but to put limits on everlasting error." How then do we get over this tendency to see the gene as totally dominant? To start with, we must drop sterile debates about obsolete dichotomies that are essentially differences without distinctions. The nature-nurture debate in relation to the origins of health and disease is one such useless dichotomy.

The concept that deficiencies and abnormalities in the environment are major factors in the origins of disease may be more acceptable to society today than the concept that we are just the result of a fixed and unchanging recipe encoded in our genes. In the brave new world of Aldous Huxley's futuristic society, there is selection of the genetic potential of the cells used to produce each fetus but, more importantly, the soup in which each fetus is grown is varied according to the need to produce a baby with a particular level of intelligence and character disposition. For future astronauts, the incubators are turned and twisted to simulate interplanetary travel; to decrease intelligence, an alcoholic womb is provided. Huxley was well aware of the importance of the environment in our earliest home in preparing us for things to come.

Programming: Education for the Future

As the society of the next millennium becomes more complex, there is a great need for better scientific education, and I do not just mean how to make the most of computers and the Internet. We all need to know and evaluate the true achievements and limitations of scientific disciplines in general. In his 1996 book *The End of Science: Facing the Limits of Knowledge*, John Horgan portrays science and scientists as burned out, finished, as having learned all there is to know that is of value. Horgan is a senior writer for *Scientific American* with a wealth of experience in a wide variety of areas of science and an enthralling ability to capture the personalities involved in generating new knowledge. But after reading his book, one might well ask which planet he is living on. A recent televised forum of Nobel laureates—winners of prizes for chemistry, physics, medicine and economics—provided a fascinating discussion of Horgan's idea that science has ended. These Nobelists poured scorn on the title and contents of Horgan's book. They repeatedly returned to the issue that, while physics is becoming more and more rarified and difficult to comprehend, we are still ignorant about our biology, about how our bodies work. To borrow Winston Churchill's words from a 1942 speech as the tide of war was changing, "This is not the end. It is not even the beginning of the end. But it is, perhaps, the end of the beginning." We certainly are not at the end of our search to understand our biology and, especially, to understand the importance of the developmental period in the womb. There is a long way to go. However, we can consider ourselves at the end of the beginning. We are definitely on the way.

Far from being at its end, biological science is going through a golden age of experimental study. Physicists may have pushed their investigations to the ultimate boundaries of comprehension and calculation. Not so the biological sciences. The energy and exuberance of the biological sciences is exhibited by the wonderful studies conducted on the intense, minute-by-minute activity within each cell; the regulation of genes by external influences, the way these genes themselves regulate cellular processes, the role of transmitters shuttling between cells as they carry on their continual dialogue, the passage of calcium and glucose across the outer membrane of each cell as they act to energize and activate, and countless other mechanisms that daily yield up their secrets End of science indeed!

In designing an experiment in biology, one puts forward a hypothesis based on previously known facts and ideas. The next step forward is dissected and questioned and finally, rather like the order to infantry to go over the top of the trench toward the enemy, the experiment is begun. Sooner, or later, data begin to come back. It is always exciting to obtain data that confirm the carefully constructed hypothesis. However, there is an equal excitement in data that show that the system works very differently from one's preconceived notions. Science is the constant modification of old ideas by new data and the subsequent challenging of these new data with fresh ideas. We will never know completely how a system works as a result of any single experiment. The new knowledge gained from each study will eventually raise new questions for which we must design new experiments. We can be sure that the field of programming will throw up new ideas that are significant for every human being, born or as yet unborn.

John Horgan's thesis that we have reached the end of science smacks of the wide and sweeping statements made by some of my favorite pontificating pundits of the past. Here are some examples: "Babe Ruth made a great mistake when he gave up pitching," "Sensible and intelligent women do not wish to vote" (attributed to President Grover Cleveland) and one of my favorites, "Heavier than air flying machines are impossible" (attributed to Lord Kelvin). Lord Kelvin, by the way, was the president of the Royal Society, the world's oldest scientific drinking club, as some have called it. He was a remarkable scientist, immortalized in physics by having a temperature scale named after him. There are three temperature scales, degrees centigrade, degrees Fahrenheit or degrees Kelvin. Brilliant scientist that he was, he was completely wrong when it came to aeronautical predictions. It is impossible to conceive of the end of science, since the very word *science*, according to my dictionary, means "knowledge acquired by study; acquaintance with or mastery of any department of learning." The trouble is, the word has become associated with boffinry and abstruseness, not knowledge or mastery of learning.

John Horgan's book is essentially an interesting collage of the views of eminent scientists he has interviewed. In her review of the book, Natalie Angier rebukes the author, rightly in my opinion, for emphasizing the ideas and views of the elderly scientists "who have entered the phase of their careers called the *philopause*." They have retired from the university or grown bored with lab work and so have taken up sterile cogitation. When I was an undergraduate at Cambridge, we attended many lectures by such eminently worn-out individuals. We used to say the speaker had reached the stage of the "whither" lecture: "Whither developmental psychology?" "Whither transplantation technology?" "Whither sociobiology?" Where's the beef? Where are the data?

Science means knowledge. Every time I see huge earth-moving equipment on the freeway, I am reminded of the old ways of producing engineering works. I see mountains of earth with antlike humans scurrying up and down with small shovels. Accelerating productivity and greater efficiency, brains rather than brawn, are characteristics of human endeavor whose relationship to scientific knowledge should be clear to all.

But what about the economic productivity that comes from good health, from knowing better how our bodies work? This aspect of biology should certainly concern economists and legislators. The vast majority of legislators have received their most senior education and training in law schools. That is appropriate in many ways because it is the legislators who make the laws. So it is important for legislators to know how the law of the land functions. By formulating good legislation, lawyers can help build a better society. But what happens when legislators make laws that affect our health? More than anyone else in our society, it would help if more lawmakers were trained to know how our bodies work, the conditions that enable our children's brains to develop optimally and how stressful situations negatively impact the health of women both before and during pregnancy. Since these effects can span generations, they affect generations of citizens and generations of economies.

The pessimist would say, "How on earth are you going to get legislators who only see as far as the next election to look to the consequences for the next generation?" Fortunately, there are legislators like Representative John Porter, a staunch supporter of the need for research, who know that we are where we are today because our parents invested in the future. Public sector interest groups should become more involved and knowledgeable about these issues. These are life-and-death matters for your children and grandchildren.

We all need knowledge about our bodies in order to take responsibility for our own health just as we have to take responsibility for our food, clothing and housing. It is all too easy to pass the blame to others when our health is impaired. Modern obstetrics in the developed world has become a battleground of recrimination when anything goes wrong. A friend of mine who is the chair of obstetrics at a major university hospital once said to me, "Modern thinking is often along the lines that unless your baby is perfect physically and has an IQ of 150, it's the doctor's fault." There is a superabundance of attorneys who will press the case for economic compensation for every adverse outcome that occurs throughout pregnancy, especially problems that occur around the time of delivery. The attorneys stand to lose little, especially when legal aid is provided. Patients who feel aggrieved also stand to lose little financially from any accusation, even when it is misplaced. Although they may not lose financially, they are the losers because they do not know the true root cause of the problems that result from suboptimal conditions before birth. The results of their lack of knowledge will pass across generations—another example of the transgenerational passage of poor health.

Every obstetrician looks after two patients, keeping a very wary eye on the mother's health as well as the baby's. It is this fascinating and complicated interrelationship between two independent individuals, together but separate, that makes the biology of pregnancy so fascinating. It is also this need to treat two patients that makes the care of complicated pregnancies so demanding. Consider the following true story. A senior obstetrician friend of mine was asked to take care of a pregnant woman with very high blood pressure. Blood pressure above the upper limit of normal pregnancy levels is a clear indication that something is wrong in the pregnancy. High blood pressure in pregnancy is accompanied by a decrease in the amount of blood flowing to the placenta. It is likely that this woman's fetus was already compromised when she first visited the obstetrician. When blood pressure is high in pregnancy, there is always the risk of complications for both the mother and fetus.

When this particular pregnant patient came to see my obstetrician colleague for the first time, she was twenty-six weeks pregnant (two-thirds of the way through) and her blood pressure was already well above normal. Her approach to pregnancy had started off badly. The first visit to an obstetrician in pregnancy should be made much earlier than twenty-six weeks, preferably by six weeks of pregnancy. The obstetrician described the dangers that the she and her baby faced to the patient and her own mother, who accompanied her.

When a pregnant woman's blood pressure is very high, the first question the obstetrician must ask is whether the baby is mature enough to survive if delivered by cesarean section. Premature babies have not yet made enough preparation of their lungs, gut, kidneys and other systems needed to function independently in the outside world. If the baby in a pregnancy in which the mother has high blood pressure has completed enough of the preparation for independent life, the best course is to deliver the baby, usually by cesarean section. When cesarean section is safe for the baby, it is always the best course for the mother. Within hours of delivery, the mother's blood pressure will be down, and the risks to her health will have greatly diminished. The obstetrician must decide whether and when it is safest for both mother and baby to get on with the delivery by cesarean section.

If the baby is not yet mature enough to survive independently of support by mother and placenta, the obstetrician must attempt to control the mother's blood pressure and wait until the baby matures a little more. The mother can help to keep her blood pressure down by taking as much rest as possible. Bed rest is an excellent aid to getting blood pressure down into the normal range. Since this woman's pregnancy was only twenty-six weeks along, my friend told the mother that he wanted her to get to thirty-two weeks and then he would start her in labor. In the meantime, she should confine herself to bed in the hospital as much as possible. He wanted to observe her continuously.

The very day the patient reached thirty-two weeks of pregnancy, she got out of bed, walked into the hallway smoking area and lit up a cigarette. She was smoking the cigarette when she experienced pronounced pain in the area of her uterus. Her high blood pressure had led to a large hemorrhage into the placenta. Since the placenta was no longer functioning properly, the baby died very quickly for lack of oxygen. There was not even time to get her to the operating room for an emergency cesarean section. When the placenta was eventually delivered, it was not a pretty sight. Blood clots in several areas of the placenta showed that there had been several small bleeding episodes before the final big one. This placenta was very much a suboptimal placenta.

A few weeks later, the patient came to her postnatal checkup with her mother and her partner. My colleague is a dedicated and sensitive obstetrician and understood the grief that can accompany the loss of a baby at any time during pregnancy. He asked the patient if there was information she needed. The patient's mother broke in aggressively, saying that the family felt it was the obstetrician's duty (the exact word used) to show (again the exact word used) why things had gone wrong. Despite the difficulty of a progressively more confrontational three-way conversation, my friend repeated the explanation of the risks he had given when he first saw the patient of how the placenta gets damaged when the mother's blood pressure is high. This damage leads to oxygen deprivation in the fetus and often fetal death. Being kind, he omitted to discuss the effects of tobacco and other negatively impacting features of the patient's lifestyle on a poorly functioning pregnancy.

The patient's mother was unsatisfied and revealed that they already had made an appointment with an attorney later that week.

The mother said that she was "unprepared to have her daughter suffer at the hands of the medical profession in the way she, the patient's mother, had done during her own pregnancies." Since a major message of this book is that problems in pregnancy can have long-term effects that only reveal themselves much later, often in subsequent generations, it is of interest that the patient's mother should have had a poor past obstetric history of her own. There are several transgenerational issues here. There is the biological one that if the patient's mother had known more about the biology of pregnancy, her daughter, the patient, might have been able to confer with her. Also, given the information we have discussed, one wonders how much of the unfortunate course of pregnancy was due to suboptimal development in this patient's own prenatal life. I have dealt with this sad story at some length because it contains biological and medical messages, ethical and societal messages, philosophical and personal messages that fittingly bring this book to a conclusion.

The biological and medical message is that our bodies function according to very strict rules. We break the rules of proper diet, exercise, rest and mental ease at our peril (and, it seems, the peril of our children). The ethical and societal message is that we get nowhere when we pass the blame for our ill health onto the very segment of the community that is trying to alleviate the problems that we have stored up for ourselves (and our future children). What is the old saying? We have seen the enemy and they are us. The philosophical and personal message suggests that we become more proactive in terms of health. We need to learn more about our own biology until we are as familiar about how our bodies work as we are about how our automobiles work. Our lives are our own responsibility. If we smoke, we imperil future generations. If we eat incorrectly, we imperil future generations. If we pollute the environment, we imperil future generations. It is not the obstetrician who is at fault for the case history I mention above. It is we as a society for failing to educate each generation in the need for the three best physicians in the world: Dr. Diet, Dr. Quiet and Dr. Happiness. I sometimes feel that these three characters have been laid off as excess to need in the downsizing of the richness of our lives as we all struggle to fulfill the fiscal bottom line.

Programming: Research for the Future

The adverse consequences of suboptimal conditions in the womb will not just disappear with education. We need research into the biological mechanisms at the basis of programming. David Barker, whose human epidemiological research I have leaned on heavily in outlining the prenatal origins of health and disease, is fond of saying that the mechanisms that govern programming will only be explained by animal research. The controversy over animal research has become more and more heated over the years. Perhaps we would have more light and less heat if each person were asked to focus on this central and fundamental question: Do you truly believe that the information we need to improve the health of humans and animals can be obtained without studying how the whole body works?

It is difficult for me to see how one can study the trans-generational effects of adverse prenatal conditions without studying several generations of animals and humans. Although much can and should be done in the test tube and on the computer, in the final analysis, we must study the whole system in its entirety. To wish that we could obtain the information without animal studies is understandable. To think that the needed information can be obtained without research that studies how animals function is to deny the complexity of the body. Animal research in pregnancy is indispensable because of the need to understand the interactions of the mother and fetus. It is reassuring to know that someone like David Barker, a clinician who has spearheaded these ideas as a result of his detailed and lengthy study on human records should so strongly support the indispensability of animal based research in the effort to understand the underlying processes.

There is a central issue on which the whole of society must adjudicate. Do we need research on living material to understand life? Do we need research on the whole organism to understand how the whole organism works? The animal rights activists will say we do not need to do research on animals. Some now say that even animal tissues must not be used. Research has made major advances in understanding of normal and abnormal biological systems as they affect our own health and the health of our children, as well as that of all animal species. If society wishes to abandon the accumulation of knowledge that will prevent and treat diabetes, infectious disease and brain damage before birth, it is society's prerogative to do so. The choice must be made with the full understanding of the consequences of what we are doing. Do not let us delude ourselves that the information we need will come in any other way. We are not yet at the position at which we can understand how the whole body works without studying the whole body. We are not yet at the position that we can understand how an otherwise externally perfect newborn baby can die of sudden infant death syndrome with no warning. To understand this tragedy, we need to know how the newborn baby adapts to an air-breathing environment after living so long in an environment in which the mother, through her breathing, her circulatory system and the placenta, takes care of the oxygen supply on the baby's behalf.

"But," you may say, "all this research has not told us everything we must do during pregnancy. Researchers cannot just tell people what we know about adverse conditions in the uterus, what epidemiologists and animal researchers have found about fetal development. It is incumbent upon researchers to tell people what they must do." The collection of knowledge inevitably precedes action. We are still in that period of time at which the available knowledge is not yet complete enough to allow physicians to give firm advice.

The carefully amassed scientific research and the epidemiological data I have presented shout out, scream to us to pay more attention and to learn more about life before birth. The biology of these events is so clear: the evidence of a critical period of programming on sexual function; the long-term effects of oxygen deficiency in the uterus on how the brain functions; the changes in growth of the thymus gland, the key organ in the neck that produces the cells that regulate our defenses against infection and alter our susceptibility to allergies; the association of heart disease and decreased liver growth in fetuses that have to alter their blood flow to protect the brain. The economic and social success of research-based knowledge from universities and noncommercial organizations are quickly forgotten. A study published in the *New England Journal of Medicine* on May 16, 1994, states that the use of artificial surfactant in the treatment of premature babies who cannot breathe properly saves up to $90 million a year in annual hospital costs. Add to that the costs of treating long-term consequences of more severe lifelong impairment that occurred before the availability of surfactant, and the savings are enormous. Since surfactant therapy first became available in 1989, the death rate from lung problems in premature babies has been reduced by more than one-third. The value of these agents was first noted in animal studies in sheep. It should be remembered that Sir Graham (Mont) Liggins' work with fetal sheep was not initially directed toward studying lung maturation. He designed his first studies with fetal sheep to work out the signals that start labor and delivery.

The history of great medical advances can be split into two major categories: development of new treatments and the introduction of preventive measures that remove the need for treatment. Some treatments also prevent complications. Thus, when treated with insulin, diabetics live longer, and suffer fewer of the complications than would occur if insulin were not available. Indeed, without insulin, the life expectancy of insulin-dependent diabetics is generally a matter of weeks from the time their pancreas fails. Treatment can help to prevent further disease, although the pancreas will never recover. The battle against infectious disease has been the larger of the two great battlegrounds of preventive medicine. The second arena has been the use of knowledge about nutrition to prevent deficiency diseases caused by the lack of vitamins and specific nutritional components.

I was recently at a scientific meeting in Vancouver, Canada, at which a researcher was asked his opinion on the mechanisms that lay behind an observation that he had recently made in the laboratory. “I haven't the remotest notion,” he answered quickly and bravely. My mind went to the story I had read many years before about Captain Cook, who explored the western coast of North America right up to and just past the current location of the Canadian-American border. In this region, around Seattle and the islands off the coast of British Columbia, Cook wrote on his charts, "Nobody knows." Not many years later, Cook's second-in-command on the earlier voyage carried out a second expedition in the same waters. He charted the coastline up from what is now the northernmost part of the western United States. Using the same charts as those used by Cook, he was able to write, "Somebody knows." The name of the captain was Vancouver.

Similarly, the search for new biological knowledge involves setting sail into uncharted waters where "nobody knows." Like the researcher whose words stick in my mind, investigators currently must often say, "I haven't the remotest notion." But if we have the will, the secrets will yield to us. We will enjoy the fascination of knowing more about how our bodies work. We will understand how the outside world that nurtures us activates our internal blueprint to make us who we are. Until we understand our biology, our development, our own brains and how they alter our behavior under different conditions, we will never understand the true roots of love, of humor, of sadness. We need to understand our own development to be at one, to be at peace with who we are, in sickness and in health. The prenatal origins of health and disease are central to our knowledge of ourselves.

The skeptic would say, "All this and still so much prenatal disease!" Research carries no guarantees. The pearl diver dives into the ocean but does not always come up with a pearl. Progress is slow.

Programming: Economy for the Future

An ounce of prevention is worth a pound of treatment. In life we always pay now or pay later. A recent article in *The Economist* entitled "Disease Fights Back" stated, "Established and curable diseases [such as resistant forms of tuberculosis] are doing more harm to people than new diseases. What is worse, their strength is growing, not fading." The article addresses issues such as the reemergence of resistant forms of tuberculosis. I would like to introduce a new concept with great economic consequences: Disease fights forward. There is a parallel between the loss of resistance and the resurgence of tuberculosis and the loss of our knowledge of what is good during pregnancy. That same comment could certainly be made about the problems of suboptimal intrauterine health.

Again *The Economist:* "In late 18th century Europe tuberculosis killed perhaps one in five. Careful use of antibiotics gradually put paid to it. After a while the world decided that the fight was over; but no-one told the tuberculosis bacillus. In New York City, spending on tuberculosis fell from $40 million in 1968 to $2 million in 1989. The cuts hit outpatient work, no one was there to ensure that the sick—often homeless drug addicts—took their medicine properly. That let resistance bloom. By the beginning of 1991 almost half of New York's cases of tuberculosis were resistant to the two main drugs previously used, and the costs of hospitalizing people with tuberculosis in the city had reached $50 million. So much for the saving in spending of $38 million between 1968 and 1989."

The need to have a concerted program in the face of nationwide and worldwide health problems as fundamental as the consequences of inadequate prenatal care that arise from the issues described in this book should be clear to all. It is too easy to shuffle off the responsibility. We can perhaps learn something from this resurgence of tuberculosis. *The Economist*: "National surveillance worked well until the 1970s. When, against advice, responsibility for this work was given to the states, the program fell apart. In 1986 just as the comeback [by the tuberculosis bacillus] was getting under way, the multi-drug-resistance unit at the Centers for Disease Control in Atlanta was closed. All told, cuts in tuberculosis programs during the 1980s saved America perhaps $200 million. According to one estimate, America spent more than $1 billion on multi-drug-resistant tuberculosis in the five years up to 1994."

One reliable source predicted that Americans would spend $600 billion on health care in 1990. That figure has undoubtedly risen significantly since then. And what portion of that figure is spent on research for prevention? The total research budget of the National Institutes of Health is about $12 billion, about 2 percent of spending on health care. As Lowell Weicker, the past president of the foundation Research! America, said, "If health is the goal, we've got to start putting up more money and putting it up front."

One of the clarion calls of the budget cutters is that we cannot saddle future generations with the debt. I agree. But if we cut the resources needed to give the next generation a healthy, relatively disease-free life, saddling our children with debt is exactly what we will be doing. The debt will be the cost of treating obesity, heart disease and mental illness. This debt will be payment for our unwillingness to improve their health at the most critical and cost-efficient time, during development. We are all threatened when cuts come. However hard-won and costly, information and preventive approaches easily disintegrate when underfunded. It is always more costly to build something than to allow it to fall away.

Programming: the Political Future

In this era of the gene dominant, there is much discussion on the ethical and political dangers that can arise from the knowledge that a particular individual has a genetic disease. There is a basic fear in some segments of the community that knowledge of genetic predisposition to a disease will adversely affect the cost or even the availability of health and life insurance. Insurance companies need to factor in everything they know about the risk of each policy. Insurers legitimately adjust health premiums according to whether the applicant smokes or is overweight or adjust automobile premiums according to how carefully or irresponsibly the applicant drives.

In the light of the knowledge provided here, will the insurance companies see a need to adjust our premiums according to the quality of our prenatal developmental programming? We have seen that there is an increased risk of heart disease in babies of low birthweight who have large placentas. The incidence of stroke is higher in babies with a normal-sized head but smaller body whose home in the womb appeared to have restricted their growth mostly in the final portion of pregnancy. Will the time come when applicants are asked to provide details of their birthweight, placental weight, length and body form at birth before they obtain a life insurance quotation? These are major social issues that flow from the notion of programming. I hope they will be vigorously debated.

Some unpleasant features will no doubt surface in the wake of the acceptance that life in the womb programs our health after birth. Somewhere there will be attorneys who will be willing to bring cases against parents on behalf of children who think they have been disadvantaged as a result of the mother's lifestyle during pregnancy. I am not completely sure that this will happen, but I would be prepared to put a little money on it. There appears to be no limit to some members of the legal profession's willingness to exploit uncertainty by supplanting it with their own certainty. I truly fear the possibility that, unless something is done about it in the laws of the land in Western countries, attorneys will tell individuals that they have a right to redress in the courts for their suboptimal beginnings.

Imagine a radio and television advertisement similar to the ambulance-chasing that goes on in the auto injury market. "Do you have high blood pressure? Are you overweight even though you are only thirty? It may be that your mother worked too hard while she was pregnant. Current medical research clearly shows that as a result of your mother's lack of good nutrition and rest, you are now programmed to have life-threatening high blood pressure, and you will probably suffer from heart disease. We have great experience in this type of case and would like to represent you because you may be entitled to damages for the suboptimal environment in which you developed before birth. Don't worry if you cannot track down your father. We realize that many fathers are not around these days, but your mother could be forced to indenture herself to you for many years. It is unfortunate that society in general no longer feels it has a role to play; otherwise, we could have sued for several times the damages that we are currently pursuing for over two hundred clients. We are indeed thinking of bringing a class-action suit against the current government. Should we do so, would you like to join it?"

We can do much about the adverse effects of the environment during pregnancy if we have the will. Providing better nutrition, removing undue stress about economic issues and providing adequate prenatal and postnatal care are all commonsense approaches for society. Many people have a fundamental aversion to any interference in the lives of pregnant women and society in general. Yet we have laws that prevent parents from battering their children. Society accepts that it has a right to enter the family circle and institute certain rules of conduct for the well-being of the young child who cannot protect herself or himself. In the developed world, we say we no longer believe in child labor. So we do reserve the right to interfere for the well-being of children.

The fetus—although in many ways resembling the abused child—is even more defenseless and is often held hostage.

Don't Blame Mom

When I have participated in discussions with lay groups on fetal development, my remarks on the potential lifelong consequences of developing in a suboptimal intrauterine environment have often been met by the remark, "Don't blame mom!" It is sad if the wish to determine the way development impacts our health is perceived as being targeted at blaming anyone, especially pregnant women. My only goal is to provide the evidence as it stands. Our biology dictates that the milestones we pass at critical periods of development will be hugely important in determining our health throughout life and our susceptibility to disease.

There are those who warn that the story told in this book will induce unnecessary guilt in parents, especially mothers. I understand that this is a real, unavoidable possibility of acceptance of the idea that prenatal development programs lifetime health. The reality of the connection has been clearly discussed throughout this book. The root causes lie in society and in past generations. The clarion call to the present generation is for more knowledge to improve the situation for children as yet unborn whose names we do not know and whose faces we will never see. The knowledge will also help us to reverse consequences of programming that adversely impact our own health.

We can, like the ostrich, bury our heads in the sand and think the connection between the health of the mother and the health of the baby does not exist. If women who wish and are trying to become pregnant continue to drink alcohol in the early weeks of pregnancy when they are as yet unaware they are pregnant and if they continue to smoke cigarettes, they ignore the connections that have been amply demonstrated between alcohol and smoking and birth defects and growth retardation.

The concept that all the blame lies with the individual parent is fundamentally unsound. There are several arguments against such a simple view. One argument has biblical proportions and needs to be understood. There is a biblical saying, "Visit the sins of the parents on succeeding generations." This is an old and very prescient comment on the ideas of transgenerational passage of health problems through mechanisms that are personal, social and environmental rather than genetic. The answer to the problems that follow from poor prenatal conditions lie with the family and society. Both have responsibilities. It is preferable to consider the issue of long-term implications of inadequate preparation for life-long good health as society's problem not just that of the individual. This sense of responsibility and accountability must match reality—our biological reality—otherwise it is a meaningless ideology.

Programming: Fatalism or Activism?

The concept of intrauterine programming of health and disease does not mean our only option is to be fatalistic, accepting whatever deck of cards we were dealt before birth. On the contrary, there is much that can be done. We may not be completely in charge of our own personal destinies, but we do have an enormous potential to influence how we live and how we die. We are the products of our lifestyles as well as the producers of those lifestyles. Although the history of our own intrauterine life is critical to the function of our vital organs, our brain, liver and pancreas, there is much that happens after birth that either improves our situation or makes it much worse.

The message is always pay now, or pay later. Pay more attention to the quality of both prenatal and postnatal development. Pay more attention to your biology; you cannot transcend it. The evidence is compelling that our prenatal and immediate postnatal history is as important as our genes in determining who we are and the health we will enjoy throughout life. Ranchers and dog breeders have known for centuries that we are a combination of nature and nurture. Since we correctly eschew the use of forced genetic selection (which probably would not work anyway), the human race should pay closer attention to the environment in which we develop. It is the major modifiable factor that determines our health throughout life. We must have the courage to face what programming means for each and every one of us, biologically, intellectually, philosophically, financially, socially and politically. It is critically important that we follow lifestyles that provide the optimal home in the womb. I present no nostrums about how to get society to change its ways.

The philosophical question arises concerning the meaning of programming in relation to free will. I do not have an answer. In his *New York Times* book review of *"The Emotional Brain,"* by Joseph Le Doux, Richard Restak, himself an author, concludes; "My sole disappointment in this engrossing and engaging book is Mr. Le Doux's failure to elaborate on some of the forensic implications of his view of the human brain. For instance, if it's true that emotions exert such a powerful effect . . . what does this mean for the idea of individual responsibility?" Those who wish to raise similar questions about programming must be patient. We do not know for certain whether changes in the programming of the central brain systems involved in stress are the only cause or even the main cause of such conditions as anxiety or depression, which markedly alter personality. The experimental evidence clearly points to a relationship of these conditions to altered brain transmitter function, but there is much to learn.

The epidemiologic research, animal studies and clinical observations of many investigators in scores of laboratories around the world clearly point to a connection between maternal nutrition and the environment in the womb and obesity in later life. However, we do not yet know whether obesity is irremediably and exclusively (which I doubt) programmed by suboptimal prenatal life. The mechanisms whereby suboptimal maternal nutrition affects the developing pancreas, liver and fetal brain are only now being unraveled. The fetus that develops a thrifty metabolism to cope with the immediate problems in fetal life may program herself or himself for trouble in later life in a society where such thrift is not only unnecessary but is quite dangerous in the setting of abundant nutrition. There is much to learn before we can answer this overarching question. But a start has been made on building the necessary firm experimental and epidemiological foundation of knowledge.

What should the information on programming persuade us to do? Should we be fatalistic about the outcome? Should we even accept that prenatal conditions in our womb markedly alter the whole of our lives? In an age when so many people are prepared to turn to the horoscope pages daily to find out how their destinies are determined, it may not seem so difficult to accept that our time in the womb, not just the astrological sign under which we were born, may influence our lives.

The evidence I have given and the ideas I have raised may not be too readily acceptable to some readers. They may consider the notion that we are prenatally programed to a major extent to be dangerous nonsense that destroys feelings of control over our individual and collective destiny. Such a biological idea also alters our view about virtue and vice. The idea that we are programmed to some extent by prenatal life has similarities to the religious doctrine of original sin. Certainly, in both situations it is accepted that we are born into this world with some fairly rigid guidelines for our lives already in place. The idea of programming modifies, not destroys, the concept of free will. To accept that programming occurs in the womb is not dangerous nonsense. The danger lies in not considering the possibility. The peril lies in not evaluating the extent and the organ systems that may be affected (including brain and behavior). If, as a result of evaluation of the data, we find the evidence compelling, we should act accordingly. Free will may not exist, but we had better behave as if it does. For those who believe in free will, then paradoxically the correct response to developmental programming is to exert that freedom of action to improve the developmental heritage of our children and maximize their capability to exert their own free will after birth and throughout life.

Programming, like all new stories, is not completely new. The concept is, however, iconoclastic. It shakes the foundations of how we look at our own emotional and physical reactions to life. Focus on environmental aspects of programming runs counter to the current obsession with the genome. Advocating the existence of programming in the womb does not decrease the importance of our genetic blueprint. There is a difference between the naysayer and the iconoclast. The iconoclast has construction in mind but must first put forward firm data to tumble the icons she or he would destroy and then replace. The icon in this instance is the concept of the gene dominant. I hope I have given you a satisfying explanation of how some prenatal influences program lifelong health. I have tried to describe what we have learned about the mechanisms. I leave it to you, the reader, to evaluate whether these ideas are not just plausible but have an existence in reality.

A fundamental distinguishing feature of the human race when compared with other animal species is its ability to take information and use it to individual and collective advantage. The evidence I have presented has been obtained by dedicated researchers throughout the world. The information is yours; it has largely been produced by your tax dollars provided through national health funding agencies. The information belongs to you. What you do with it is your business. I just wish you and your children a healthier life and a better understanding of who we are and of the strengths and limitations of our biology. Do with this information what you will, but wonder at how we are made; for as the psalmist says, we are “fearfully and wonderfully made.”

There is a measure of pain in the beauty of the biological concept that developmental programming can modify our health and well-being throughout life. Just as Darwinism shook the nineteenth century from its complacent view that God has worked it all out for us and there is nothing for us to do, so the idea that we can influence our fate, in this case our children’s health and that of subsequent generations, imposes limitations on us and defines obligations for the future. Freud had the same disquieting effect on how we view ourselves. The idea that our health throughout life is programmed in a major way must alter how we view ourselves.

Deeper knowledge about programming will enable us to understand ourselves better and bring this knowledge to bear on problems of health and disease. Polio was not conquered by building a better iron lung. The iron lung provided treatment for the symptoms, it just kept the patient breathing. It did not prevent or even greatly lessen the progress of the disease. Prevention, the best cure, followed detailed understanding of the biology of the virus and the ability to produce an effective vaccine. Only then was polio finally overcome. As we improve understanding of the way our bodies work and piece together the origins of health and disease, our lives and those of our children and our children's children will be less troubled by illness that lessens their potential and their enjoyment of this beautiful world in which we live.

There are two major reasons that stimulated me to write this book. First, I would like to think that some readers have explored new territory, previously unknown to them about their biological origins. It is these origins that make us who we are. The details of our prenatal origins influence us just as much as, if not more than, the homes in which we grow, the towns in which we live, the people who we meet and like or dislike, the schools we attend and the jobs we perform. Second, when we survey the vista that makes us who we are and how we respond to the world and people about us, knowledge of our own biology, especially our early development, is as important to our knowledge of the world we live in as places we have been and people we have known. "Perhaps the roses really want to grow, the vision seriously intends to stay. If I could tell you, I would let you know."

FURTHER READING AND NOTES

CHAPTER 1. THE PRENATAL ORIGIN OF HEALTH AND DISEASE

Challenges, choices and consequences: Fetal life is lived by a set of biological rules that often differ from the rules that operate in life after birth. Babies in the womb are not just miniature adults. They have very different tasks to perform than they do after birth. Fetuses must live for the present while at the same time planning for a future of which they have no experience. In *Life Before Birth: The Challenges of Fetal Development* (W. H. Freeman, 1996), I have described many of the challenges fetuses face during normal development. I also described how the fetus makes difficult choices in suboptimal conditions.

Fetal responses to lack of oxygen: Specialized cells in the nervous system monitor oxygen levels in the fetal blood. When the delivery of oxygen to the fetal brain falls below the required level, fetuses shut down the blood supply to less important organs such as their skin, gut and muscles of the limbs and increase the supply to their heart, brain, adrenal glands and placenta. This redistribution of blood is a very clever trick, similar to what happens if an adult hemorrhages from a stomach ulcer. An adult in shock from hemorrhage looks ashen because the blood supply to the skin has been drastically reduced. Redistributing blood to the brain and heart at the expense of the liver, gut and other fetal organs is a clever choice in the short term. However, when the compensation continues for a lengthy period, growth of the deprived organs slows as a consequence of cutting down their blood supply. As a result, a growth-retarded baby may have a relatively normal-sized head accompanied by reduced abdominal girth. The challenge to the growing body may exact a long-term price as a consequence of making these choices that are beneficial in the short run.

The interested reader will find a large number of studies that describe how fetuses centralize their blood supply in times of need. Many of them are reviewed in an excellent book, *Fetus and Neonate: Physiology and Clinical Applications—The Circulation* 1 (1993): 1–438, (ed: Hanson, M., et al., Cambridge University Press); Itskovitz, J., et al., "Effects of cord compression on fetal blood flow distribution and O_2 delivery," *Am. J. Physiol.* 21 (1987): H100–H109; Jensen, A., et al., "Effects of reducing uterine blood flow on fetal blood flow distribution and oxygen delivery," *J. Dev. Physiol.* 15 (1991): 309–323; Cohn, H. E., et al., "Cardiovascular responses to hypoxemia and acidemia in fetal lambs," *Am. J. Obstet. Gynecol.* 120 (1974): 817–824; Jensen, A. and Berger, R., "Fetal circulatory responses to oxygen lack," *J. Dev. Physiol.* 16 (1991): 181–207.

Ten principles of programming. My list of ten major principles of programming is not meant to be exhaustive. However, together, these principles show that to provide every child with the best start in life, it is necessary to understand the importance of development during life before birth. These ten principles also help us to know more about how we should live our lives to best fit the style of preparation we completed during life before birth.

The Barker hypothesis of prenatal programming: For a detailed summary of the data from Dr. Barker and his research group at the Medical Research Council Environmental Epidemiology Group at the University of Southampton as well as other investigators worldwide, see the second edition of his book, *Mothers, Babies and Health in Later Life* (Churchill Livingstone, 1998). For his contribution to developing these new ideas, David Barker was elected a Fellow of the Royal Society in 1998.

The value of a responsive genome: The ability of the genome (the term for all the genes we inherit from our parents) to respond to prenatal environmental challenges and insults is clearly advantageous to postnatal survival of the individual. Regardless of whether any specific prenatal modification of development is beneficial, a responsive rather than a fixed and unresponsive genome will provide opportunities for natural selection to modify development to produce individuals with characteristics that reflect the effect of the environment on the genome. The flexibility provided by this opportunity for the genetic program to respond to the environment gives greater chances for the species to adapt to changing environments by producing a different phenotype.

It is important to distinguish phenotype from genotype: The phenotype of an individual is that individual's ultimate body construction and function. Each one of us has a particular phenotype achieved as a result of the interaction of our genotype (another term for genome) and the environments in which we developed and have lived throughout our lives. Species with a responsive genome will produce offspring with a broader range of phenotypes.

Fetal learning and behavior: Dr. Peter Hepper from Queen's University, Belfast, Northern Ireland, and other psychologists have extensively studied the behavior of the fetus and newborn baby. From their work they have provided clues on how the baby undergoes transitions—often rapidly—through stages of maturation of brain and behavior.

The TV soap opera *Neighbours* is very popular in Britain. Peter Hepper used ultrasound to observe fetuses of mothers who regularly watched this program. By thirty-seven weeks of pregnancy, the babies clearly were responding to the theme tune by increasing their body movements. When these same babies were tested two to four days after birth, they stopped moving and paid attention. So their response to the music had changed in the transition from fetal to newborn life. By twenty-one days of life, the babies had ceased to respond to the *Neighbours* theme music. The babies' behavioral response was not a response just to any music since when Peter Hepper played the tune backward, the babies did not respond at any time. These studies show that babies have a limited ability to retain sound and other memories of challenges to which they were exposed in the uterus.

Exposing the fetus to garlic when mothers eat large quantities late in pregnancy results in the ability of the baby to detect garlic in early life. Babies are born with considerable learning ability that allows them to make attachments to their mother. It is very important for babies to have familiarity and recognition for the structure of life around them. However, the learning that occurs at this time appears to be poorly retained. See also notes in chapter 9. Hepper, P. G., "Fetal memory: Does it exist? What does it do?" *Acta Paediatr. Suppl.* 416 (1996): 16–20.

Newborn milestones: T. Berry Brazelton has written extensively about the spurts of development that occur over the first years of life after birth. He has focused attention on this period as providing very important windows, or touch points, to understand the development of behavior. These milestones are described in his book *Touchpoints* (Addison-Wesley, 1992). We also need to be aware that we pass more biological milestones during life before birth than we do after we are born.

Sexual differentiation of the brain: For a fuller discussion of the effects of male hormones on the maturing brain, see chapter 9, and also *Life Before Birth: The Challenges of Fetal Development* (W. H. Freeman, 1996), page 124; Swaab, D. F. and Hoffman, M. A., "Sexual differentiation of the human hypothalamus in relation to gender and sexual orientation," *Trends in NeuroSciences* 18 (1995): 264–270; Barraclough, C. A., "Production of anovulatory, sterile rats by single injections of testosterone propionate," *Endocrinology* 68 (1961): 62–67.

Structure of DNA: In 1954, Crick and Watson put forward the concept that our genes are made like two strings of pearls wound around each other. There are only four different types of individual pearls, or bases, to use their chemical name. The bases are paired so that a link is present between one base on each string as the two strings wind around each other. These links hold the two strands together. The four bases are adenine, thymine, guanine and cytosine. Adenine on one string always pairs against thymine, and guanine with cytosine. When a cell divides, the two strings separate. As a new double string is made, each base can only pair off with its specific partner base. As a result an exact copy of the original double string will be made by pairing the specific bases on the two single strings. Thus, the genetic blueprint can be preserved from cell to cell and generation to generation. The precise pattern of bases on the string carries the code that tells a cell which proteins it should make. Proteins have two fundamental functions in the cell: They are the structural building blocks of cells, so inadequate production of proteins leads to poorly structured bodies; and proteins are enzymes that regulate the rate of synthesis and degradation within cells. As a result of these two functions, the way the genes produce specific proteins in each cell type will control the level of activity of that cell. In its nucleus, every cell has every one of the same 100,000 genes that constitute our heritage. However, as cells differentiate to undertake specific functions they focus on producing just a few specialized proteins—the ones they need to carry out their specialized activities. See also chapter 3 "Notes." Darnell, J. E., "RNA," *Scientific American*, 253 (1985): 68–87.

Palmistry and dermatoglyphics: Perhaps fortune-tellers know more about some features of our bodies than biologists. One study followed up 139 men and women who were born in Sharoe Green Hospital in Preston, England, from 1935 to 1943. The number of whorl patterns was greater on the fingers of people who were thin at birth. This fascinating paper also describes a longer palm in individuals with long thin hands. High blood pressure in later life was associated with increased numbers of whorls on the fingertips as well as thin palms. Similar studies have been conducted in India and on Japanese Americans in Hawaii. In a study from Scotland Yard, the coordinating police center in Britain, whorls were shown to be commoner on the right hand than the left. Godfrey, K. M., et al., "Relation of fingerprints and shape of the palm to fetal growth and adult blood pressure," *Br. Med. J.* 307 (1993): 405–409.

A link between fingerprints and eugenics: Sir Francis Galton (1822–1911) first introduced the use of fingerprints into forensic science as an aid to catching criminals. Galton is often considered as one the first proponents of eugenics. The science of eugenics aims to improve the biological capabilities of humans by selecting premium parents. As the *Encyclopedia Britannica* states, Galton "tended to underestimate the role of the social environment." Needless to say, he was totally ignorant of the critical and significant effects of the prenatal environment on human performance and on health and disease throughout life. I wonder what Galton would have thought about the environmental as opposed to genetic causes of changes in fingerprints.

Galton also had another interest that can be related to prenatal programming. The *Encyclopedia Britannica* notes, "His investigations of . . . sterility arising from marriage with heiresses (who as sole issue of unprolific parents might tend themselves to be infertile) are of particular importance." The principles of programming can be invoked to explain the relative infertility of heiresses, often the single child of the wealthy parents. It is possible to propose that the mother of the heiress provided a suboptimal beginning to life in the womb, and that is why she produced only one child. If that female child was growth-retarded and herself had a small uterus, then she may be more likely to have trouble conceiving. In addition, this sole female child may have a resetting of the hormone systems that control her reproductive cycles. Such a scenario would fit with transgenerational passage of body functions from mother to daughter.

Progression to rational treatments: For a very readable account of the transition from Greco-Roman medicine based on authority, speculation and superstition to modern evidence-based medicine, see *Science and the Quiet Art* by David Weatherall (W. W. Norton, 1995).

The position of diabetes in the death scorecard: The developed world is experiencing an epidemic of diabetes. *USA Weekend* published a death score card, which places diabetes sixth in the list of causes of death of women (33,130 deaths in 1995) and eighth among men (26,124 deaths in 1995). The relative contributions of genes and the environment to this recent increase in diabetes are hotly debated. There are several places in this book at which this debate is addressed, but see particularly chapter 7. In 1995, heart disease accounted for 374,849 deaths in women of all ages, cancer for 256,844 and strokes for 96,428. In men, heart disease accounted for 262,714 deaths, cancer for 281,611 and strokes for 61,563. "Who's Healthier," *USA Weekend,* Jan. 2–4 (1998): 4–7.

Cellular sociology: Cells in organs form a society similar to any human town or village. Cells in the body talk to each other by a variety of different mechanisms. The study of cellular biology could be called cellular sociology. There are basically four distinct ways cells talk to each other: via nerves, hormones, and paracrine and autocrine regulatory chemicals. Nerves carry out long- distance communication via fibers that are hardwired between the two cells that are conversing. Endocrine communication is wider ranging. Endocrine cells secrete hormones directly into the bloodstream. Examples are insulin in the case of the pancreas or thyroxine from the thyroid gland in the neck. Once in the blood, the hormone can circulate freely to nearly all the cells in the body. The major exceptions are cells in the brain. Most cells in the brain lie behind a barrier through which many hormones cannot pass. When the hormone passes cells that have surface receptors for the hormone, the hormone attaches to a receptor and is taken into the cell. Hormones either stimulate or inhibit their target cell. Paracrine communication is more intimate. Paracrine regulatory chemicals are secreted by cells into the fluid surrounding them. They then act to alter the function of their immediate neighbors, either increasing their activity or inhibiting it. The molecules that carry the paracrine message do not have to get into the bloodstream to have their effects. Like neighbors, cells communicating in a paracrine fashion talk across the garden fence. Autocrine regulatory molecules are secreted by cells and then act on the membranes of the same cell that released them. Several aspects of these methods of cell talk are considered in chapter 4 of *Life Before Birth: The Challenges of Fetal Development* (W. H. Freeman, 1996).

Correlation and causation: Stephen Jay Gould has written extensively about the misuse of statistical relationships. See *Full House* (Three Rivers Press, 1996) and *The Mismeasure of Man* (W. W. Norton & Co., 1981).

Tobacco as a risk factor for cancer: David Weatherall writes in *Science and the Quiet Art* (W. W. Norton, 1995), "In October 1989 the World Health Organization convened a consultative group on tobacco-related mortality and some of its frightening conclusions were published in the spring of 1992 . . . annual deaths from smoking in the developed countries alone numbered about 0.9 million in 1965 and are predicted to reach approximately 2.1 million in 1995 . . . half these deaths will be of persons in the age range of thirty-five to sixty-nine." This book contains an interesting history of the work that lead to the indictment of tobacco as a major cause of cancer. There is more information about mechanisms by which smoking creates an unfavorable environment in the womb in chapter 8. The several whammies that cigarette smoking delivers to the developing fetus are considered in detail in the chapter entitled "Baby on Board—Don't Abuse" in *Life Before Birth: The Challenges of Fetal Development* (W. H. Freeman, 1996).

The placenta as a supply line between fetus and mother: The many functions of the placenta are discussed in chapter 5 of *Life Before Birth: The Challenges of Fetal Development* (W. H. Freeman 1996). Although the placentas of different animal species differ greatly in shape and complexity, the placenta plays similar roles in all species. Because the placenta has to perform the functions of a lung, gut and kidney for the fetus, regardless of the species, much has been learned from the comparative studies on the placenta in many species. The placenta grows to almost its full size very early in pregnancy. Growing a good placenta is a major key to good prenatal development.

The words *congenital* and *genetic* are too often confused and misused: The word *congenital* refers to a condition that is present at birth. Articles by writers who should know better declaim that such and such a condition is genetic *because* the condition is present at birth. The presence of an abnormality at birth does not tell us that the abnormality is genetically controlled. A condition that is present at birth does not have to be inherited from the parents. For example, the deformed facial features and mental retardation of a baby exposed to alcohol during development in the womb is a congenital condition. This condition is called fetal alcohol syndrome (FAS). FAS is discussed at some length in chapter 8. The abnormalities that occur in FAS are present at birth. They are clearly not caused by the genes. If the baby had not been exposed to alcohol during development, the condition would not occur.

Chapter 2. The Dutch Hunger Winter

The ill-fated British paratroop airdrop at Arnhem in eastern Holland: British paratroopers were dropped into the Arnhem area on

September 17, 1944, in an attempt to seize a strategic bridge across the Rhine river. For an account of this episode in the Second World War, see W. Warmbrunn in *The Dutch under German Occupation 1940–1945* (Stanford University Press, 1963).

Lifelong health consequences of the Dutch Hunger Winter: A major effort is currently under way to study the lifelong consequences of being a fetus during the Dutch Hunger Winter. Women in Holland who were nutritionally deprived during the winter of 1944–1945 gave birth to babies who were more likely to be of lower birthweight. Their babies were also more likely to suffer from obesity, diabetes and schizophrenia in later life. Ravelli, G. P., et al., "Obesity in young men after famine exposure in utero and early infancy," *N. Engl. J. Med.* 295 (1976): 349–353; Ravelli, A. C. J., et al., "Glucose tolerance in adults after prenatal exposure to famine," *Lancet* 351 (1998): 173–177.

Studies in rats show that there is transgenerational passage of the effects of poor nutrition during fetal life: Much can be learned about the effects of poor nutrition on many aspects of lifelong health from two classic reports, one published as early as 1975. In these studies, rats were maintained on either adequate or marginally deficient protein diets for twelve generations. The malnourished group of rats were adversely affected in many ways when compared with rats receiving adequate nutrition. In the malnourished rats, growth retardation was ten times as high, sexual maturation was delayed and several key organs including the kidneys and brain, were smaller than rats who had received a normal diet. Young rats in the malnourished group had increased random exploratory activity. It was more difficult to attract and keep their attention. There is an eerie similarity to attention hyperactivity disorders that are too often seen in young boys and girls. The study states, "In situations demanding a choice the animals were very excited, emitted loud squeals and tried to escape from what was clearly a stressful situation . . . casual examination of the malnourished adults revealed a rather small, badly groomed, excitable rat without gross abnormalities." Rehabilitation of rats from the twelfth generation exposed to malnutrition was attempted by feeding the mothers a normal diet at one of three times: during pregnancy, from immediately after they delivered or after they had weaned their babies. The only group to recover their weight completely were the pups of mothers who were rehabilitated during pregnancy. Most, but not all, the behavioral and learning deficits disappeared after three generations of maternal rehabilitation. Stewart, R. J. C., et al., "Twelve generations of marginal protein deficiency," *Brit. J. Nutr.* 33 (1975): 233–253; Stewart, R. J. C., et al., "The effect of rehabilitation at different stages of development of rats marginally malnourished for ten to twelve generations," *Brit. J. Nutr.* 43 (1980): 403–412.

There is information from the Dutch Hunger Winter that shows the transgenerational passage of poor nutrition in human pregnancy: Dr. Lambert Lumey, working both at Columbia University in New York and at the Academic Medical Center in Amsterdam, studied the outcome of pregnancy in 1,808 daughters of the Dutch Hunger Winter born between January 1, 1944, and June 30, 1946. Most of these mothers had spent different parts of their own lives as fetuses exposed to the Dutch Hunger Winter. Those who had not been exposed at all acted as controls against which to compare the effects of food deprivation. When mothers had spent the first six months of their own fetal life during the famine, their own babies were smaller than the babies of the mothers not exposed to the famine. If the exposure to malnutrition in the womb occurred only during the final third of pregnancy, the mothers did not have smaller babies. Lumey, L. H., "Decreased birthweights in infants after maternal in utero exposure to the Dutch famine of 1944-1945," *Paediat. Perinat. Epid.* 6 (1992): 240–253.

Studies conducted immediately after the Second World War on the effects of wartime starvation in Holland: Clement Smith's two classic reports are well worth reading as a medical history of a little-known effect of war. Smith, C. A., "The effect of wartime starvation in Holland upon pregnancy and its product," *Am. J. Obstet. Gynecol.* 53 (1947): 599–608; Smith, C. A., " Effects of maternal undernutrition upon the newborn infant in Holland (1944-1945)," *J. Pediatr.* 30 (1947): 229–243.

Effect of poor nutrition on the early growth of the placenta: The single most important requirement in early pregnancy is the correct growth of a placenta that will function efficiently throughout the whole period of fetal development. There are many studies that have shown that early nutritional deprivation results in increased placental growth. This overgrowth of the placenta appears to be an attempt to increase transfer of nutrients and oxygen to the fetus. Pregnancy lasts 150 days in sheep. Drs. Faichney and White were among the first to show the effects of moderate dietary restriction in early pregnancy on the growth of the placenta. They restricted the diet of pregnant ewes from the fiftieth to the hundredth day of pregnancy and then provided an adequate diet in the rest of the pregnancy. This diet resulted in the production of a large placenta and the birth of a large lamb. Since this early observation, these results have been thoroughly confirmed. Information is now needed on the mechanisms that promote this increased growth of the placenta. In many pregnant women, the function of the placenta is less than adequate for a variety of reasons, and knowledge of the ways in which the placenta tries to compensate for poor nutrition may provide opportunities to help the growth-retarded baby. Faichney, G. J. and White, G.A., "Effects of maternal nutritional status on fetal and placental growth and on fetal urea synthesis in sheep," *Aust. J. Biol. Sci.* 40 (1987): 365–377.

Under nutrition during fetal development can result in either obesity or leanness in later life: Dr. Gian Carlo Ravelli and colleagues at the Academic Medical Center in Amsterdam studied 300,000 nineteen- year-old men who were exposed as fetuses to the Dutch famine. If the famine occurred during the last third of the babies' prenatal life or in the early postnatal period, the men were less likely to be obese when they grew up. The explanation may be that when food deprivation occurs during the late developmental stages when fat cells are forming or dividing, an individual will have fewer fat cells throughout life. In sharp contrast, if the food deprivation occurred during the first half of fetal life, the opposite effect was noted. There was a higher incidence of obesity in later life in men who were in the early months of development during exposure. The authors suggest that when the food deprivation occurs early, appetite centers in the baby's brain are reset, resulting in an excessive food intake in later life. See number four of our principles of programming. Ravelli, G. P., et al., "Obesity in young men after famine exposure in utero and early infancy," *N. Engl. J. Med.* 295 (1976): 34.

The effects of prenatal malnutrition on babies who were born during the siege of Leningrad, now renamed Saint Petersburg: Unfortunately, information available on babies born during the Leningrad siege lacks the babies' birthweights. For this reason, conclusions on the lifelong adverse effects on babies who underwent their prenatal development during the siege will never be as powerful as the information on the Dutch Hunger Winter. John Yudkin and his colleagues have studied adults who were born during the Leningrad siege. They came to the following conclusions regarding the key lifetime health messages from this epic struggle: "In this study intrauterine exposure to malnutrition was not associated with glucose intolerance [which reflects a tendency to diabetes] . . . [However] obesity and blood pressure were more strongly related in subjects exposed to intrauterine malnutrition than in subjects either unexposed to malnutrition or exposed to malnutrition only as infants." Stanner, S. A., et al., "Does malnutrition in utero determine diabetes and coronary heart disease in adulthood? Results from the Leningrad siege study, a cross sectional study," *Brit. Med. J.* 315 (1997): 1342–1349.

Male fetuses are more at risk during development than female fetuses: The proportion of males in the general population decreases at each stage of life. At conception, males comprise 56 percent of the population; in the first five years of life males, are 51 percent; below thirty years of age, males are 50 percent; between fifty and fifty-four years of age, males have dropped to 49 percent, or less than half of the population for the first time; over sixty-five years of age, men comprise only 41 percent of the population; over eighty-five, males have dwindled to 29 percent; and only 18 percent of centenarians are male. "Who's Healthier," *USA Weekend* Jan. 2–4 (1998): 4–7.

CHAPTER 3. DETECTIVE STORIES

Small pieces of information whose significance originally went unnoticed may often provide the critical clue: The knowledge that DNA contains only four different bases, cytosine, guanine, thymine and adenine, had been available to biochemists for some time when the Austrian born American biochemist Erwin Chargaff demonstrated that the number of cytosine bases in DNA exactly matches the number of guanine bases and that the number of adenine and thymine bases also match each other. At the time he made this observation, Chargaff was blissfully unaware that he had found the key to DNA's twisting double helix structure. It was left to Francis Crick and James Watson to understand the significance of this pairing. They made the equal content of cytosine and guanine and the similar equal content of adenine and thymine the basis of their revolutionary new idea of how the two helical chains of DNA wound around each other in a way that allows them to separate and duplicate themselves at the time of cell division. Crick and Watson argued that since adenine and thymine were matched, they were probably paired opposite each other. Similarly, guanine and cytosine must be paired up against each other. It was from this new use of old knowledge that Crick and Watson were able to go on to the fundamental idea that DNA is made up of two strands with one base present on one strand of DNA and the other matching base on the opposite strand. They proposed that, as the two strands of the DNA molecule wound themselves around each other, the bases were the glue that held the strands together. Once this relationship was apparent, determining the structure of the double helix could proceed rapidly. See also notes to chapter 1 and David Weatherall in *Science and the Quiet Art* (W. W. Norton, 1995).

Mothers, Babies and Health in Later Life by David Barker (Churchill Livingstone, 1998), is an excellent compendium of David Barker's own papers and the detailed work on programming.

Intelligence and the quality of life before birth: David Barker's early paper makes it quite clear that a multitude of factors affects human intelligence. Until we have a better understanding of the normal development of the brain, it will be very difficult to apportion the relative roles of nurture and nature, the environment and the genes, in determining who we are and how we perform throughout life. The debate is not helped by sloppy science such as portrayed in Richard Herrnstein and Charles Murray's book *The Bell Curve* (Free Press, 1994) and other attempts to demonstrate that intelligence is all in our genes, all hereditary. For a lively discussion of many of the issues raised in *The Bell Curve,* see *The Bell Curve Debate,* edited by Russell Jacoby and Naomi Glauberman (Times Books, 1995). The best estimates of the contribution of the genes and the environment is that they contribute in roughly equal amounts. You can take your pick from all the various calculations on this tendentious subject. The numbers run from 40 to 60 percent for each. Barker, D. J. P., "Low intelligence: Its relation to length of gestation and rate of foetal growth," *Br. J. Prev. Soc. Med.* 20 (1966): 58–66; and Herrnstein and Murray's *The Bell Curve: Intelligence and Class Structure in American Life* (Free Press, 1994). See also "Notes" for chapter 9.

The importance of the study of the physiology of life before birth to the care of human babies, both before and after birth: The progress in building the epidemiologic story in support of prenatal programming shows the importance of continuity in any scientific discipline. Much of the work that has helped to elucidate the concept of programming has come from studies on pregnant animals. The sheep has been the major animal to be studied and has provided critical, life-saving information that is widely used in the neonatal intensive care unit. The rigorous scientific study of the fetus began in Cambridge, England, in the 1930s in the laboratory of Sir Joseph Barcroft, who many consider the founder of the study of fetal physiology. Barcroft was born in 1872 in Ireland of Quaker stock. He died in 1947. For a short biography of Barcroft, see the loving dedication by Donald Barron in *Fetal and Neonatal Physiology,* Proceedings of the Sir Joseph Barcroft Centenary Symposium, ed: Comline, R. S., et al. (Cambridge University Press, 1973).

Barcroft's ideas and methods were taken across the Atlantic to laboratories in the United States following a serendipitous event in

1935. Donald Barron, a young American student, had recently arrived at the Physiological Laboratory at Cambridge University to study the passage of electrical signals along nerve fibers with Sir Bryan Matthews. One day, while walking on the Downing site, where the science laboratories are located in Cambridge University, Barron saw an elderly, white-coated scientist trying to cajole a pregnant sheep through a door. Being young and eager to help, Barron went to the researcher's assistance, and together, they coaxed the sheep into Barcroft's laboratory. The senior scientist and young student struck up an acquaintance. One thing led to another, and Barron developed a lifelong interest in fetal development. Barron returned to Yale and was the pioneer force behind the American school of fetal physiology. Two of Barron's students, Giacomo Meschia and Frederick Battaglia, were among the leaders of the next generation, taking the discipline west from Yale to Denver. The fourth generation now carries on the work in Denver under Dr. William Hay and at many other sites in America, Australasia and Europe. There is transgenerational passage of function in science, too, that is not genetically based.

The difficulty of proving correlation from human epidemiologic studies: Human development is a continuum. Each step is based on what has gone before. Thus, even though a correlation may be shown between two events, each of those events can be correlated to other events. It may be that both of the correlated events are caused by a separate third event that occurred earlier than both. Even when two lifetime events are correlated, the cause may be just one part of one event. When we can show that heart disease is correlated with early development, it is important to find out which phase of early development and what are the mechanisms. One of the major contributions from the Southampton data has been to focus attention on the prenatal period. Prior to the work of David Barker and his colleagues, most researchers considered the critical periods in determining lifelong health were all postnatal. See Barker, D. J. P., et al., "Infant mortality, childhood nutrition, and ischaemic heart disease in England and Wales," *Lancet* 1 (1986): 1077–1081.

The devil is in the details: The use of well-collected

epidemiologic data is clearly seen in the studies mentioned in this chapter. The value of the conclusions from epidemiological studies depends on the detail and clarity of the record database. The outcomes of pregnancies occurring around the time of the Dutch Hunger Winter can be related to the period of pregnancy during which the mother, and hence her baby, were undernourished. The Dutch studies showed that the final third of pregnancy is the single most important third as far as overall growth is concerned. However, the greatest effects were always seen in the babies who were deprived throughout the full period of their development. Their heads were the smallest. They were also the shortest and weighed the least. The value of different human epidemiologic studies depends on the selection of the individuals studied. When, for example, only patients who are in a hospital are studied, the population has already selected itself and may not be truly representative of the world at large. In contrast to the detailed Dutch data, the data on babies born during the siege of Leningrad lacks detail on birthweights and other important features, which makes the follow up of individuals much less rewarding. See also chapter 2 "Notes" on the Dutch Hunger Winter.

CHAPTER 4. TRANSGENERATIONAL ORIGINS OF HEALTH AND DISEASE: DISEASE FIGHTS FORWARD

Diabetes, the wasting disease: Under normal circumstances, the body does not waste glucose by passing it out in the urine. If normal amounts of glucose are present in the blood, the kidney is quite able to reabsorb all the glucose that is filtered out of the blood when the urine is formed. However, when blood glucose levels rise above a certain threshold, the kidney's reabsorption mechanism is overwhelmed, and glucose begins to appear in the urine. Testing for glucose in the urine is one of the easiest ways to diagnose diabetes. The name *diabetes* comes from the Greek word meaning "to flow through" and refers to the large amount of urine that is formed. The full name of the disease that occurs when the body produces insufficient amounts of insulin is *diabetes mellitus*. *Mellitus* comes from the Greek word for "sweet" and refers to the presence of much sugar in the urine, which gives it a sweet taste.

By itself, this loss of glucose from the body is not critically damaging. However, the loss of energy sources results in an increase in appetite, so diabetics eat more. The sinister aspect of the loss of glucose in the urine is not the actual amount of glucose lost. The danger to the body is the reason behind the loss, namely the inability of the majority of cells in the body to take up the glucose they need to maintain normal function. However, there is an unwanted side effect of a large amount of glucose in the urine. As glucose appears in the urine in larger and larger amounts, glucose drags water out of the body with it. As a result, the uncontrolled diabetic is constantly passing urine and, if untreated, diabetics can become fatally dehydrated.

Without enough insulin in their blood to pack away the glucose into the cells, the brain of a diabetic will function efficiently in the short term because the nerve cells do not need insulin to allow them to take up glucose. However, insulin-deficient individuals cannot pump glucose into their muscle and fat cells. If the insulin deficiency occurs during development, many developing organs will suffer. When these cells are deprived of their energy sources, they have to burn other fuels, fat and protein. If diabetics burn too much protein, there won't be enough left to grow normally. Indeed, in a real crisis, young diabetics may have to put growth processes into reverse and break down some tissues that they have just built up. The burning of too much fat is also not a good idea. Unless there is some glucose to burn, fat burned by itself produces acids that smell like rotten apples and increase the acidity of the blood. Untreated, a completely insulin-deficient diabetic will die of increased levels of acid in the blood, wasting and dehydration.

Glucose tolerance tests enable the physician to determine whether a patient's body is using glucose correctly: Normality of the body's ability to regulate the amount of glucose in the blood is evaluated by how high the blood glucose will rise following the administration of a standard amount of glucose. This is called a glucose tolerance test. If the amount of insulin secreted in response to the sudden load of glucose in the body is deficient, the amount of glucose in the blood will rise abnormally high. If the cells in the body are resistant to the action of insulin, the glucose levels may be abnormally high even if normal amounts of insulin are secreted. Both of these abnormalities can exist in humans. They may be mild or severe. The extent of the damage to the pancreas caused by exposure of the fetus to the consequences of untreated maternal diabetes can be tested by challenging the offspring with a glucose tolerance test.

The key role of the fetal pancreas during development: One of the best examples of the way in which the functions of hormones in the fetus differ from the functions in the adult is the critical role of insulin in regulating growth in the fetus. The elegant studies of Dr. Abigail Fowden at Cambridge University and other investigators in the United States, Australia and New Zealand, primarily studying the sheep fetus, have demonstrated that growth hormone plays a minor role in regulating growth before birth. Fowden, A. L., "The role of insulin in prenatal growth," *J. Dev. Physiol.* 12 (1989): 173–182; Fowden, A. L., et al., "The effects of insulin on the growth rate of the sheep fetus during late gestation," *Q. J. Exp. Physiol.* 74 (1989): 703–714; Fowden, A. L., "Endocrine regulation of fetal growth," *Reprod. Fert. Dev.* 7 (1995): 351–363.

The remarkable ability of the placenta to pass nutrients to the fetus: The placenta has a wide range of transport capabilities. Some molecules are actively transported across from the mother to the fetus by energy-consuming reactions. A good example is how the placenta provides the iodine that fetuses need to make their own supplies of the hormone thyroxine. Thyroxine crosses the placenta poorly, so fetuses must make thyroxine for themselves. Other compounds such as glucose have special carriers, called transporters, which facilitate their passage through the placenta. As glucose crosses from mother to fetus, the placenta uses some of the glucose for its own energy needs. The efficiency with which the placenta passes glucose from mother to fetus varies between species. The horse placenta is very efficient, the sheep less so. Primates, including humans, are more like the horse than the sheep. For a general review of the functions of the placenta, see chapter 5 of *Life*

Before Birth: The Challenges of Fetal Development by Peter W. Nathanielsz (W. H. Freeman, 1996).

Reduction in the numbers of blood vessels that form in an organ during fetal life will determine the function of that organ for a whole lifetime: The lifelong effect of formation of fewer blood vessels in an organ during development is an example of principle four in our list of principles of programming. The investigators from the Catholic University at Louvain in Belgium showed that when rats were fed the normal amounts of calories together with only half the normal amount of protein throughout pregnancy, there was a dramatic reduction in the number of blood vessels that developed during fetal life in the pancreas of their pups. Snoeck, A., et al., "Effect of a low protein diet during pregnancy on the fetal rat endocrine pancreas," *Biol. Neonate* 57 (1990): 107–118.

The pups of pregnant rats fed a low protein diet during pregnancy modify the preparations that occur in their livers during fetal development: When pregnant rats are fed a low-protein diet throughout pregnancy, key enzymes in the liver of their pups are permanently altered. Low-protein diets probably affect the fetus by changing the populations of different cell types in the liver—principle number four of our ten principles of programming. Hales, C. N., et al., "Fishing in the stream of diabetes: From measuring insulin to the control of fetal organogenesis," *Biochem. Soc. Trans.* 24 (1996): 341–350; Burns, S. P., et al., "Gluconeogenesis, glucose handling, and structural changes in livers of the adult offspring of rats partially deprived of protein during pregnancy and lactation," *J. Clin. Invest.* 100 (1997): 1768–1774.

When there are high levels of glucose in the mother's blood, glucose crosses the placenta to the fetus and damages the developing fetal pancreas: The cells in the pancreas that produce insulin are very sensitive to excessive challenge during their development. The pancreas of the babies of both diabetic rats and diabetic women shows similar signs of damage. Fortunately, diabetes in human pregnancy can be very carefully controlled with insulin to avoid these damaging effects on the fetal pancreas. Aerts, L., et al.,

"Rat foetal endocrine pancreas in experimental diabetes," *J. Endocrinol.* 73 (1977): 339–346.

The critical importance of developing the correct apparatus for air breathing by the lungs: The microscopic air sacs in our lungs are the place where oxygen finally gets close enough to our blood vessels to enter our bloodstream. Just like small balloons, air sacs tend to collapse due to the tension in their walls. The pressure in small bubbles is greater than in large bubbles, so small air sacs will tend to empty into larger ones. The lung produces surface-active chemicals to equalize the pressures in the air sacs of different sizes so that all the air sacs stay open. The ability of fats to maintain small bubbles is a general physical principle. It is even crucial to baking a light, airy loaf. When shortening is added to the dough, it provides the necessary fats. During baking, the fat from the shortening spreads itself over the bubbles of air in the bread so that the small bubbles maintain a low pressure. "The Science of Baking," *The Economist* (1996): 77.

Diabetic babies have problems producing the necessary surface active molecules, so they are more prone to problems with breathing immediately after birth. For more on the development of the fetal lungs, see chapter 6 of *Life Before Birth: The Challenges of Fetal Development,* Peter W. Nathanielsz (W. H. Freeman, 1996).

Transgenerational passage of diabetes across generations of rats by non-genetic mechanisms: The profound impact of the studies of Dr. Andre Van Assche and Dr. William Oh and their colleagues in Belgium and the United States has yet to register on the thinking of biologists and physicians in the evaluation of the relative effects of genetic inheritance and prenatal environmental effects in causing diabetes. I often think that Lamarck must be rolling in his grave. What he would have given for this information in support of his ideas on the transgenerational passage of acquired characteristics. These studies open new vistas on the ability of environmental effects to carry over from generation to generation. They provide truly revolutionary concepts that will alter our approach to health and disease. Van Assche, F. A., et al., "Long-term effect of diabetes and pregnancy in the rat," *Diabetes* 34 (1985): 116–118;

Holemans, K., et al., "Evidence for an insulin resistance in the adult offspring of pregnant streptozotocin-diabetic rats," *Diabetologia* 34 (1991): 81–85; Gelardi, N. L., et al., "Glucose metabolism in adipocytes of obese offspring of mild hyperglycemic rats," *Pediat. Res.* 28 (1990): 641–645; Gelardi, N. L., et al., "Evaluation of insulin sensitivity in obese offspring of diabetic rats by hyperinsulinemic-euglycemic clamp technique," *Pediat. Res.* 30 (1991): 40–44; Oh, W., et al., "Maternal hyperglycemia in pregnant rats: Its effect on growth and carbohydrate metabolism in the offspring," *Metabolism* 37 (1988): 1146–1151; Oh, W., et al., "The cross-generation effect of neonatal macrosomia in rat pups of streptozotocin-induced diabetes," *Pediat. Res.* 29 (1991): 606–610.

The maternal passage of susceptibility to diabetes in Pima Indians: The Pima Indians have lived in the Sonoran Desert area of the southwestern United States and northern Mexico for more than 2,000 years. For the last thirty years, the National Institute of Diabetes and Digestive and Kidney Disease, one of the National Institutes of Health, has been studying the incidence of diabetes and obesity among the Pima Indians. One-half of adult Pima Indians suffer from diabetes. Of these diabetics, 95 percent are overweight. The average age at which a Pima Indian becomes diabetic is thirty-six years. In white Americans, onset of diabetes usually occurs at about sixty years of age. Since the Pimas are a highly intermarried society, many investigators have jumped to the conclusion that the high prevalence of diabetes must be due to genetic transmission of diabetes. In 1962, the geneticist James Neel proposed that survival of the Pimas through periods of famine was made possible because they have a thrifty gene that helps them to store fat in times of plenty for use in times of shortage. Those who support the thrifty genotype hypothesis claim that it explains obesity in modern Pimas by proposing that while the gene helped individuals survive in times of famine, it leads to obesity in modern times where food is plentiful and little exercise is taken.

Those who favor the thrifty genotype hypothesis point to the differences between the Arizonan Pimas and their close relatives, the Pima's who live in the Sierra Madre of northern Mexico. In one small study, less than 10 percent of the Mexican Pimas suffered from diabetes. In addition, obesity was not a problem for the Mexican Pimas. One of the leading researchers in this field is quoted as saying, "We've learned from this study of Mexican Pimas that if the Pima Indians of Arizona could return to their traditions, including a high degree of physical activity and a diet with less fat and more starch, we might be able to reduce the rate, and surely the severity, of unhealthy weight in most of the population. . . . However, this is not as easy as it sounds because of factors such as genetic influences that are difficult to change."

The contrary view is put by David Pettit, also of the NIH. He says, "We know there is a non-genetic cause of diabetes, the diabetic intrauterine environment, which poses problems for the child that extend well beyond those apparent at birth. . . . It's a vicious cycle. Children whose mothers had diabetes during pregnancy have a higher risk of becoming obese and getting diabetes at a young age. Many will have diabetes . . . by the time they reach child-bearing years, thus perpetuating the cycle. . . . The challenge for the future is to see if it's possible to achieve diabetes control good enough to prevent the developing fetus from recognizing that the mother has diabetes. If we can do that, the rate of diabetes in the next generation is likely to decline, an achievement that would benefit not only the immediate children but future generations." *The Pima Indians: Pathfinders for Health*, a booklet published by the National Institutes of Health (publication number 95–3821).

CHAPTER 5. GROWTH IN THE WOMB: SIZE IS NOT EVERYTHING

The environment in the womb constrains the growth of the fetus: In the 1930s, Walton and Hammond crossed Shetland ponies and Shire horses and observed the size of the foals. This remains a classical investigation on the extent to which the size and nutrients available within the womb will permit the developing baby to develop to her or his full genetic potential. Walton, A. and Hammond, J., "The maternal effects on growth and conformation in Shire horse-Shetland pony crosses," *Proc. R. Soc. Lond.* 125 (1934): 311–335.

Embryo transfer studies are a better approach to investigating the effects of maternal constraints on fetal growth: The genetic makeup of the embryos in the Shire-Shetland and Shetland-Shire crosses is clearly different. The transfer of embryos of similar genetic makeup to mothers of different size and nutritional background is a much more powerful way to investigate the maternal constraints to growth. One interesting small study of pregnancies following ovum donation in women also showed that the birthweight of the baby was correlated with the birthweight of the recipient and not the donor. The authors conclude that "the environment provided by the human mother is more important than her genetic contribution to birthweight." Brooks, A. A., et al., "Birth weight: Nature or nurture," *Early Human Dev.* 42 (1995): 29–35; Youngs, C. R., et al., "Investigations into the control of litter size in swine: III. A reciprocal embryo transfer study of early conceptus development," *J. Anim. Sci.* 72 (1994): 725–731.

When the ratio of the weight of the placenta to the weight of the baby is high, that is evidence that the attempts are being made at compensation: Babies born at high altitudes weigh less than babies born at sea level. One Peruvian study compared babies born in Lima (altitude 500 feet) and in Rio Pallanga (altitude 15,100 feet). The ratio of the placental weight to birthweight in firstborn babies was 0.14 in Lima and nearly half as much again, 0.20 in babies born in Rio Pallanga. Put another way, babies born in Lima weighed an average of 3.37 kilograms (7.4 pounds) and their placentas weighed 474 grams (1.04 pounds). At the high altitude of Rio Pallanga, the babies' birthweight was reduced to an average of 2.92 kilograms (6.4 pounds), but their placentas weighed a whopping 581 grams (1.28 pounds), or over 100 grams more than the placentas of babies born at sea level. Kruger, H., et al., "The placenta and the newborn infant at high altitudes," *Am. J. Obstet. Gynecol.* 106 (1970): 586–591.

The placenta is our only throwaway organ: For nearly nine months during the development of each of us in the womb, the placenta was our lung, obtaining oxygen from mother; our gut, obtaining food; our kidneys, removing waste products. In addition, the placenta produced an enormous array of hormones. Despite these numerous critical activities on our behalf, the placenta's role was over at the time of birth and we threw away our placentas and took on the responsibilities ourselves. For more details on the development of the placenta, see chapter 6 of *Life Before Birth: The Challenges of Fetal Development*, Peter W. Nathanielsz (W. H. Freeman, 1996).

Country folklore about the placenta: George Evans writes in Chapter 16 of his book *The Pattern under the Plough: Aspect of the Folk-Life of East Anglia* (Faber and Faber, 1966): "there were a number of interesting East Anglian practices relating to cattle; they were similar to practices in other regions and they should be recorded if only because they illustrate the principles that underlie these practices everywhere. The first is the placing of a cow's afterbirth [placenta] on a thorn-bush. The same custom was practised with sows and mares. In clearing up after the birth the horseman or stockman took the placenta and threw it over a white-thorn, usually on a remote part of the farm where it remained until it had rotted away. The dynamic of this belief is pure contagious magic. While the placenta was on the thorn-bush there would be an unbreakable link between the animal and the bush; the thorn-bush was the *quickset* which as its name implies is always abundantly alive. This would ensure that the animal would still remain *quick* or fertile and would breed again next season; or alternatively, that the offspring of this particular birth would grow into a fine foal or calf, which was only a different application of the same principle."

"This belief was also held in East Anglia; and the writer recalls a Cambridgeshire woman giving a warning about the disposal of the placenta: 'You got to be very careful to bury it deep enough so the dogs won't get hold of it.' A district nurse in Suffolk has noticed a reluctance, especially in country areas. to burn the placenta. Burying is the accepted way of disposing of it, chiefly—she believes—because this has always been the practice, and probably not because many people believe in the continuing link between the mother and the severed part of her. But even in this apparently neutral practice the old principle of contagious magic persists in the suggestion that the best place to bury the placenta is under a grapevine."

A growing teenage mother competes with her baby for essential nutrients: Some recent animal studies throw light on some of the problems of teenage pregnancy. Dr. Jacqueline Wallace and her colleagues from Aberdeen in Scotland have developed a highly controlled model to study the way a growing mother's tissues may compete during pregnancy with those of her developing baby. She uses embryo transfer techniques to implant very similar embryos from adult sheep in the womb of adolescent sheep. This way, like Dr. Stephen Ford in his pig embryo transfer studies, Dr. Wallace can be sure that factors in the embryo are not the cause of any differences between the different groups of adolescent ewes she studies. She divides her pregnant adolescent ewes into two groups. During the first two thirds of pregnancy, she feeds one group a diet calculated to maintain their normal adolescent growth pattern. The other group is fed so that they grow rapidly. Rapid growth of the mother is accompanied by a decreased fetal and placental weight when compared with the ewes who grow at their normal rate. There are other problems with pregnancy in the rapidly growing adolescent ewes. They are more likely to deliver prematurely and they have less milk to feed their newborn lambs after birth. Wallace, J. M., et al., "Nutrient partitioning and fetal growth in rapidly growing adolescent ewes," *J. Reprod. Fertil.* 107 (1996): 183–190.

The many important functions performed by the fetal adrenal gland: The adrenal gland is essential to survival during life after birth. The various adrenal steroid hormones control the body's response to stress challenges and regulate the composition of our body fluids. Normal function of the baby's adrenal gland before birth is essential to normal maturation of many vital fetal organs, particularly the lung, kidneys and gut. The fetal adrenal gland also plays a key role in the processes that initiate labor and delivery. See chapter 12 of *Life Before Birth: The Challenges of Fetal Development,* Peter W. Nathanielsz (W. H. Freeman, 1996).

Two-way conversation between the fetus and the placenta: Early in pregnancy, fetuses that are short of nutrients send signals to the placenta to stimulate it to grow and work harder. The placenta also sends signals to the fetus. Several members of the prostaglandin group of molecular messengers are produced in the placenta, which secretes them into the umbilical vein. In the umbilical vein, prostaglandins pass from the placenta to the fetus and alter many fetal functions such as the breathing movements fetuses make to prepare for life after birth. Prostaglandins are also secreted from the maternal side of the placenta into the uterine vein. In pregnant sheep, the amount of prostaglandins produced by the placenta increases when the mother is undernourished. In this situation it is likely that the placenta is sending messages—encoded as prostaglandins—to both mother and fetus. Fowden, A. L., et al., "Nutritional control of respiratory and other muscular activities in relation to plasma prostaglandin E in the fetal sheep," *J. Dev. Physiol.* 11 (1989): 253–262; Fowden, A. L., et al., "The nutritional regulation of plasma prostaglandin E concentrations in the fetus and pregnant ewe during late gestation," *J. Physiol.* 394 (1987): 1–12.

Another interesting hormone produced by the placenta is corticotropin releasing hormone (CRH). CRH was first found in the brain by Drs. Wylie Vale and Roger Guillemin. The best-known function of CRH is to control the brain's responses to stress stimuli (see chapter 6). Placental CRH is secreted into both the maternal and fetal blood. Some researchers hold the view that when CRH is secreted into the maternal blood, it plays a role as a signal to both normal birth at the correct time as well as to starting the birth process early when premature birth occurs (see chapter 10). McLean, M., et al., "A placental clock controlling the length of human pregnancy," *Nature Medicine* 1 (1995): 460–463; Hobel, C. J., et al., "Maternal stress as a signal to the fetus," *Prenatal and Neonatal Med.* 3 (1998): 116–120.

The various specialized areas of the brain develop at different times in different species: The brain is the most complex organ in the body. There are well described spurts in the growth of the different brain regions at different times during prenatal development. As a result, suboptimal conditions in the womb will have varied effects on the brain depending on when they impact development.

Researchers who study brain development in prenatal and young animals are demonstrating that deficits from prenatal exposure to toxic materials such as lead are sometimes very subtle. Dobbing, J., et al., "Comparative aspects of the brain growth spurt," *Early Hum. Dev.* 3 (1979): 79–83; Davison, A. N., et al., "Myelination as a vulnerable period in brain development," *Br. Med. Bull.* 22 (1996): 40–44.

Nutritional deprivation at one stage of development may increase life span, while food shortages at other times in life may shorten life: Male offspring of pregnant rats who are fed a low-protein diet live a significantly shorter life than the male offspring of rats fed a normal diet. In contrast, lifespan of the males is increased if protein deprivation is restricted to the immediate postnatal period. Dr. Hales and his colleagues at Cambridge University in England combined prenatal protein restriction with excellent nutrition after birth aimed at producing catch-up growth by accelerating the growth of the newborn pups. Plentiful food postnatally did allow the pups of underfed mothers to catch up with the weight of pups from mothers who had been fed normally during pregnancy. However, the effect of forcing the pups to catch up by feeding them more after birth was remarkable. Forcing catch-up growth shortened lifespan by two months when compared with control pups from normally fed mothers. Translated into a human life span at the age of sixty, two extra months of rat life are equivalent to fifteen years. Principle number seven of our ten principles states that attempts to reverse the consequences of programming may have their own unwanted consequences. These studies did not investigate the cause of the early death in the rats that were forced to grow fast after birth. However, as mentioned below, rapid growth after birth may increase the risk of cancer. Hales, C. N., et al., "Fishing in the stream of diabetes: From measuring insulin to the control of fetal organogenesis," *Biochem. Soc. Trans.* 24 (1996): 341–350.

High birthweight is associated with a higher than normal risk of breast cancer: There may be unwanted outcomes when babies grow faster in the womb than their optimal rate. High birthweight has been associated with an increased risk of breast cancer. This is especially true for women who get breast cancer at an early age, in distinction to those whose cancer begins later in life. It has been suggested that the rapid growth in the womb is a response to higher-than-normal estrogen levels in the mother's blood. Estrogen is known to enhance the blood supply to the uterus, and this may provide the basis of the accelerated growth of the baby. When the baby is a female, the maternal estrogens may alter the number of cells growing in the developing baby's breast. This is an example of principle number four of our ten principles of programming. Michels, K. B., et al., "Birthweight as a risk factor for breast cancer," *Lancet* 348 (1996): 1542–1546; Sanderson, M., et al., "Perinatal factors and risk of breast cancer," *Epidemiology* 7 (1996): 34–37.

Ovarian cancer may be related to rapid weight gain in infancy: In a study of 5,585 women in Hertfordshire in the United Kingdom, David Barker and colleagues noted that the 41 women who died from ovarian cancer were almost a pound heavier at the age of one year than those who did not die of ovarian cancer. In contrast, the birthweights of those who died of ovarian cancer were no different from other women in the study. The researchers conclude that ovarian cancer may be linked to altered brain secretion of the hormones that control the function of the ovary resulting from prenatal setting of the system at an abnormal level. This altered setting of a feedback system may result from a permanent change in the receptors in the part of the brain that controls reproduction. Resetting of the production of brain hormones of the stress axis has been clearly demonstrated following maternal stress as discussed in chapter 6. Barker, D. J. P., et al., "Weight gain in infancy and cancer of the ovary," *Lancet* 345 (1995): 1087–1088.

Humans are growing larger with each generation: British men have been growing taller with every generation. Men between twenty-five and thirty-five years of age are more than 15 centimeters taller in 1998 than at the turn of the century. This represents an increase of one centimeter a decade. Women have increased their height by a little under half a centimeter a decade. The article that reported these numbers in the London *Sunday Times* (March 29, 1998) listed the following possible explanations for the continued growth: better nutrition, fewer infectious diseases in childhood and improved housing conditions. Better maternal nutrition was not discussed. In this article, as in so many others, the importance of prenatal development is consistently ignored.

CHAPTER 6. PRENATAL SETTING OF STRESS LEVELS

Why Zebras Don't Get Ulcers: This excellent book by Dr. Robert Sapolsky describes the way stress acts on our bodies. Dr. Sapolsky has made fundamental contributions to our knowledge of how the brain, endocrine system and body interact in normal and stressful situations. His book is published by W. H. Freeman (1994). *Dorland's Medical Dictionary,* 26th Edition (W. B. Saunders, 1974).

The placenta contains an enzyme that is responsible for protecting the fetus from maternal cortisol: Cortisol produced by the mother can cross the placenta. In order to protect the fetus from being too heavily impacted by changes in maternal cortisol, the placenta contains an enzyme that inactivates cortisol by converting it to cortisone. This enzyme is unable to convert all the cortisol that crosses the placenta. Abnormally high levels of cortisol or synthetic steroids in the maternal blood can adversely affect the development of the fetus. Edwards, C. R. W., et al., "Dysfunction of placental glucocorticoid area: Link between fetal environment and adult hypertension," *Lancet* 34 (1993): 355–357; Benediktsson, R., et al., "Glucocorticoid exposure in utero: New model for adult hypertension," *Lancet* 341 (1993): 339–341; Langley-Evans, S. C., et al., "Protein intake in pregnancy, placental glucocorticoid metabolism and the programming of hypertension in the rat," *Placenta* 17 (1996): 169–172.

Receptors in the brain measure the amount of steroid hormones circulating in the blood and turn on or turn off their production as appropriate: In an elegantly organized feedback system, receptors at various sites in the brain monitor the amount of cortisol (corticosterone in the rat) circulating in the blood. At any one moment, the strength of feedback depends on two factors: the amount of cortisol in the blood and the number of receptors on the surface of the monitor cells that are available to bind cortisol. When the amount of cortisol in the blood rises above the level the body wants, the negative feedback increases, and the production of cortisol is slowed until the blood level drops to the correct level for the current situation. It's just as in your hot water system; the water is not heated to a level above which you set the temperature level because when that temperature you set is reached, the heater is switched off. The critical monitor cells are in the hippocampus, hypothalamus and pituitary. When they bind with cortisol, these receptors act to switch off the system. They act as if they improve the sensitivity of the thermostat. The more receptors, the smaller the amount of cortisol necessary to switch the system off. Anything that depletes the number of receptors makes it more difficult for the circulating cortisol to switch the whole system off. If the level of receptors decreases, more corticotropin releasing hormone (CRH) is secreted by the brain. CRH stimulates more adrenocorticotropin (ACTH) secretion by the pituitary. As a direct result, more cortisol is secreted by the adrenal until finally there is a high enough level of cortisol in the blood to bind enough receptors to switch off the production of CRH and ACTH. But the system is switched off at a higher circulating level of cortisol. High levels of corticosterone, the rat cortisol equivalent, are necessary and beneficial for the rat for short periods at times of acute stress, but consistently elevated corticosterone levels have been shown to be very damaging to the brain and other organs. Rats who have higher baseline corticosterone concentration throughout the twenty-four-hour day age faster than normal rats. A shorter lifespan is a rather fundamental negative effect of too much stress hormone secretion, a consequence most of us would prefer to avoid.

In stressful situations the mother's stress steroids cross the placenta and play a critical role in programming the fetal stress responses: A group of French researchers from the University of Bordeaux conducted a key study that shows clearly that stress responses in the mother can program the later stress responses of her offspring for the whole of their lives. When pregnant rats are restrained, their adrenal glands produce more corticosterone, the rat equivalent of the human stress steroid, cortisol. Some of the corticosterone crosses the placenta into the fetus and permanently reduces the number of receptors that bind corticosterone in key parts of the fetal brain. When the pups whose mothers were stressed during their pregnancy grow up, they have an abnormally high release of stress steroids in response to stressful challenges. In a separate study, the investigators showed that the programming effect on the developing brain was due to corticosterone from the mother. The researchers removed the adrenal glands from pregnant rats before they were stressed. As a result, the mothers' steroid levels did not rise and the long-term consequences to the pups did not occur. In a clinching study, they showed that if large amounts of adrenal steroids are given to the pregnant rats whose adrenals had been removed, then the pups were affected in later life. This final test shows that the stress of the mother exerts its effects on the fetus through the passage of adrenal stress hormones across the placenta to the fetus. Barbazanges, A., et al., "Maternal glucocorticoid secretion mediates long-term effects of prenatal stress," *J. Neurosci.* 16 (1996): 3943–3949.

Effects of early life exposure to bacterial toxins: Dr. Michael Meaney and his colleagues in Montreal have shown that exposure of newborn rats to bacterial toxins on the first day of life has a very similar effect on the rat's response to stress in later life as stress exposure of the mother in late pregnancy. In both situations, the pups show an increased response to stress in later life. Meaney's findings point to the very close connection between the stress system and our immune responses. It remains to be seen how the exposure of the developing brain to agents that stimulate the immune and stress systems produce these permanent effects on stress responses. These effects of bacterial toxins appear to be different from the exposure of rats to other challenges at this stage of life and much more research is necessary to unravel all the complexities. Shanks, N., et al., "Neonatal endotoxin exposure alters the development of the hypothalamic-pituitary-adrenal axis: Early illness and later responsivity to stress," *J. Neuroscience* 15 (1995): 376–384.

Maternal care plays a key role in programming hormone responses to stress throughout life: Licking and grooming of rat pups by their mother in early life alters the level of activity of the pups' stress systems in later life. When rat pups receive extensive maternal care, their stress systems function at a lower level in later life. Similar effects have been shown in macaque monkeys. Liu, D., et al., "Maternal care, hippocampal glucocorticoid receptors, and hypothalamic-pituitary-adrenal responses to stress," *Science* 277 (1997): 1659–1662; Meaney, M. J., et al., "Effect of neonatal handling on age-related impairments associated with the hippocampus," *Science* 239 (1988): 766–768; Ladd, C. O., et al., "Persistent changes in corticotropin-releasing factor neuronal systems induced by maternal deprivation," *Endocrinology* 137 (1996): 1212–1218; Coplan, J. D., et al., "Persistent elevations of cerebrospinal fluid concentrations of corticotropin-releasing factor in adult nonhuman primates exposed to early-life stressors: Implications for the pathophysiology of mood and anxiety disorders," *Proc. Natl. Acad. Sci. USA* 93 (1996): 1619–1623.

Our internal circadian clocks: The use of powerful molecular biology techniques has shown that a cellular circadian clock is present in very primitive organisms such as flies, fungi and plants. If organisms made up of just a few cells have clocks, it should not be surprising that mammals have similar regulatory mechanisms. Each one of us has our own rhythm idiosyncrasies. Some people are morning people, others are evening people. Morning people are very different from night owls. Although we do not yet know why these two types of people are so very different, the answer may well come from a better understanding of the function of two genes, *per* (per is an abbreviation for period, since something that is rhythmic repeats after a fixed period) and *tim* (short for timeless). Each gene produces a protein. The proteins produced by the per and tim genes combine together to turn the genes off. If there were only one protein that switched its own gene off by a classical negative feedback, the situation would just plateau at a stable level at the setpoint of the feedback, like regulating the temperature at a constant level in your hot water heater. Since there are two genes, the duration of each cycle of the clock will be determined by the rate of production and association of their protein products. The manufacture, combination and breakdown of the proteins regulates the oscillation backward and forward that produces the circadian rhythm within an individual cell. Dunlap, J. C., et al., "The genetic and molecular dissection of a prototypic circadian system," *Prog. Brain Res.* 111 (1996): 11–27; Takahashi, J. S., "The biological clock: It's all in the genes," *Prog. Brain Res.* 111 (1996) 5–9.

Resetting of the cortisol stress axis has wide implications in later life: Dr. David Phillips and his colleagues traced 1,157 baby boys born in Hertfordshire in England between 1920 and 1930. The researchers knew the birthweights of these individuals who were men in their sixties and seventies when the researchers located them. Dr. Phillips measured the amount of cortisol in their blood and related the cortisol level to their blood pressure and ability to deal with a load of glucose. In support of the concept of prenatal programming, they found that plasma cortisol was highest in those men who had been the smallest babies at birth. Similarly, those who had been the smallest babies were least able to deal with a load of glucose. The researchers suggest that prenatal programming of the steroid stress axis may be one mechanism that results in high blood pressure and increases an individual's likelihood of being intolerant to glucose in adult life. Phillips, D. I. W., et al., "Elevated plasma cortisol concentrations: A link between low birthweight and the insulin resistance syndrome?" *J. Clin. Endocrinol. Metab.* 83 (1998): 757–760.

Differences between prenatal and postnatal programming in the rat: The long-term effects of postnatal experience on lifetime setting of the stress axis are more complex than the effects of prenatal exposure. Since the rat brain is developing much faster after birth than before, it will not be surprising that the experimental findings from altering the system after birth are more complex than changes before birth. Many of the structures that develop after birth in the rat develop before birth in human babies. Thus, any corresponding changes in human babies are likely occur before birth. The overall message of programming of the stress axis around the time of birth is, however, the same. The setting of the adrenal system can be altered permanently by alterations in exposure to adrenal steroid hormones in critical periods of early development.

The importance of correct setting of the brain-pituitary-adrenal system: The evidence is very powerful that disorders of mood involve the brain-pituitary-adrenal system. During episodes of depression, the amounts of cortisol circulating in the blood is increased and the pituitary and adrenal glands are enlarged. CRH concentration in samples taken from the cerebrospinal fluid, the fluid that surrounds the brain and spinal cord, are elevated during depression. In spontaneous remission or following successful treatment of depression with Prozac, these indices of increased activity of the adrenal stress axis have returned to normal. Permanently altered feedback on the CRH-producing nerve cells in the hypothalamus could account for these changes. This interesting story points to the importance of correct alignment and setting of the brain-pituitary-adrenal system. To have a healthy brain, it is clearly necessary for the activity of all levels of the adrenal system to be set at an appropriate level. Of course, the interesting question remains whether changes outside the norm are associated with creativity or criminality, altruism or aggression. The final synthesis is likely to show that both internal and external factors are critical. However, it is very clear that permanent resetting of the whole system is a feature of great importance in both animals and humans. Stout, S. C., et al., "Stress and psychiatric disorders," *The Neurosciences* 6 (1994): 271–280; Musselman, D. L., et al., "Adrenal function in major depression," *The Endocrinologist* 5 (1995): 91–96.

CHAPTER 7. HEART DISEASE, OBESITY AND DIABETES

Dean Ornish's Program for Reversing Heart Disease (Random House, 1990). This book, and others like it, full of advice on what to do to keep a failing heart in good condition, are about closing the stable door after the horse has bolted.

The epidemiology of a suboptimal environment in the womb and heart disease, obesity and diabetes in later life: An excellent resource for much of the information that indicates that heart disease, obesity and diabetes are programmed prenatally can be found in David Barker's book, *Mothers, Babies and Health in Later Life* (Churchill Livingstone, 1998).

Relationship of poor nutrition during the mother's own childhood and heart disease and stroke in her own children: When young girls are undernourished, their bones grow poorly. If an X-ray examination of the pelvis of mothers shows that the bones of her pelvis are smaller than they should be, there is a high likelihood that her uterus will also be small and that, while early growth of her baby may be normal, late in pregnancy, the baby's growth may be compromised by lack of space. Death from stroke in later life is associated with a low birthweight for the head size of the baby as well as a low placental weight in relation to the size of the baby's head at birth. Both the low birthweight to head size and the relatively small placental size show that growth was compromised in the uterus and that compensatory mechanisms occurred to protect the head. These investigators showed that in contrast to the increased incidence of death from stroke in these babies that tried to compensate for prenatal growth problems, coronary heart disease was higher later in life in babies whose prenatal growth was impaired for reasons other than failure of their placenta to grow properly. Martyn, C. N., et al., "Mothers' pelvic size, fetal growth, and death from stroke and coronary heart disease in men in the UK," *Lancet* 348 (1996): 1264–1268.

Relationship of maternal body weight to heart disease in later life: A study carried out in Mysore, India, showed that babies of mothers with a low body weight have a higher chance of suffering from heart disease in later life. The highest incidence of heart disease in later life occurred in people who were less than 2.5 kilograms (5.5 pounds) in weight at birth and whose mothers weighed less than 45 kilograms (99 pounds). Stein, C. E., et al., "Fetal growth and coronary heart disease in South India," *Lancet* 348 (1996): 1269–1273.

The association of low birthweight and heart disease and stroke in later life holds for women as well as men: There is strong evidence that women who were small at birth are also at greatest risk to suffer from heart disease or stroke in later life. One large study analyzed the health records of 121,700 nurses in the United States whose overall health had been followed since 1976. In this study, too, low birthweight was associated with heart disease in later life. Rich-Edwards, J. W., et al., "Birthweight and risk of cardiovascular disease in a cohort of women followed up since 1976," *Brit. Med. J.* 315 (1997): 396–400.

The Harvard Health Professionals Follow-up Study showed a higher incidence of high blood pressure and diabetes in men who had a low birthweight: One Harvard study that involved 22,693 men concluded that "men with low birthweight were at significantly higher risk for high blood pressure and diabetes." This relationship held even after correcting for obesity, which itself predisposes to both high blood pressure and diabetes. Curhan, G. C., et al., "Birth weight and adult hypertension and diabetes mellitus in U. S. men," *Am. J. Hypertens.* 9 (1996): 11 Abstract.

Swedish study conludes that failure to realize growth potential in utero is associated with high blood pressure in later life: The conclusion of a Swedish follow-up of 1,333 men of known birthweight was that "failure to realize growth potential in the uterus [as indicated by being light at birth but tall as an adult] is associated with raised adult blood pressure. Impaired fetal growth may lead to substantial increases in adult blood pressure among only those who become obese." The final sentence again shows how life before birth increases a susceptibility that can be reversed by a good nutritional lifestyle. Leon, D. A., et al., "Failure to realize growth potential in utero and adult obesity in relation to blood pressure in 50 year old Swedish men," *Br. Med. J.* 312 (1996): 401–406.

The mother's weight in pregnancy and coronary heart disease in later life are associated, according to a report from Finland: The conclusion from this study gives strong support to the Barker Hypothesis that the origins of heart disease are prenatal. The conclusion also sounds a hopeful note. "These findings suggest a new explanation for the epidemics of coronary heart disease that accompany Westernisation. Chronically malnourished women are short and light and their babies tend to be thin. The immediate effect of improved nutrition is that women become fat, which seems to increase the risk of coronary heart disease in the next generation. With continued improvements in nutrition, women become taller and heavier; their babies are adequately nourished; and maternal fatness no longer increases the risk of coronary heart disease which therefore declines." Forsén, T., et al., "Mother's weight in pregnancy and coronary heart disease in a cohort of Finnish men: Follow up study," *Brit. Med. J.* 315 (1997): 837–840.

The same issue of the *British Medical Journal* has an editorial by Nevin S. Scrimshaw, director of the United Nations University Food and Nutrition Program for Human and Social Development (pages 825–826), that reads, "Most human embryos have the potential for a long and healthy life. From the moment of conception, however, adverse environmental forces limit this potential. Intrauterine growth retardation due to poor maternal malnutrition is an important factor; but so are diet at all ages, cigarette smoking, a sedentary lifestyle, and the use of drugs, and others.

"The Barker group's findings have made it clear that preventive measures should begin with improving the nutrition and health of women to prevent damage to their fetuses. This will require attention to the risk factors for low birthweight before pregnancy since nutritional supplements during pregnancy are inadequate. Moreover, for a long and healthy life, good nutrition and lifestyle are necessary throughout the entire life span. While not all individuals have the same genetic potential for avoiding premature degenerative disease, their chances of doing so can be dramatically improved by good nutrition and health practices from womb to tomb."

The father's social class influences the incidence of cardiovascular disease in men in midlife: The British Regional Heart Study has shown that the sons of manual workers have a higher incidence of heart disease than the sons of white-collar workers. In the words of the authors, "The higher risk of non-fatal . . . heart disease seen in men whose father's social class was manual suggests that socioeconomic status early in life has some persisting influence on ischemic heart disease risk in adult life." Wannamethee, S. G., et al., "Influence of fathers' social class on cardiovascular disease in middle-aged men," *Lancet* 348 (1996): 1259–1263.

The rate of postnatal growth may also affect an individual's susceptibility to high blood pressure: Low birthweight babies who grow fast in early life have higher blood pressure when they are adults than babies who have the same birthweight but do not grow fast. This is a reminder of the fascinating observation by Dr. Nicholas Hales that force-feeding growth-retarded rat pups will shorten their life span. During life in the womb, babies set themselves an optimal growth rate that suits them best to the prenatal conditions in the womb. If the quality and quantity of food available is changed after birth, there may be dire consequences. The programming of our metabolism is like setting the cruise control of our body's engine. Once the design process is finished, it is very difficult to change the speed that is optimal for the design. Hales, C. N., "Fetal and infant growth and impaired glucose tolerance in adulthood: The 'Thrifty Phenotype' hypothesis revisited," *Acta Paediatr. Suppl.* 422 (1997): 73–77.

Size at birth is related to both noninsulin dependent diabetes and insulin concentrations in Swedish men at age fifty to sixty: Reduced growth before birth was associated with an increased risk of diabetes and resistance to the action of insulin in a group of 1,333 Swedish men. Lithell, H. O., et al., "Relation of size at birth to non-insulin dependent diabetes and insulin concentrations in men aged 50–60 years," *Br. Med. J.* 312 (1996): 406–410.

High incidence of diabetes on Nauru: The tiny island of Nauru lies just south of the equator in the Pacific Ocean. It is a little over six miles across and has a population of less than 6,000. Prior to the Second World War, the inhabitants of Nauru led a subsistence existence. After the war, they became affluent as a result of phosphate mining by Australian and American companies. The incidence of diabetes in Nauruan islanders increased dramatically when nutrition improved. This sequence of events supports the thrifty phenotype concept in which individuals who develop a metabolism that helps them survive in times of food shortage are more likely to suffer from diabetes when their food intake increases dramatically. Now that the level of affluence allows young women to have better nutrition during their own growth and in pregnancy, the incidence of diabetes in Nauru has decreased. These findings show that there is hope that as we understand about programming, we will be able to improve the health of tomorrow's children. Hales, C. N., "Non-insulin-dependent diabetes mellitus," *Br. Med. Bull.* 53 (1997): 109–122; Dowse, G. K., et al., "Decline in incidence of epidemic glucose intolerance in Nauruans: Implications for the 'Thrifty Genotype,'" *Am. J. Epidemiol.* 133 (1991): 1093–1104.

High carbohydrate diets early in pregnancy suppress placental growth: Pregnant women who eat high-carbohydrate diets in early pregnancy have smaller placentas than women who eat a more balanced diet. The effect of high carbohydrates is especially marked if the dietary protein intake is low. This important observation speaks loudly to the need for adequate and balanced nutrition in pregnancy if adverse programming effects are to be avoided. Godfrey, K., et al., "Maternal nutrition in early and late pregnancy in relation to placental and fetal growth," *Br. Med. J.* 312 (1996): 410–414; Godfrey, K. M., "Maternal regulation of fetal development and health in adult life," *Eur. J. Obstet. Gynecol.* 78 (1998): 141–150.

One of the many functions played by cortisol secreted by the fetal adrenal gland is to regulate the development of blood vessels: Cortisol plays a multitude of roles in preparing the fetus for the challenges of life after birth. When a fetal sheep is infused with cortisol-like steroids, there is a marked rise in fetal blood pressure. These findings support the view of many investigators that much of the detrimental effect of maternal nutrition results from the increased secretion of cortisol by the mother when she is short of food. The cortisol crosses the placenta in greater amounts than usual and alters the normal program of development of many fetal functions, including the blood vessels. Derks, J. B., et al., "A comparative study of cardiovascular, endocrine and behavioural effects of betamethasone and dexamethasone administration to fetal sheep," *J. Physiol.* 449.1 (1997): 217–226.

Low protein intake during pregnancy leads to high blood pressure in later life: Dr. Simon Langley-Evans and his colleagues at Southampton University have undertaken an extensive series of studies in rats that show that a diet that is low in protein during pregnancy programs the rat pups growing in the womb to have a higher blood pressure in later life. They have clearly shown that the maternal adrenal gland is involved in the programming. The current explanation is that the stress of the poor diet during pregnancy results in increased production of steroids by the mother. These steroids then cross the placenta and program the fetal blood pressure regulating system. Edwards, C. R. W., et al., "Dysfunction of placental glucocorticoid barrier: Link between fetal environment and adult hypertension?" *Lancet* 341 (1993): 355–357; Langley-Evans, S. C., et al., "In utero exposure to maternal low protein diets induces hypertension in weanling rats, independently of maternal blood pressure changes," *Clin. Nutr.* 13 (1994): 319–324; Langley, S. C., et al., "Increased systolic blood pressure in adult rats induced by fetal exposure to maternal low protein diets," *Clin. Sci.* 86 (1994): 217–222; Langley-Evans, S. C., et al., "Maternal protein restriction influences the programming of the rat hypothalamic-pituitary-adrenal axis," *J. Nutr.* 126 (1996): 1578–1585; Langley-Evans, S. C., et al., "Protein intake in pregnancy, placental glucocorticoid metabolism and the programming of hypertension in the rat," *Placenta* 17 (1996): 169–172.

Blood clotting factors that are increased in men can be related to birthweight and growth during the first year of life: An increase in blood clotting factors is one mechanism by which reduced early growth may predispose to later heart disease. Since clotting factors are produced by the liver, altered levels may reflect an imbalance of the different cell types in the liver caused by growth retardation in the womb. This is an example of our fourth principle of programming, namely that a suboptimal situation in the womb may lead to structural changes in developing organs, which then lead to an imbalance of specialized cell types. Barker, D. J. P., et al., "Relation of fetal and infant growth to plasma fibrinogen and factor VII concentrations in adult life," *Br. Med. J.* 304 (1992): 148–152.

A Danish study shows that when only one of a pair of identical or nonidentical twins has diabetes, the diabetic twin is more likely to have a lower birthweight than the nondiabetic twin: This very important paper from Denmark reminds us that twins do not grow under equal conditions in the womb. The authors conclude that "the association between low birthweight and non-insulin-dependent diabetes in twins is at least partly independent of genotype and may be due to intrauterine malnutrition." Poulsen, P., et al., "Low birth weight is associated with NIDDM in discordant monozygotic and dizygotic twin pairs," *Diabetologia* 40 (1997): 439–446.

What can we learn about the inheritance of diabetes from twin studies? One Danish study investigated the relationship of birthweight differences between twins and the incidence of noninsulin dependent diabetes mellitus (NIDDM] in both identical twins and nonidentical twins who were of the same sex. The study focused on twins that were discordant for NIDDM. The twins with NIDDM, whether a member of an identical or nonidentical pair, had lower birthweights (by 270 grams; 0.59 pounds) than their cotwin who was not affected by NIDDM. The relationship held even after the identical and nonidentical twins were separated out. Phillips, D. I. W., et al., "Can twin studies assess the genetic component in type 2 (non-insulin-dependent) diabetes mellitus?" *Diabetologia* 36 (1993): 471–472.

There is a tendency for concordance rates of diabetes in identical twins to drop as more studies are conducted. In one recent study, concordance for NIDDM was only 33 percent. When identical and nonidentical twins were compared, there was no significant difference in the concordance of NIDDM and only a weak significance in the concordance of NIDDM and impaired glucose tolerance combined. The authors conclude that NIDDM is probably the result of a complex set of factors including nongenetic components. Vaag, A., et al., "Etiology of NIDDM: Genetics versus pre- or postnatal environments? Results from twin studies," *Exp. Clin. Endocrinol. Diab.* 104 (1996): 181–182.

Data obtained from twins needs very careful analysis. One leader in the field of twin data was later exposed as a complete fraud: William Broad and Nicholas Wade's book *Betrayers of the Truth: Fraud and Deceit in the Halls of Science* (Simon and Schuster, 1982) is a must read for all those who wish to know about the scientific process. The authors touch on so many points fundamental to the scientific method. When discussing Cyril Burt's fraudulent data on identical twins, they point to the need for replication in discovery. "One reason, of course, for the tolerance of error [in Burt's work] was that most of the psychologists who used Burt's . . . results did not try to replicate them." I have already addressed the fallacies in *The Bell Curve.* It is of interest that Broad and Wade remind us, "Arthur Jensen [from Stanford University] made considerable use of Burt's findings in his 1969 article in the *Harvard Educational Review,* a furiously debated tract in which he argued that since the genetic factor determines 80 percent of intelligence, programs of compensatory education addressed to lower class black and white children were useless and should be scrapped. Burt's twin data were relied upon even more heavily by Richard Herrnstein [the same Herrnstein of *The Bell Curve*] . . . in the *Atlantic* arguing that social class is based in part on inherited differences in intelligence."

Broad and Wade go on to explain that it was left to the Princeton University psychologist, Leon Kamin, to expose Burt. Kamin noted that Burt's correlation coefficient in IQ of identical twins reared together was 0.944 in three different studies. Too good to be true. In addition, Burt's supposed colleagues and coinvestigators whose names appeared on some of his papers, Miss Howard and Miss Conway, did not exist.

The mother's blood pressure during pregnancy affects fetal growth: A study in England has associated a rise in the mother's blood pressure during pregnancy with slowing of fetal growth. We have seen how babies who fail to grow to their full potential have a greater susceptibility to higher blood pressure in adult life. If this study is confirmed, this effect is yet another example of possible transgenerational effects in daughters of mothers who have high blood pressure during pregnancy. Churchill, D., et al., "Ambulatory blood pressure in pregnancy and fetal growth," *Lancet* 349 (1997): 7–10.

The children of the Dutch Hunger Winter have impaired ability to pack glucose away into their cells (referred to as glucose intolerance): In a study involving 702 Dutch babies born between November 1, 1943, and Feb 28, 1947, Dr. Anita Ravelli and her colleagues concluded that those babies who suffered exposure to poor nutrition in the womb as a result of the Dutch Hunger Winter were less able to deal with a typical glucose tolerance test given to identify diabetics. They state, "Poor nutrition in utero may lead to permanent changes in insulin-glucose metabolism [function], even if the effect on fetal growth is small. This effect of famine on glucose tolerance is especially important in people who become obese." We have seen that there is a higher tendency for individuals to become obese if they were undernourished when they were in the womb. Ravelli, A. C. J., et al., "Glucose tolerance in adults after prenatal exposure to famine," *Lancet* 351 (1998): 173–177.

The thrifty phenotype: The thrifty phenotype hypothesis proposes that poor prenatal growth in the womb leads to a decreased ability to secrete insulin from the pancreas in adulthood. We have seen how poor nutrition during life before birth can permanently lower the blood supply to the pancreas. In addition, there are changes in the way the pancreatic cells take up glucose in rats that were growth-retarded at birth. The proponents of the thrifty phenotype concept consider these changes in pancreatic function to be adaptive responses to protect the growth of the brain and aid the survival of the young in situations after birth in which food may be short. Hales, C. N., "Non-insulin-dependent diabetes mellitus," *Br. Med. Bull.* 53 (1997): 109–122.

The thrifty genotype: Some researchers disagree with the concept that the explosion of diabetes that is affecting the developed world can be explained by prenatal development of a thrifty phenotype. According to this alternative view, there have been periods in human evolution when famine would have selected individuals with genes that conferred a thrifty metabolism on individuals who possessed these genes. According to this thrifty genotype view, these thrifty genes would be more prevalent in areas where the population has been repeatedly exposed to the challenge of food shortage, such as Nauru. When food becomes plentiful in these areas, the incidence of diabetes rises. Supporters of the thrifty genotype view must explain the very rapid changes in the incidence of diabetes, first an increase and now a decline, over just fifty years or so. The explanation offered is that the severity of the epidemic of diabetes has removed (i.e., killed) a large segment of the population that has the thrifty genes. However, given the ability of modern medicine to keep diabetics alive, it is impossible that a change in the gene pool could have taken place so quickly. Dowse, G. K., et al., "Decline in incidence of epidemic glucose intolerance in Nauruans: Implications for the 'Thrifty Genotype,' " *Am. J. Epidemiol.* 133 (1991): 1093–1104; Neel, J. V., "The thrifty genotypc revisited," in *The Genetics of Diabetes Mellitus*, ed: Köbberling, J. and Tattersall, R., Serono Symposium No. 47 (Academic Press, 1982): 283–293.

A sea change in medical science: Stomach ulcers are caused by a bacterium not by stress: Helicobacter is a bacterium that colonizes the stomachs of up to 95 percent of people in some parts of the world. The bacterium has been shown to be the cause of most stomach ulcers. Not so many years ago, surgeons were unanimous and confident that the only real cure for a stomach ulcer was to cut out the ulcerated stomach tissues. Now stomach ulcers are being treated with antibiotics. There is even a promising test for infection with helicobacter that utilizes the way the bacteria use the common compound urea. This breath test is certainly much less trying than the old tests for ulcers that involved swallowing copious volumes of compounds that could be seen on an X-ray. Much current research involves the study of how this simple organism can cause conditions that used to result in extensive and debilitating surgery. Those who are interested in this astonishing story could follow up many aspects in the proceedings of a recent international conference reported in the December 1997 supplement of *Gastroenterology* volume 113; Fox, J. G. and Lee, A., "The role of helicobacter species in newly recognized gastrointestinal tract diseases of animals," *Lab. Anim. Sci.* 47 (1997): 222–255.

Chapter 8. Environmental Influences in the Womb

The remarkable insight of Aldous Huxley in his novel *Brave New World*: Some books are perennial sources of wisdom. One such book is *Brave New World,* first published in 1932. This classic book tells of a future in which different types of humans are mass-produced in numbers required for different positions in society. Embryos are grown in hatcheries by Bokanovsky's process and tended by scientists dressed in "white, their hands gloved with pale corpse-colored gloves." Eggs produced in the fertilization room are grown in special broths and budded until ninety-six buds are produced from each embryo. The buds are then placed in incubators. In the book, the director of the Central London Hatchery and Conditioning Center describes the process "Two, four, eight, the buds in their turn budded; and having budded were dosed almost to death with alcohol . . . thereafter—further arrest being generally fatal—[they are] left to develop in peace."

Production of large lambs by manipulation of the early cell division phases: Local factors in the developing embryo's environment will alter the proportion of cells that participate in the production of the fetus and placenta. Walker, S. K., et al., "The production of unusually large offspring following embryo manipulation: concepts and challenges," *Theriogenology* 45 (1996): 111–120; Walker, S. K., et al., "Culture of embryos of farm animals," *Embryonic Development and Manipulation in Animal Production,* ed: Laria, A. and Gandolfi, F. (Portland Press, 1997): 77–92; Kleemann, D.O., et al., "Enhanced fetal growth in sheep administered progesterone during the first three days of pregnancy," *J. Reprod. Fertil.* 102 (1994): 411–417; Sagan, C., *The Demon-Haunted World; Science as a Candle in the Dark* (Ballantine, 1996).

In different seasons of the year, the fetal sheep adjusts the preparations for the time to be born: Dr. John Bassett and his coworkers at Oxford University gave me the answer to my concerns over the wide variation of the hormone prolactin in the blood of fetal sheep. They showed that fetal lambs due to be born in the spring had about half a microgram of prolactin in a liter of blood. Fetal lambs due to be born in the fall had four hundred times that amount of prolactin in their blood, around two hundred micrograms in a liter of blood. The pattern of the changes in concentration in the mother's blood was very similar. The parallel between the mother's and the fetal blood might seem immediately to show that the prolactin passes easily across the placenta so that the baby's and the mother's concentrations rapidly equalize. Some things are not that simple. Several studies have shown that the prolactin molecule is too large to cross the placenta. So what is the explanation? As days shorten in the winter, the mother's brain secretes more of the hormone melatonin. Melatonin inhibits the production of prolactin. Since melatonin is small enough to go across the placenta, fetal prolactin production is also inhibited. Prolactin stimulates wool growth. Melatonin is a timekeeper, telling the fetus that the days are shortening or lengthening in the world outside the womb. The fetus can then make the right preparation, growing more wool if he is to be born in the fall, less if he is to be born in the spring. Bassett, J. M., et al., "Photoperiod: An important regulator of plasma prolactin concentration in fetal lambs during late gestation," *Q. J. Exp. Physiol.* 73 (1988): 241–244.

In the Gambia, the season of the year in which you are born may well affect your resistance to infection throughout life: Children born during the harvest season in the Gambia in West Africa have nearly 50 percent more likelihood of living to the age of forty-five than children born during the rainy season, which is referred to as the hungry season by Gambians. The commonest time of death in individuals born in the rainy season is between fifteen and forty-five years of age. In infancy, there is no difference in survival of individuals born in the rainy or the harvest season. Andrew Prentice, Sophie Moore and Tim Cole propose that "certain environmental stresses related to the season of birth have permanently programmed the immune system in a way that first appears at puberty and which becomes amplified with age." Prentice, A., et al., "Birth, life and death in rural Africa," *MRC News* 77 (1998): 12–16.

Some would like to suggest that all we have to do to produce people with perfect health is to mix together the best genes and then repeatedly clone the same individual: Sharon Begley wrote an excellent and balanced piece on cloning in *Newsweek* when the Dolly controversy erupted. In addition to clearly describing how Ian Wilmut did his work, she points out the need to consider the important role that the environment plays in determining who we are. Here I quote, "The incidence of schizophrenia doubled among Dutch

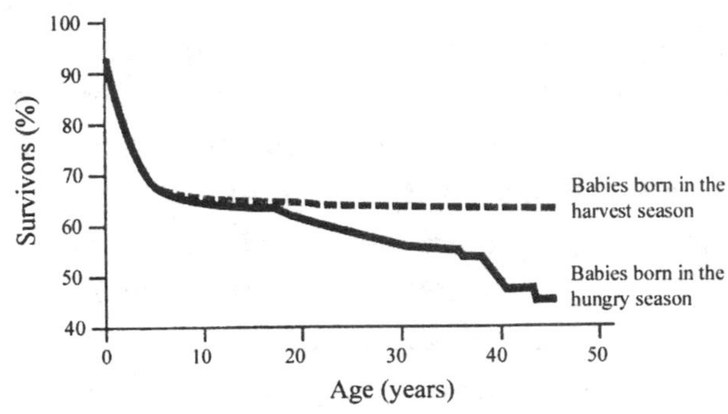

FIGURE 1

In the country districts of Gambia in West Africa there is a great difference in life expectancy for babies born in the harvest season and babies born in the dry season.

children born in the Netherlands' 'winter of famine' during World War II. Maternal malnutrition can trigger the disease. But a clone of one of these children, a genetic duplicate, might evade schizophrenia if borne by a woman who ate normally during pregnancy." Begley, S., "Little lamb, who made thee?" *Newsweek* (March 10, 1997): 53–60; Campbell, K. H. S., et al., "Sheep cloned by nuclear transfer from a cultured cell line," *Nature* 380 (1996): 64–66.

Alcohol exposure before birth produces significant differences in the lines on the palms of the two hands: We saw in chapter 1 that alterations in the whorls on the fingertips occur in growth retarded babies. In one study, thirty-one individuals known to have been exposed to high levels of alcohol during life in the womb had a greater difference in the ridges on their palms than thirty-one individuals who had not been exposed to alcohol prenatally. So again we must wonder what the palmist can see or thinks she or he can see. Wilber, E., et al., "Dermatoglyphic asymmetry in fetal alcohol syndrome," *Biol. Neonate* 64 (1993): 1–6.

Effects of maternal alcohol consumption on the developing fetal brain: Alcohol crosses the placenta freely. When alcohol is consumed, fetal blood levels rise as rapidly as the maternal levels, and within one hour, the amount of alcohol in the baby's blood is the same as the amount in the mother's blood. It takes about twelve hours for the alcohol to be cleared from the baby's and the mother's blood. Of great concern is the observation from studies in pregnant sheep that alcohol remains in the amniotic fluid for several hours after the fetal and maternal blood are free of alcohol. The amniotic fluid appears to act as a reservoir for alcohol. All of these observations in sheep have parallels in the limited human data and the extensive data from other species such as the guinea pig.

Alcohol redirects the amount of blood flowing to different parts of the fetus. Most importantly, alcohol decreases the amount of blood flowing to the fetal brain. This is a very dangerous state of affairs. If the mother who drinks alcohol also smokes, the amount of oxygen in her blood and the blood of the fetus will be even further decreased. So the baby is exposed to multiple whammies. There is both less blood going to the baby's brain and less oxygen in that blood.

It has been shown that alcohol increases the production of prostaglandins in the human placenta and in the fetal sheep brain. As a result, fetal breathing movements and fetal REM sleep are suppressed. Both of these effects of alcohol on the fetus are undesirable. REM sleep is critical to normal development of the brain, and when fetal breathing is decreased, the lungs do not grow properly. Brien, J. F., et al., "Effects of alcohol (ethanol) on the fetus," *J. Dev. Physiol.* 15 (1991): 21–32.

The eyes are a window on the effects of alcohol on the brain: Using an ophthalmoscope, it is possible to see the optic nerve as it enters the back of the eye. This is the only place in the body at which

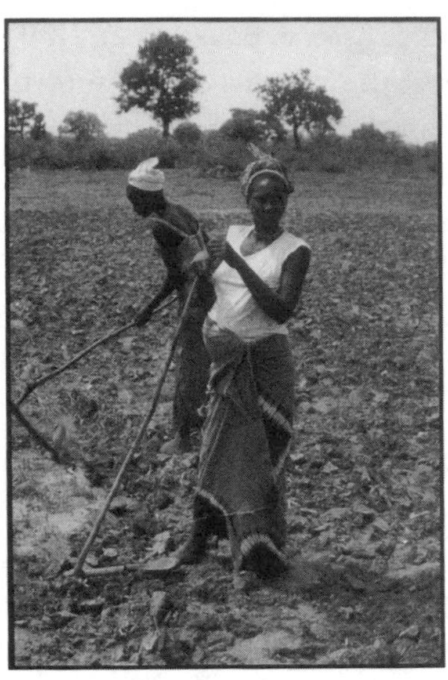

FIGURE 2

In Gambia, as in many other countries, pregnant women work in the fields. Their special needs during pregnancy are often ignored.

it is possible to see nerves directly. It is also possible to see the arteries that feed the optic nerve. Following exposure to alcohol during fetal life, the size of the optic nerve may be reduced as much as 50 percent and the arteries around the nerve become tortuous. Strömland, K., "Ocular involvement in the fetal alcohol syndrome," *Surv. Ophthalmol.* 31 (1987): 277–284.

Fetal alcohol syndrome [FAS]: FAS was first described in France in 1968 by Lemoine and colleagues. The landmark papers from the United States followed in 1973. Some researchers working in the field of FAS have called it the only known 100 percent preventable birth defect. The overall incidence of FAS in the United States ranges from 1 to 3 per 1,000. However, the incidence can rise as high as 10.7 per 1,000 in some groups of Southwestern Plains Indians. The lifetime cost of a typical FAS baby has been calculated as nearly $600,000 for each child affected. Cost estimates for the United States are difficult to make because of the difficulty in diagnosis and the existence of all ranges of level of effect. The estimated cost has been placed as high $9.7 billion a year. Regardless of whether this is a gross overestimate, the costs in terms of lowered quality of life and increased risks to society from deviant behavior are high. Jones, K. L. and Smith, D. W., "Recognition of the fetal alcohol syndrome in early infancy," *Lancet* 2 (1973): 999–1001; Jones, K. L., et al., "Pattern of malformation in offspring of chronic alcohol mothers," *Lancet* 1 (1973): 1267–1271; Sokol, R. J., "Significant determinants of susceptibility to alcohol teratogenicity," *Ann. N. Y. Acad. Sci.* 477 (1986): 87–102.

Chronic exposure to low oxygen during the critical last third of gestation in the rat alters sexual behavior: Although the fetus has marvelous powers of survival in poor conditions during life in the womb, we have seen time and time again that the compensations the fetus makes carry a price—principle number six of the ten principles of programming. Researchers in California have shown that when male fetal rats develop in an environment of roughly half the usual amount of oxygen in the mother's blood for the last third of pregnancy, there are problems with sexual behavior when the rats grow up. Hermans, R. H. M., et al., "Altered adult sexual behavior in the male rat following chronic prenatal hypoxia," *Neurotoxicol. Teratol.* 15 (1993): 353–363.

The placenta as a drug tsar and environmental policeman: In most species, the placental barrier is very thin, but barrier it is, nevertheless. The fact that the barrier is there has many important consequences for the fetus. To some extent, the barrier prevents the passage of toxic chemicals to the fetus. Sadly, the barrier is far from complete. Drugs that cause fetal abnormalities will cross the placenta and harm the fetus. Drugs of abuse cross from mother to fetus with ease. Indeed, once in the blood of the fetus, the structure of many drugs both legal and illegal is changed to compounds that are not able to pass back across the placenta from the baby's body to mother. As a result, the levels of these altered drug forms build up in the baby. Some of these compounds produced within the baby may be even more toxic than the original drug. As a result, they have pronounced adverse effects. When it comes to drugs—prescription or otherwise—the best rule is "in ignorance, abstain."

Smoking causes growth retardation: In a section in the article "Tobacco and Health" Anne Charlton addresses "Children and Smoking: The Family Circle." She writes "Children and adult's smoking can form a 'family circle.' Young women and their male partners who are less well-educated and less affluent are most likely to smoke during the woman's pregnancy. The harmful effects on the fetus, including low birthweight and increased risk of respiratory diseases, are carried forward into childhood." Babies born to mothers who smoke heavily were on average 441 grams (0.97 pounds) less than babies born to those who smoked very moderately. We should not forget that this decrease in weight is twice the average decrease noted in the Dutch Hunger Winter. "Tobacco and health," *Br. Med. Bull.* 52 (1996): 90–107.

Deprivation of rapid eye movement sleep can lead to abnormal development: Twenty years ago, Dr. Majid Mirmiran from the Netherlands Institute for Brain Research showed that REM sleep deprivation of newborn rats just from the age of seven to twenty-one days of life led to abnormal behavior patterns, particularly exploration and sexual mating behavior when the rats reached adulthood. Again we see how an early event programmed brain function in later life. Corner, M. A., et al., "Does rapid-eye-movement sleep play a role in brain development?" *Prog. Brain Res.* 53 (1980): 347–356.

The effects of contractures (uterine hugs) on the developing fetus: In studies in a large number of species including sheep, rats, monkeys, baboons and cows, several research groups throughout the world have shown that the muscle in the wall of the womb is not quiet during pregnancy. Throughout pregnancy, intermittent bouts of activity of the uterus occur that last several minutes. This type of muscle activity is very common in muscle of the nonvoluntary type that makes up the uterus. The muscles that drive our limbs are called voluntary muscles because they are dependent on signals from the brain via the nerves for their activity. If the nerve to a limb muscle is accidentally severed, the muscle will be paralyzed. The muscles of the gut, the heart and the uterus are very different. They continue to contract without any outside influences. True, the nerves to the heart will slow our heartbeat down or speed it up, but the heart will beat at its own appointed rhythm without the need of any help from the nerves.

Throughout pregnancy in sheep, a burst of activity occurs in the uterus about every half hour and lasts three to fifteen minutes. These events are very different from the contractions that occur at the time of birth. So when we first observed them in pregnant sheep, we called them *contractures* to distinguish them from labor and delivery *contractions.* In monkeys and baboons, the pattern of contractures is slightly more frequent than in sheep. They are likely to be the same events that women feel in late pregnancy. In pregnant women, they are named after the British physician, John Braxton Hicks, who first described them in 1872.

Because the fetus almost completely fills the womb in late pregnancy, contractures squeeze the fetus. Measurements of the chest of the lamb during a contracture in late pregnancy show that the front-to-back dimension of the fetal lamb's chest can decrease by as much as a third during a contracture. Tom Kirschbaum from Albert Einstein Hospital calls contractures an intrauterine hug. We know that the baby is switching in and out of different sleep states. Contractures are one of the major factors that determine how the fetus slips in and out of different patterns of sleep states. See chapter 6 and 13 of *Life Before Birth: The Challenges of Fetal Development,* Peter W. Nathanielsz (W. H. Freeman, 1996).

Chapter 9. You Are Your Brain

"You are your brain" is a statement I have heard repeatedly over the years from Dick Swaab, the director of the Netherlands Institute for Brain Research. His constant reminder of the central role of the brain in our lives has great value in focusing our attention on the critical importance of early brain development for health throughout life. The importance of protecting the development of the brain and limiting the price that may be paid in doing so is key to good health throughout life.

The visual system has been used extensively to study the developing brain: The interplay of genetic factors and activity of the developing neurons is fundamental to normal brain development. Shatz, C. J., "The developing brain," *Scientific American* September (1992): 61–67.

When fetuses are mature enough to take on the challenges of the world outside the womb, they send signals from the brain to the placenta to start the birth process: The story of how the fetus signals to the mother is told in chapter 12 of *Life Before Birth: The Challenges of Fetal Development,* Peter W. Nathanielsz (W. H. Freeman, 1996).

The fetus has very well-developed methods of protecting the blood supply to the brain in times of oxygen lack: See the "Notes" for chapter 1.

A poor-protein diet during pregnancy in rats permanently modifies the brain's stress response axis: See chapter 6 and "Notes" for chapter 8.

The cumulative harmful effect of generations of malnutrition on brain function: Maintaining pregnant rats on a marginally deficient protein diet for twelve generations revealed important information on brain development (see "Notes" for chapter 2). Pups born in the malnourished colony were ten times more likely to be growth-retarded, and their brains were about 5 percent smaller. Some parts of the brain such as the cerebellum, the area of the brain that controls fine movement and balance, were as much as 10 percent smaller. Stewart, R. J. C., et al., "Twelve generations of marginal protein deficiency," *Br. J. Nutr.* 33 (1975): 233–253; Stewart, R. J. C., et al., "The effect of rehabilitation at different stages of development of rats marginally malnourished for ten to twelve generations," *Br. J. Nutr.* 43 (1980): 403–412.

The search for the gene for schizophrenia: John McGrath, David Castle and Ron Murray conclude an article with the following comments: "Overall, the case that prenatal influenza causes schizophrenia is far from proven, but has sufficient credibility to merit further research. . . . The focus of research is therefore likely to move to biological and experimental studies." McGrath, J., et al.,

"How can we judge whether or not prenatal exposure to influenza causes schizophrenia," *Neural Development and Schizophrenia*, ed: Mednick, S. A. and Hollister, J. M., (Plenum Press, 1995: 203–214); Jones, P., "The early origins of schizophrenia," *Br. Med. Bull.* 53 (1997): 135–155; Ezzell, C., "Of multiple minds over the genetics of schizophrenia," *J. NIH Res.* 7 (1995): 25–27.

The Bell Curve (Free Press, 1994), by Richard Herrnstein and Charles Murray, makes some very provocative claims on its jacket. The prediction is made that the book is "certain to ignite an explosive controversy. Herrnstein and Murray break new ground in exploring the ways that low intelligence, independent of social, economic or ethnic background, lies at the root of many of our social problems. The authors also demonstrate the truth of another taboo fact: that intelligence levels differ among ethnic groups. This finding is already well-known and widely discussed among psychometricians and other scholars. . . . Our public policy refuses to acknowledge the proofs of human difference, or to deal with its consequences." These statements are perniciously constructed. Of course no one can disagree that, at this precise moment in time, given the conditions in which different ethnic groups live, intelligence levels differ among ethnic groups. However, to understand causation, we must pose three critical questions: Is intelligence a simple single factor? How do we quantify intelligence? Most importantly, are these differences in intelligence due to nature or nurture? The way Herrnstein and Murray cunningly set up their argument, they provide as a given, undebatable, incontrovertible fact that these differences are "independent of social, economic or ethnic backgrounds." The authors pay no attention to differences between individuals and ethnic groups caused by prenatal programming determined by the conditions that exist in the womb.

Herrnstein and Murray write, "We are content, in other words, to say that heritability of IQ falls somewhere within a broad range and that, for purposes of our discussion, a value of 0.6 plus or minus 0.2 does no violence to any of the competent and responsible recent estimates." What a statement. They are saying that heritability of intelligence lies somewhere between being responsible for 40 to 80 percent of the variation in intelligence. That is quite a gap from being relatively less important than environmental factors (40 percent) to being responsible for 80 percent of the variation. Such a wide range hardly helps us in deciding whether nature of nurture is more important in determining intelligence.

The authors again: "Finally, and most surprisingly, the evidence is growing that whatever variation is left over for the environment to explain [i.e., 40 percent of the total variation, if the heritability is taken to be 0.6], relatively little can be traced to the shared environment created by families. It is, rather, a set of environmental influences, mostly unknown at present, that are experienced by individuals as individuals. The fact that family members resemble each other in intelligence in adulthood as much as they do is very largely explained by the genes that they share rather than the family environment they shared as children." Nothing about the home in the womb.

In *The Bell Curve*, there is a small boxed story of a study with relatively small numbers in which the children born to German women and fathered by American servicemen after the Second World War were studied. Only 264 children of black servicemen and 83 children of white servicemen were studied. There were no overall differences in IQ. This finding is compatible with the idea that environment is important in the controversy over racial differences in blacks and whites. However, since the fathers were unknown, there are many factors that could not be analyzed. However, the maternal prenatal environment is likely to be similar in these 347 children born to German women.

In the chapter on "Raising Cognitive Ability," Herrnstein and Murray mention six important policy issues. The first is the need for more research. They note that research must be focused, long term, free from bureaucratic intervention, insensitive to what is politically correct and directed only at the truth. Most important of all, these authors single out the need for "insights into the physiological basis of intelligence." The other issues are nutrition, investment in schooling, preschool programs and adoption. While I applaud the call for more research (which does show that the authors accept that we do not know everything we need to know), nowhere do they mention the need for better prenatal care.

The publication of *The Bell Curve* was one of those remarkable occasions when one book immediately led to the production of a flood of books for and against Herrnstein and Murray's central thesis. The contention proposed in *The Bell Curve* is that intelligence is predominantly inherited and independent of the environment, either in the womb or after birth. One of the central complaints of those who disagreed with Herrnstein and Murray, the authors of *The Bell Curve,* was that the authors were guilty of oversimplification. These critics hold that there are several forms of intelligence and that Herrnstein and Murray place their whole thesis on the central and unique importance of the IQ test. The many critics of *The Bell Curve* say that intelligence is too complex to be defined that rigidly or simply. See also *The Bell Curve Debate,* edited by Russell Jacoby and Naomi Glauberman (Times Books, 1995).

The Bell Curve jacket also contains the following statement: "We are not indifferent to the ways in which this book, wrongly construed, might do harm. . . . But there can be no real progress in solving America's social problems when they are misperceived as they are today. What good can come of understanding the relationship of intelligence to social structure and public policy? Little good can come without it." I could use exactly the same words to describe the concepts I have put forward here that show a clear link between prenatal programming and how we perform intellectually and in other aspects of our lives. My fundamental criticism of Herrnstein and Murray is that they have fallen prey to gene myopia and have failed to see the firm biological data that show that we can do much to improve performance in our complex society by improving nutrition and social structure and public policy.

Correcting the balance on the heritability of IQ: One recent report in *Nature* makes two major conclusions. First, "The shared maternal environment may explain the striking correlation between the IQs of twins." The report notes that the major milestones in brain growth take place in the womb or in the first year of life, since the brain reaches 70 percent of its final weight by the end of the first year of life. It is also noted that IQ is correlated with birthweight. The concluding statement is, "Our analysis suggests that it will be important to understand the basis for these maternal effects if ways in which IQ might be increased are to be identified." Devlin, B., et al., "The heritability of IQ," *Nature* 338 (1997): 468–471; Goldenberg, R. L., et al., "Pregnancy outcome and intelligence at age five years," *Am. J. Obstet. Gynecol.* 175 (1996): 1511–1515; McGue, M., "The democracy of the genes," *Nature* 388 (1997): 417–418.

There are critical periods of development at which sex hormones modify the function of the brain: In human development, there are peaks of sex hormones at three stages of development that differ between male and female fetuses. These are during the first half of pregnancy when the genitalia form, around the time of birth and finally at puberty. Dick Swaab and his colleagues at the Netherlands Institute for Brain Research have shown that several structures in the male brain contain more neurons and are larger than the same structures in the female brain. He proposes that the surges in male sex hormones during development protect the male brain from the programmed cell death that takes place in these structures in the brains of females. Dick Swaab has shown that one collection of brain cells, the bed nucleus of the stria terminalis, is larger in males than in females and is smallest in transsexuals. This is the first indication that there are anatomical differences that relate to sexual preference rather than just plain sexual makeup (or the genetic complement). There are problems in the use of words like *sex* and *gender* because they have different meanings for different people.

Sexual differentiation of the brain is one of the best examples of prenatal programming. Much of the differentiation of sexual behavior occurs before birth. The expression of these changes in different structures in the brain may not appear until after birth. This is another excellent example of the critical importance of life in the womb. Swaab, D. F. and Hofman, M. A., "Sexual differentiation of the human hypothalamus in relation to gender and sexual orientation," *Trends in NeuroSciences* 18 (1995): 264–270; Kimura, D., "Sex differences in the brain," *Scientific American* (September, 1992): 119–125.

The passage of sound through the uterus to the baby: Throughout life in the womb, the fetus is subjected to many influences. Sound penetrates the uterus easily, especially low-frequency sound in the frequency range of the father's voice. The ease with which we all clutch at straws that might improve performance is shown by the recent wish of the governor of Georgia, Zell Miller, to buy a classical music tape or CD for every child born in Georgia. Gripped by a story in *Time* magazine that the brain is very plastic in its early years, Miller proposed to enhance the development of the intelligence of the youth of Georgia by making them listen to classical music. Even researchers who had shown that playing the piano improved the spatial abilities of young children responded negatively. The governor was not, however, daunted, and his office reported that they hoped to have the program up and running by April 1, 1998, a very appropriate date. See also chapter 1. "Mozart for Georgia Newborns," *Science* 279 (1998): 663.

CHAPTER 10. BORN TOO SOON, BORN TOO LATE

The baby normally links the timing of birth to adequate maturation for life outside the womb: Extensive research over the last twenty years has shown that when the baby is mature enough to take on the challenges of the world outside the womb, the fetal brain sends out hormonal signals to begin the birth process. There are considerable parallels in the mechanisms that the fetal lamb and the fetuses of other species use to start the birth process. During the last days of pregnancy, the fetal sheep adrenal gland secretes more and more cortisol. The cortisol travels in the fetal blood to the placenta and instructs the placenta to convert the steroid hormone progesterone to estrogen. This clever system simultaneously removes progesterone, whose blocking activity maintains pregnancy and increases the level of estrogen, a hormone that stimulates many of the processes needed to start labor. McDonald, T. J. and Nathanielsz, P. W., "Bilateral destruction of the fetal paraventricular nuclei prolongs gestation in sheep, " *Am. J. Obstet. Gynecol.* 165

(1991): 764–770; Liggins, G. C., "Adrenocortical-related maturational events in the fetus," *Am. J. Obstet. Gynecol.* 126 (1976): 931–941.

Primate placentas, including monkey and human placentas, lack the enzymes required to convert progesterone to estrogen. Thus human and monkey fetuses have to adopt a different strategy during the final days of pregnancy. As the time of birth approaches, the primate fetal adrenal gland secretes more and more of a different type of steroid, androgen. The androgen travels in the fetal blood to the placenta and is converted to estrogen. Thus the uterine muscle in both pregnant sheep and pregnant primates is exposed to more and more stimulation by estrogen until labor begins. Mecenas, C. A., et al., "Production of premature delivery in pregnant rhesus monkeys by androstenedione infusion," *Nature Medicine* 2 (1996): 443–448; Nathanielsz, P. W., chapter 12, "A Time To Be Born," in *Life Before Birth: The Challenges of Fetal Development* (W. H. Freeman, 1996).

Although the fetus determines the duration of pregnancy, under normal circumstances the mother determines the precise time of the day or night she goes into labor. The mother's brain produces more of the hormone oxytocin at nighttime and signals to the uterus to start contracting. Honnebier, M. B. O. M. and Nathanielsz, P. W., "Primate parturition and the role of the maternal circadian system," *Eur. J. Obstet. Gynecol.* 5 (1994): 193–203.

Transfer of embryos from different breeds of sheep shows that the genetic make up of the fetus determines the length of pregnancy: Dr. David Kitts from British Columbia and Gary Anderson from the University of California at Davis have provided strong evidence for the fetal regulation of the duration of pregnancy. They transferred either embryos of breeds of donor sheep who have a relatively short pregnancy or embryos from donor sheep with a longer duration of pregnancy to recipient ewes. Ewes receiving the embryos from the donor breed with short lengths of pregnancy delivered earlier than those receiving embryos whose period of development in the womb usually takes longer. Kitts, D. D., et al.,

"Temporal patterns of Δ4 C-21 steroids in coexisting, genetically dissimilar twin lamb fetuses throughout late gestation," *Endocrinology* 14 (1984): 703–711; Kitts, D. D., et al., "Studies on the endocrinology of parturition: Relative steroidogenesis in coexisting genetically dissimilar ovine fetuses, concomitant with the temporal patterns of maternal C_{18} and C_{19} steroids and prostaglandin F2α release," *Biol. Reprod.* 33 (1985): 67–78.

There is debate as to the exact nature and origin of the fetal signal that starts the birth process: While most researchers now accept the view that the fetus gives orders to the mother to start the birth process and thus end pregnancy, there is still much to learn about how normal labor begins. Dr. Caroline McMillen and her research group from Adelaide, Australia, have put forward the concept that the fetus gradually becomes more and more stressed as the placenta becomes less and less able to provide for the growing baby's needs. These researchers propose that, as a result of this nutritional stress the fetus starts to produce more cortisol. While fetal stress may contribute to some forms of premature birth, many researchers feel that the fetus normally is quite at ease in the womb. To quote a major authority in this field of research, Dr. John Challis from Toronto, Canada, "Survival of our species depends upon birth. The idea that birth depends upon the creation of an adverse environment that is not good for fetal growth, that is not good for fetal development, that is not good for neuronal structure, doesn't make sense to me. Biology is smarter than that." In "Let Me Out" by Gary Hamilton, *New Scientist,* January 10, 1998.

Maternal stress may act as a signal to begin the birth process prematurely: Several investigators have suggested that the hormones produced by a stressed mother may result in an early labor. These researchers have tried to find a connection between psychosocial factors that affect pregnant women and premature birth. Concentrations of corticotropin releasing hormone in the mother's blood rise in late pregnancy. The levels of this key stress hormone rise earlier in women who are at risk for premature birth. Dunkel-

Schetter, C., "Maternal stress and preterm delivery," *Prenatal and Neonatal Med.* 3 (1998): 39–42; Hobel, C. J., et al., "Maternal stress as a signal to the fetus," *Prenatal and Neonatal Med.* 3 (1998): 116–120.

Normal labor and delivery involve more than just the contraction of the womb: A set of carefully orchestrated changes must occur for safe delivery of the baby. In addition to good contraction of the muscular layers of the womb, the mother's cervix must dilate to provide an adequate exit for the baby, and the membranes around the fetus must rupture. Only after the membranes have ruptured and the fluids around the fetus have escaped can the baby begin to breathe air properly.

Premature babies are at great risk for a variety of complications*:* Modern medical technologies are keeping more and more low birthweight babies alive. There are many severe complications that face these babies in the early weeks of their tiny lives. The incidence of complications is very high in very low birthweight babies—babies less than 1500 grams (3.3 pounds). In this group of premature babies, 40 percent will suffer from bleeding into the brain, 24 percent will be affected by blood-borne infections and 8 percent will have major problems with their digestive tract. Hack, M., et al., "Very-low-birth-weight outcomes of the National Institute of Child Health and Human Development Neonatal Network, November 1989 to October 1990," *Am. J. Obstet. Gynecol.* 172 (1995): 457–464.

"Miracle in Iowa" . . . so reads the cover of *Time* magazine for December 1, 1997: Dramatic advances in techniques to assist human reproduction made possible the pregnancy in which the seven McCaughey septuplets were conceived. Unfortunately, assisted reproductive techniques to improve fertility are resulting in an epidemic of pregnancies with two or more babies—so-called multiple pregnancies. The survival of all seven very premature McCaughey babies was made possible by the training and skill of dedicated pediatricians and nurses in the neonatal intensive care unit. These health care professionals provided the support these babies would normally have experienced for several more weeks in the womb. For example, the baby in the intensive care unit does not have a placenta. In the womb, the placenta acts as a fetal lung, exchanging oxygen with the mother's blood. The placenta plays the role of a gut for the fetus, carrying nutrients to the baby. The placenta also acts as the baby's kidneys, removing waste products from the baby's blood. In the neonatal intensive care unit, machines have to look after these vital functions. Nathanielsz, P. W., *Life Before Birth: The Challenges of Fetal Development* (W. H. Freeman, 1996, chapter 5).

The same *Time* magazine article provides several cautionary tales. For example, it reminds us of the early deaths of two of the famous Canadian Dionne quintuplets born in 1934. There are many long term consequences of prematurity that often occur following the multiple births produced by the new assisted reproduction methods. The unfortunate consequences of these problems are often lost in the wonder at these miraculous births and the survival of the babies during the immediate period after birth (*Time* magazine, December 1, 1997).

Europeans and Americans place very different values on prenatal care: Throughout Europe there are mechanisms directed at providing financial and other resources to the pregnant mother before, as well as after delivery. Without support, pregnancy may be a major physical and psychological stress for the mother, instead of being a perfectly normal biological process. The sources of support available in many European countries are not within the culture in the United States. In many circles in the United States, any thought of support to pregnant mothers is seen as "socialist," provision of welfare and even an interference with the private rights of the individual to look after her own life. Why this cultural difference?

Dr. Emile Papiernik, from Maternité Port-Royale Baudelocque in Paris, is one of the leading researchers in obstetric care in Europe. He has researched the origins of the European caregiving approach to pregnancy. He traces much of the attitude back to 1895, when an obstetrician in France, Dr. Adolph Pinard, became concerned about the high rate of prematurity in young, unmarried women in the sweat shops of Paris. The young laundresses had to continue working throughout their pregnancy. Their work involved much physical effort, lifting drapes and other damp laundry. Dr. Pinard advocated less hard physical work during pregnancy as a means to reduce premature labor. In doing so, he was a pioneer of concern in society for pregnant women. There is little doubt that excessive, unrelenting physical activity during pregnancy is harmful for both mother and baby. "100 Ans de Puériculture à Port-Royal," ed: Papiernik, E. and Relier, J.-P. (1995).

It ought to be very easy to sell better health care to Americans on the basis of long-term benefits for the health of our children. But if we cannot do that, perhaps people will be persuaded by the argument that the economic payback will be significant and rapid.

The remarkable increase in allergies over recent years may have a partial explanation in the conditions under which we develop during life before birth: High birthweights and staying in the womb one or two weeks longer than normal may set up an individual's immune system to be more susceptible to allergies in later life. This extraordinary connection may seem to stretch our credulity. However, as with other examples of programming, biologists can propose very precise cellular mechanisms that provide strong links.

The thymus gland in the neck has an important job to do in late fetal life, processing the baby's immune cells as they develop. The thymus undergoes very marked changes in the last few days of life in the womb. The underlying biology of programming tells us that critical events in the baby's development need to proceed in a very precise order. When the developing fetus gets the order of events wrong for any reason, the ratio of the different types of cells in different organs in the body may be changed permanently. Allergies are more likely to occur when there are changes in the proportions of different types of immune cells in the blood. Shaheen, S., "Discovering the causes of atopy," *Brit. Med. J.* 31 (1997): 987–988;

Godfrey, K. M., et al., "Disporportionate fetal growth and raised IgE concentration in adult life," *Clin. Exper. Allergy* 24 (1994): 641–648; Olesen, A. B., et al., "Atopic dermatitis and birth factors: historical follow up by record linkage," *Brit. Med. J.* 31 (1997): 1003–1008.

Promising tests may help predict prematurity: One major key to preventing and treating premature delivery is to develop tests that can be used early in pregnancy to identify women at risk. The other need is to find effective treatments for women who have been diagnosed as being at risk for premature delivery. The measurement of the molecule fibronectin in the secretions in the cervix and vagina can tell the obstetrician when the fetal membranes are beginning to separate too early from their attachment to the uterine wall. Lockwood, C. J., et al., "Fetal fibronectin in cervical and vaginal secretions as a predictor of preterm delivery," *New Engl. J. Med.* 325 (1991): 669–674; Peaceman, A. M., et al., "Fetal fibronectin as a predictor of preterm birth in patients with symptoms: A multicenter trial," *Am. J. Obstet. Gynecol.* 177 (1997): 13–18.

As described above, normal labor occurs when the placenta begins to produce more estrogen. Several interesting studies have shown that when estrogen levels in the mother's saliva rise too soon, premature birth is more likely to occur. Darne, J., et al., "Increased saliva oestradiol to progesterone ratio before idiopathic preterm delivery: a possible predictor for preterm labour," *Brit. Med. J.* 294 (1987): 270–272; McGregor, J. A., et al., "Salivary estriol as risk assessment for preterm labor: A prospective trial," *Am. J. Obstet. Gynecol.* 173 (1995): 137–142.

As we learn more about normal and premature birth, other methods of predicting premature birth may become available. Dr. Roger Smith, from Newcastle, Australia, and other groups of investigators have focused on the possibility that the placenta acts as a clock, secreting more and more corticotropin releasing hormone as labor approaches. According to these researchers, if the levels of corticotropin releasing hormone in the mother's blood rise too soon, it is an indication that the mother may go into premature labor.

McLean, M., et al., "A placental clock controlling the length of human pregnancy," *Nature Medicine* 1 (1995): 460–463.

"As More Tiny Infants Live, Choices and Burden Grow." This is the title of an article by Elisabeth Rosenthal in the New York *Times* of September 29, 1991. The long-term handicap and the moral, ethical and economic dilemmas posed by prematurity all show how critical it is that society summons up the will to deal with the problem of prematurity, the most serious complication of pregnancy.

The economics of preterm delivery: Dr. Jeannette Rogowski writes, "Due to the large size of expenditures for the care of low birth weight infants, interventions that reduce premature births and thus the number of infants with low birthweights have the potential to produce significant economic savings. This will accrue primarily during the first year of life for the infant." This rapid return should be appealing to all administrators at the state and federal levels. "For infants with birthweights over 750 grams, a shift in birthweight of 500 grams at birth saves $28,000 in first year medical costs [in 1987 dollars]. . . . The economic burden of low birthweight is borne heavily by public sources of funding. This is both due to public health insurance for the poor and low-income children as well as to government funding of developmental care and special education needs. However, private health insurers also share in the cost, not only for the children they insure but due to cost shifting onto private patients due to charity care and low reimbursement rates from other payers such as Medicaid. Similarly, medical providers bear some of the economic burden to the extent that they incur losses. The families of the children may also bear a considerable burden for the costs of low birthweight due to such factors as the special expenditures for the care of the children. Society as a whole loses when children are born with conditions that could have been preventable but that result in increased morbidity and mortality."

Dr. Rogowski is saying quite clearly that we all are losers when a baby is born prematurely. Rogowski, J. A., "The economics of preterm delivery," *Prenatal and Neonatal Med.* 3 (1998): 16–20.

How effective is home monitoring of contraction of the womb for women at risk of preterm labor? There are several companies that rent equipment for monitoring the activity of the uterus in a home situation. One Kaiser Permanente study conducted at thirty clinics in northern California compared how well a pregnancy progressed and was completed in women who had daily contact with a nurse, with or without home monitoring, against the pregnancy outcome in women who had weekly contact with the nurse alone with no home monitoring. The study concluded that, "Women who have daily contact with a nurse, with or without home monitoring of uterine activity have no better pregnancy outcomes than women who have weekly contact with a nurse." Dyson, D. C., et al., "Monitoring women at risk for preterm labor," *N. Engl. J. Med.* 338 (1998): 15–19.

Home uterine activity monitoring is certainly ill-advised in normal pregnancy. As long ago as 1993, the U. S. Preventive Services Task Force from the Office of Disease Prevention and Health Promotion clearly stated, "There have been no controlled trials of home uterine activity monitoring in normal pregnancies [pregnancies with no risk factors for preterm labor]. In view of the cost of home uterine activity monitoring and the poor evidence that it is efficacious in high-risk pregnancies, the [task force] recommends against the use of home uterine monitoring in normal pregnancy." U. S. Preventive Services Task Force, "Home uterine activity monitoring for preterm labor," *JAMA* 270 (1993): 369–376.

Women with gum disease have a higher risk of delivering low birthweight babies and having premature labor: One small clinical study concludes that women with gum disease may have as great an increase in the risk of giving birth to a premature baby as women who smoke. Bacteria in the mouth secrete toxins that can activate contraction of the womb. Good health throughout childhood and regular visits to the dentist by young girls are thus part of prenatal care many years later. Offenbacher, S., et al., "Periodontitis-associated pregnancy complications," *Prenatal and Neonatal Med.* 3 (1998): 82–85.

Stress and ethnic factors are independently associated with preterm labor: The National Institute of Child Health and Human Development has a nationwide Maternal-Fetal Medicine Units Network to plot trends in diseases that affect the health of the nation's children. This network undertook a detailed study to determine whether the stress associated with poor psychosocial conditions in pregnancy were linked to prematurity and low birthweight. The study concluded, "Stress was associated with spontaneous preterm birth and low birthweight even after adjusting for maternal demographic and behavioral characteristics. Black race continues to be a significant predictor of spontaneous preterm birth, fetal growth restriction, and low birthweight even after adjustment for stress, substance abuse, and other demographic factors." Copper, R. L., et al., "The preterm prediction study: Maternal stress is associated with spontaneous preterm birth at less that thirty-five weeks' gestation," *Am. J. Obstet. Gynecol.* 175 (1996): 1286–1292.

African Americans and Mexican-Americans have a higher risk of preterm delivery: A 1986 study reported that black Americans were nearly twice as likely to have a preterm delivery as white Americans. The risk was even higher for very premature babies. This study from northern California concludes, "Research on the causes of the large ethnic differences in preterm delivery may provide insights into the etiology [cause] of preterm birth in general. Rather than being causal, ethnicity may be a surrogate for other unknown risk factors for preterm birth. The relationship between preterm labor and other factors such as stress, physical activity, poverty, and failure to recognize the symptoms of early labor merits additional attention." In this conclusion, the authors are indicating that preterm labor may not result from genetic causes but rather the environmental factors that affect African- and Mexican-Americans more than white Americans. Shiono, P. H. and Klebanoff, M. A., "Ethnic differences in preterm and very preterm delivery," *Am. J. Public Health* 76 (1986): 1317–1321.

The National Commission for Infant Mortality and Birthweight published its report for 1985 in May 1988: This short report makes compelling reading on the indirect costs of infant mortality, the indirect costs of disabilities of low birthweight children, and foregone federal taxes. The opening sentence of the summary states: "Infant mortality—babies who are born alive but die before their first birthday—is one of the best indicators of the overall health of a society." In reflecting the health of society, infant mortality rates tell us many things. The rate at which babies die in the first year of life is a very clear indication of how well they were nurtured in the womb. Each unacceptable infant death tells us about the health of young women, the quality of medical care and the willingness of all of us to invest in the future. Chu, R. C., "1985 indirect costs of infant mortality and low birthweight," *Nat. Comm. Prev. Inf. Mort.* May 1988: 1-5.

CHAPTER 11. BACK TO THE FUTURE

Genetic engineering of the human race to improve human health is not only more difficult to perform but may not be as successful as preventive action to improve the home in the womb: Few would agree to society introducing genetic engineering to improve our health and well-being. In contrast, society has much it can do to improve the health of mothers before, during and after pregnancy and thereby improve the health of their children.

The designation genetic is often incorrectly used for conditions that are congenital: One major error common in both the lay and scientific communities is the constant failure to distinguish between genetic and congenital. It is so common to hear or read that such and such a condition is genetic because it is present at birth. The presence of a condition at birth certainly does not show that the feature is genetically controlled. We must never forget that the environment in the womb has been working on the baby's genetic potential for nine months.

What dietary advice do we give a woman during pregnancy? Two independent studies, one by Dr. Keith Godfrey and his colleagues and the other by Dr. Campbell and colleagues, have clearly shown that the balance of carbohydrate and protein in the mother's diet is critical to fetal and placental growth. Low-protein, high-carbohydrate diets were associated with small placentas and high blood pressure in the offspring at the age of forty. Strikingly, the babies of mothers who had a high animal protein diet and a low carbohydrate diet also developed high blood pressure in later life. These findings have significant parallels with the studies in pregnant rats that show that low-protein diets during pregnancy lead to high blood pressure in the offspring in later life. Whether these diets produce their effects through changes in placental growth or wether the growth of the placenta is just another feature of the altered diet remains to be decided. One thing is certain: the observations make it critical that more research is done to determine the best mix of food that a mother eats during pregnancy. Ravelli, G. P., et al., "Obesity in young men after famine exposure in utero and early infancy," *N. Engl. J. Med.* 295 (1996): 349–353.

Lamarck was not completely wrong: Lamarck's failing was that he just did not submit the concept of transgenerational programming of lifelong health to scientific study, and he didn't consider the influence of conditions in the womb. The transgenerational passage of diabetes from mother to daughter rat and then on over several generations has clearly demonstrated effects not directly due to genes. This work on the transgenerational passage of health and disease does not undermine Darwinism and modern molecular genetics. However, knowledge of these effects of the environment during development in the womb does introduce a whole new exciting dimension and area of study. To date, the cellular mechanisms underlying these transgenerational effects are poorly understood. More information is needed on how environmental influences bring about programming of cellular function and how these effects are transmitted across generations.

Disease fights forward: An article in the *Economist* on May 20, 1995, was entitled *"Disease Fights Back."* However, the story of this book shows that in truth, disease fights forward. In the last thirty years we have learned so much about how we develop, but there is so much more exciting and valuable knowledge to be revealed.

Continued search for more evidence on the fetal and childhood origin of adult disease: It is the nature of progress that new ideas must be tested in the crucible of established knowledge. The mechanisms that underlie programming of human health and disease are complex and multifactorial. Some investigators remain of the opinion that trends in disease seen in different populations are largely, if not solely, due to environmental and social causes. For such an opinion see Joseph, K. S., and Kramer, M.S., "Review of the evidence on fetal and early childhood antecedents of adult chronic disease," *Epidemiologic Reviews* 18 (1996): 158-174.

INDEX